W9-CCT-234

IF YOU ARE LIVING WITH DIABETES, YOU ARE NOT ALONE.

In the United States, nearly 24 million people—almost 8% of the population—have diabetes, and 1.6 million people are diagnosed every year.

IF YOU ARE LIVING WITH DIABETES, WHAT YOU EAT IS THE KEY TO GOOD HEALTH.

THE DIABETES COUNTER, 4th Edition

is your one-stop guide for managing diabetes and reducing complications. This one-of-a-kind book provides carbohydrate, calorie, sugar, fiber, and fat counts for thousands of foods—all the information you need to count carbs and set up a healthy eating plan. Use this reliable meal-planning guide to customize your diet to your likes and dislikes, your culture, and your life's demands.

Managing diabetes has never been easier!
It's up to you.

The
DIABETES
COUNTER

Fourth Edition

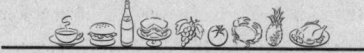

Karen J. Nolan, Ph.D.
and Jo-Ann Heslin, M.A., R.D.

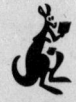

POCKET BOOKS
New York   London   Toronto   Sydney

Pocket Books
A Division of Simon & Schuster, Inc.
1230 Avenue of the Americas
New York, NY 10020

Copyright © 1991, 2003, 2007 by Annette Natow and Jo-Ann Heslin
Copyright © 2011 by Karen Nolan and Jo-Ann Heslin

All rights reserved, including the right to reproduce this book or portions thereof in any form whatsoever. For information, address Pocket Books Subsidiary Rights Department, 1230 Avenue of the Americas, New York, NY 10020.

This Pocket Books paperback edition January 2011

POCKET and colophon are registered trademarks of Simon & Schuster, Inc.

For information about special discounts for bulk purchases, please contact Simon & Schuster Special Sales at 1-866-506-1949 or business@simonandschuster.com.

The Simon & Schuster Speakers Bureau can bring authors to your live event. For more information or to book an event, contact the Simon & Schuster Speakers Bureau at 1-866-248-3049 or visit our website at www.simonspeakers.com.

Cover photo by Image Source

Manufactured in the United States of America

10   9   8   7   6   5   4

ISBN 978-1-4165-6668-7

For
Our families
Who support us through every project

ACKNOWLEDGMENTS

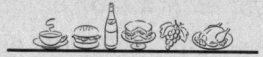

For all her continuous support and help, our agent, Nancy Trichter.

For her suggestions and editing skills, Sara Clemence.

For all her patience, comments and questions, our favorite reviewer, Jean Schwarsin.

Without the tireless cooperation of Stephen Llano and the production department at Pocket Books, *The Diabetes Counter*, Fourth Edition, would never have been completed.

A special thank you to our editor, Micki Nuding.

And, we would like to thank all of our readers for their suggestions and questions. Your input helps us to provide you with the most useful information.

The regulation of the diet is the most important consideration in the treatment of diabetes mellitus. . . . While certain general principles in regard to diet for diabetes can be laid down, each patient presents an individual problem. . . .

Mary Swartz Rose, Ph.D.
Feeding the Family
The Macmillan Company, 1919

CONTENTS

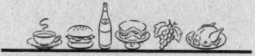

INTRODUCTION

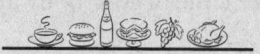

You've just been told that you have diabetes.

OR

Someone close to you has diabetes.

OR

Your doctor said you have risk factors that increase your chance of getting diabetes in the near future.

Every 24 hours, 4,100 new cases of diabetes are diagnosed in the United States. At first, most of these people feel devastated. Having to change the way you eat, and being told to lose weight, exercise, and take medication is overwhelming. But there is good news. Diabetes is a condition over which you, as an individual, have a lot of control. And the more control you exercise, the healthier and more complication-free your life will be. Most important, you can look forward to a very long life.

There is no question that being diagnosed with diabetes is a jolt—emotionally, physically, and even socially. It is a condition that requires constant attention and modifications in how you lead your life. It isn't unusual to feel down. If you do, discuss your feelings with your doctor. Depression can be caused by feeling that you can no longer control your body and your life. But you can.

With some adjustments life will be normal again, and sooner than you think. Initially it is going to take work on your part and a commitment to follow your doctor's orders. The payoff is that your body will respond, in ways that may amaze you, to your new diet, exercise, and medication plan.

UNDERSTANDING DIABETES

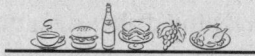

What Is Diabetes?

When you have diabetes, there is too much sugar in your blood. After you eat, your food is broken down into a sugar called *glucose*, which is carried by your blood to cells throughout your body. *Insulin*, a hormone, helps the glucose move from the bloodstream into cells, where it is burned as energy to keep your body functioning. People with diabetes either don't make enough insulin or their cells don't recognize insulin. The result in both cases is that glucose in the bloodstream can't get into cells to be used for energy, and instead builds up in the blood.

What Causes Diabetes?

In most cases, it's your genes. In the United States, almost 8% of the population (close to 24 million people) have diabetes. It's estimated that a person born in 2000 has a 1 in 3 chance of developing diabetes in their lifetime. But the good news—are you getting the pic-

3

ture, that there is always good news?—is that lifestyle choices can alter the action of your genes. Just because you carry the risk for diabetes doesn't mean you will get diabetes. People who stay slim, exercise regularly, don't smoke, and eat generally healthy diets decrease their odds of developing diabetes no matter what their genetic profiles say. And people with diabetes can control the condition, and in some cases even reverse it, with lifestyle changes.

YOU SHOULD KNOW

1.6 million new cases of diabetes
are diagnosed every year.
6 million people have diabetes and don't know it.
It is projected that more than 44 million
Americans will have diabetes by 2034.
It is important to be tested.

What Puts a Person at Risk for Diabetes?

The risk of developing diabetes increases with each of the following that apply to you.

- Being 45 or older
- Being overweight
- Having a parent or close relative with diabetes
- Being African American, American Indian, Asian American, Pacific Islander, or Hispanic/Latino American
- Having had diabetes during pregnancy

- Giving birth to a baby weighing more than 9 pounds
- Having high blood pressure
- Having high cholesterol
- Having high triglycerides
- Exercising very little or not at all
- Having polycystic ovary syndrome (a disorder affecting the female reproductive system)
- Having dark, thickened skin around the neck or armpits (acanthosis nigricans)
- Having a history of blood vessel disease
- Having higher than normal blood glucose levels at previous screenings

---

YOU SHOULD KNOW

Knowledge Is Power

The more you know about diabetes,
the better you can take care of yourself
and the healthier you will be.

What Are the Symptoms of Diabetes?

Diabetes often goes undetected for a long time because many people have no symptoms—or they ignore symptoms because they seem harmless. See your doctor if you experience any of the following problems.

- Being very thirsty
- Needing to urinate frequently

- Being very hungry
- Unexplained weight loss
- Feeling tired and weak
- Blurry vision
- Cuts and bruises that heal very slowly or do not heal at all
- Tingling or numbness in your hands or feet
- Recurring or hard-to-heal infections
- Annoying itching

How Is Diabetes Diagnosed?

Your doctor can screen for diabetes when you have blood tests. Everyone over the age of 45 should be screened. If everything is normal, screenings should be repeated every 3 years. Younger individuals need to be tested earlier if they have a number of the risk factors noted earlier. Children who are overweight should be tested periodically, too.

YOU SHOULD KNOW
Screening Tests for Diabetes

Random Blood Glucose—*Your doctor checks your blood glucose without regard to when you last ate. A normal result is less than 200.*

Fasting Blood Glucose—*Your doctor tests your blood after you have not eaten for at least 8* *hours. Results below 100 are normal. Between 100 and 125 you have a condition known as prediabetes, which signals your risk of developing diabetes in the future. If the results are 126 or higher, the test is usually repeated on another day. If the numbers stay high, this confirms a diagnosis of diabetes.*

Oral Glucose Tolerance Test—*Your blood is tested in the morning after you have not eaten for at least 10 hours, than it is tested a second time 2 hours after you drink a sweetened beverage. Results of 139 or below are normal. Between 140 and 199 you have prediabetes. Results over 200 indicate diabetes. Some doctors repeat the results on another day just to confirm the diagnosis.*

How Do I Manage My Diabetes?

Diet, exercise, and medication all play roles in managing diabetes. Once you're diagnosed, your primary care doctor will help you organize your health care team, a group of health professionals who help manage all aspects of your condition. The most important member of the team is YOU. Only you know how you feel. You will be the first to notice any problems. And you will set the pace for what you are willing and able to do. The rest of the team depends on you to be honest and to thoroughly report on your home care.

YOUR HEALTH CARE TEAM

Health Professional	Seen How Often	To Help You With
Primary Care Doctor	Every 3 months	Providing general care Monitoring blood sugar Refering you to other specialists
Certified Diabetes Educator (CDE) May be a nurse or dietitian with special training in diabetes management	As needed	Putting your drug, diet, exercise, and daily care plan in place Managing problems such as sick days Answering all questions about your self-care routine
Registered Dietitian (RD) May also be a CDE	As needed	Setting up a meal plan tailored to your treatment goals and personal choices
Eye Doctor	Yearly	Monitoring the health of your eyes Preventing and treating complications from diabetes

(*continued*)

Health Professional	Seen How Often	To Help You With
Podiatrist	As needed	Caring for your feet and lower legs
		Treating corns, calluses, sores
Dentist	Twice yearly	Monitoring the health of your mouth
		Preventing or treating gum disease and infections

TYPES OF DIABETES

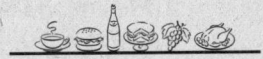

Diabetes—or more correctly, *diabetes mellitus*—is a group of similar conditions all resulting in the same outcome—too much sugar in the blood.

Why one person develops diabetes and another does not is the result of a complicated interaction between genes and environment. Researchers classify diabetes into 4 main groups—type 1, type 2, pregnancy diabetes, and "from other causes." This last group accounts for a very small percentage of cases in which the development of diabetes is usually secondary to another condition, like Down syndrome.

Type 2

This is by far the most common form, accounting for a whopping 90% to 95% of people with diabetes. The number of people with this condition is increasing daily, and experts believe that as time goes on, more and more people—even children—will develop type 2 diabetes due to being overweight and inactive. Couple this with the fact that our population is aging (type 2 is most common in those over 30), and the number of new cases could be overwhelming.

YOU SHOULD KNOW

Approximately 50% of men and 70% of women who develop type 2 diabetes are overweight. Weighing less could delay the onset of the disease—and in some cases prevent diabetes entirely.

With type 2 diabetes, your body is unable to use the insulin it produces. The cells don't recognize insulin and it doesn't enter cells to deliver the glucose needed for energy. To try to get around this problem, the pancreas, which makes insulin, produces more. At first this works, but after a while the pancreas gets exhausted from all the extra work and loses its ability to make enough insulin.

Type 2 is managed by lifestyle changes, diet, weight loss, and, when needed, medication and possibly insulin. In some cases the disease can be reversed with careful attention to diet, exercise, and weight control.

Type 3 Diabetes
New research shows that the memory loss in Alzheimer's disease could be caused by a new type of diabetes where there is both too little insulin in the brain and the brain cannot use the insulin effectively.

Type 1

In the past, this form of diabetes was called *juvenile diabetes* because most people developed it in childhood or early adulthood, but it can occur at any age. Only 5% to 10% of people with diabetes have type 1. It develops when something happens to destroy the cells in the pancreas that produce insulin. A person with type 1 cannot make any insulin and must supply it daily by injection, through an insulin pump, or in a newly approved inhalable form. The amount of insulin taken daily must be balanced with diet and exercise. There is no known way to prevent type 1, and it cannot be reversed.

Pregnancy Diabetes

Gestational diabetes mellitus occurs only during pregnancy and usually disappears after the baby is born. Being overweight or having a family history of diabetes can increase a woman's risk. To prevent problems, all pregnant women are tested for diabetes. If their blood sugar levels are too high, they are taught to adjust their food intake and may be given insulin until their baby is delivered. Having pregnancy diabetes increases a woman's risk of developing type 2 diabetes in the next 5 to 10 years.

YOU SHOULD KNOW

Treating pregnancy diabetes is not only important to the health of the mother but also reduces the risk for childhood obesity. Pregnant women with untreated diabetes have an 82% higher risk of having a child who is overweight by ages 5 to 7.

Complications

Regardless of the type, when diabetes is not well controlled you are at risk for complications—heart disease, stroke, eye disease, kidney disease, nerve damage, gum disease, tooth loss, and even amputations. It's a pretty scary list. But, as we said before, with the bad news comes some really good news. *Serious complications are not inevitable.*

YOU SHOULD KNOW

Diabetes Is a Serious Condition
Terms such as "a touch of diabetes," "mild diabetes," or "my sugar is a little high" shouldn't be used because they minimize a serious health problem.

The key to being healthy and avoiding complications from diabetes is working with your health team to keep your blood sugar down, your blood pressure down, your blood fats low, and taking your medication or insulin as prescribed.

- Keeping blood sugar levels within the normal range can reduce the risk of eye, kidney, and nerve problems by as much as 40%.

- Reducing your systolic blood pressure (the top number) by 10 reduces the risk for all complications by 12%.

- Lowering blood fats (triglycerides and cholesterol) can reduce the risk of heart disease and stroke by 20% to 50%.

- Visiting your eye doctor regularly can reduce the risk of vision problems by 50% to 60%.

- Visiting your podiatrist regularly can reduce the amputation rate by 45% to 85%.

The most important thing you need to know about diabetes is that you are in control. By keeping your condition under control, you control your risk for complications and serious health problems.

YOU SHOULD KNOW

**Diabetes and Heart Disease
Are Closely Linked**

*There is a positive side to this connection.
What benefits the heart—a healthy diet, exercise,
and good medical care—also helps to prevent
and delay the onset of type 2 diabetes.
Be good to your heart.*

A Word About Prediabetes

Prediabetes, also known as metabolic syndrome, is not a disease but a cluster of symptoms that doubles your risk for heart disease and quadruples your risk for diabetes. It is estimated that 57 million adults and 2 million teenagers in the United States have prediabetes. Over age 60, 40% have prediabetes. If we don't reduce the incidence of prediabetes soon, there could be a major increase in heart disease and type 2 diabetes over the next 20 years.

YOU SHOULD KNOW

Research Has Shown . . .

Eating less meat and fatty food and more salads and cooked vegetables reduces the risk of developing type 2 diabetes.

The guidelines for prediabetes were set by experts so they could catch and treat as many people as possible to prevent more serious problems like heart attack, stroke, and type 2 diabetes.

Having 3 of the following risk factors classifies you as someone with prediabetes.

- Being 30 or more pounds overweight. For men this usually means having a waist larger than 42 inches and for women having a waist greater than 35 inches.

- Having HDL cholesterol of less than 40 for men and less than 50 for women.

- Having triglycerides of 150 or higher after fasting, or above 400 without fasting.

- Having a blood pressure of 130/85 or higher, or being on high blood pressure medication.

- Having a blood sugar level of 100 or higher after fasting, or 140 or higher 2 hours after eating (these values are higher than normal, but not high enough for a diagnosis of diabetes).

If untreated, people with prediabetes are likely to develop diabetes within 10 years. Without treatment, women tend to progress from prediabetes to diabetes faster than men. But this is not inevitable. With treatment and lifestyle changes, prediabetes can be reversed and may never develop into diabetes.

YOU SHOULD KNOW

If you have prediabetes, losing 5% to 7% of your current weight and walking 2.5 hours a week can reduce your risk of developing diabetes by 58%. For people over age 60, the risk goes down over 70%.

SETTING YOUR WEIGHT LOSS GOALS

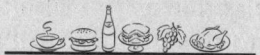

How Much Weight Do I Have to Lose to Control My Diabetes?

Your health care team will help you set your specific weight loss goals, but any weight loss is beneficial—even a few pounds can be significant. A loss of between 10 and 20 pounds, which can be accomplished in 3 to 4 months, will improve type 2 diabetes remarkably. Your blood sugar will drop, your cholesterol and triglycerides will go down, you'll have more energy, and you'll look and feel better. You may even find you're able to reduce or possibly eliminate medication.

How Much Should I Weigh?

There are many ways to determine your best weight or target weight, including weight charts, equations, even guesstimates. Your doctor, diabetes educator, or dietitian can help you with this step. But a very easy way to "guess" at a good target weight is:

Multiply your weight at age 20 by 1.2
For example, if you weighed 135 pounds in your early 20s
$$135 \times 1.2 = 162 \text{ pounds}$$

Your target weight should be 162 pounds or less. This may not be as thin as you wish to be, but it is a reasonable goal to shoot for and will give you health benefits.

YOU SHOULD KNOW

10% Is Great!

Losing 10% of your body weight—15 pounds for someone who weighs 150 pounds, 20 pounds for a person weighing 200 pounds, or 30 pounds if the scale tips in at 300 pounds—is all that is needed to significantly improve your health.
Lose 10% of your current body weight and you'll have:
Lower blood sugar
Lower blood pressure
Improved cholesterol levels
Better sex

How Many Calories Should I Eat Every Day?

As with target weight, your doctor may give you a daily calorie intake to aim for. But, here's a way to determine for yourself how many calories to eat each day.

First, you need to know your target weight, which you can get by using the equation above. Second, select an activity factor that fits your current activity level.

1. Your target weight is ____.
2. Your activity factor is ____.
   20 = Very active men
   15 = Moderately active men or very active women
   13 = Inactive men, moderately active women and
      people over 55
   10 = Inactive women, repeat dieters, seriously
      overweight people
3. Target Weight × Activity Factor = Calories needed
   each day

For example, if your target weight is 162 and you are an inactive woman (factor 10), you need about 1600 calories a day.

$$162 \text{ pounds} \times 10 = 1620 \text{ calories}$$

Eating about 1600 calories each day will guarantee weight loss because you are getting only enough calories to support your target weight, not your current heavier weight. Couple this calorie intake with some added exercise and the pounds will come off even faster.

YOU SHOULD KNOW
Your Weight Loss Goals

Your target weight is ____.

Your daily calorie intake is ____.

Why Is Exercise So Important?

Daily exercise helps to control your blood sugar and maintain your target weight. Everything counts— walking around window shopping, gardening, doing housework, bowling.

- Try to be active every day.

- Aim for 30 minutes of activity each day; you can accumulate this by doing short periods of activity (10 minutes or less) throughout the day.

- Start walking—even short walks count, like from the edge of the parking lot or up and down the aisles of the supermarket.

LET'S TALK ABOUT FOOD

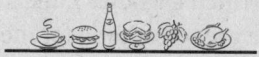

We know that when you are first diagnosed, it's overwhelming. There are so many things to manage—your weight, your blood sugar, your food, your medication, how much you exercise. So when it comes to food, let's take it slowly. We'll go step by step, and before you know it, you'll be a pro at planning meals and choosing the right foods.

The first question everyone asks is, "What can I eat, now that I have diabetes?" The simple answer is "everything." No foods are off limits. It's the time you eat and how much you eat that you need to watch.

Meal Planning

At first, the idea of planning all your meals and snacks can be stressful. Relax. It isn't that hard. Start slowly. First, become accustomed to regular serving sizes, which are probably smaller than what you now eat. Stick with the smaller, regular sizes as often as you can. Next, work on spacing meals and snacks throughout the day and try to keep to this schedule daily. Then, work on making the best selections each time you eat.

That will probably involve counting calories and car-

21

bohydrates. In the beginning, counting carbs is smart because it will help you learn a great deal about the foods you eat, and you'll become very skilled at making choices. Your Certified Diabetes Educator or Registered Dietitian will be a great resource for meal planning and carb counting. We'll help get you started with both, as well.

Meal Planning Hints

Do: Eat regular meals and aim for the same amount of food at about the same time each day.

Choose regular serving sizes.

Eat moderately sized meals.

Choose foods with carbohydrate and fiber at each meal and each snack.

Choose foods low in fat.

Bring food with you so you don't miss a meal or snack.

Go easy: On foods containing sugar.

On foods containing saturated fat.

On alcohol.

Don't: Skip meals or snacks.

Overeat.

YOU SHOULD KNOW

When researchers compared people who ate on an irregular schedule to those who ate meals at regular times each day, they found that those with regular meal patterns had lower blood sugar, lower cholesterol, and lower LDL (bad) cholesterol.

As we said earlier, you are the most important part of your health care team. Only you can decide what you can and will do to manage your diabetes.

The American Diabetes Association (ADA) recommends the following approach to managing diabetes:

Lose weight, if needed.
Be active daily.
Eat a healthy diet.

Lifestyle changes are not one-size-fits-all. The ADA further recommends you need to consider:

Your life circumstances
Your culture
Your heritage
Your food likes and dislikes
Your willingness to make changes

Let's look at some good advice for healthy living, which works whether or not you have diabetes. If you haven't paid too much attention to what you ate or how much you exercised in the past, these guidelines will help you begin to make better choices.

Carbohydrates

Paying attention to carbohydrates is important. With diabetes, your body has a limited ability to use carbs. It is important to eat the right kind, in the right amount, spaced out between meals and snacks.

- Include whole grain breads and cereals, fruits, vegetables, and lowfat milk in your meals and snacks.

- Keep track of the amount of carbohydrates you eat each day; include carbs at every meal and snack.

- It's OK to use low calorie and no calorie sweeteners.

- It's OK to eat sugar and foods containing sugar, but eat small amounts and count sugar in each day's total carbohydrate amount.

- Eat sugar and sugary foods with meals or snacks, not alone.

Fat

It is important to pay attention to fats, too. Having diabetes increases your risk for heart disease. Eating the right fats can help you control this risk.

- Eating less fat overall will help you lose weight and reduce your cholesterol.

- Eat more of the foods that contain "good" (monounsaturated) fats like olive oil, canola oil, seeds, nuts.

- Eat moderate amounts of the foods that contain

polyunsaturated fat, including margarine, corn oil, vegetable oil, salad dressing.

- Eat less of the foods that contain saturated fat like meat, whole milk, butter, cheese.

Regular Serving Sizes

Most of us have portion perceptions that are out of whack—what we think of as a "normal" portion of food, whether we make it at home or eat it in a restaurant, is often much larger than it should be. At first, use measuring cups, measuring spoons, or a kitchen scale to get used to the size of a normal portion. The following information will help you get started.

What Is a Serving?

Food	Serving Size
Breads, cereals, high carb foods	
bread	1 slice
roll, bun, or pita pocket	½
crackers	4 to 6
tortilla	1 (6 inches across)
cereal, cooked	½ cup
cereal, ready-to-eat	¾ cup
rice, cooked	⅓ cup
pasta, cooked	½ cup
popcorn	3 cups
Vegetables and fruits	
raw or cooked vegetables	½ cup
raw or cooked leafy greens	1 cup

(continued)

green peas	*½ cup*
beans	*¼ cup*
potato	*1 small*
mashed potatoes	*½ cup*
french fries	*10 pieces*
fresh fruit	*1 small*
banana	*½ regular or 1 very small*
dried fruit	*2 tablespoons*
canned fruit	*½ cup*
juice	*½ cup*

Milk, yogurt, cheese

nonfat or lowfat milk	*1 cup*
nonfat or lowfat yogurt	*1 cup*
cheese	*1 oz or 1 slice*
cottage cheese	*½ cup*

Meat, poultry, fish

cooked	*3 to 4 ounces*
egg, cooked	*1*

Fats

butter or margarine	*1 teaspoon*
cream cheese	*2 tablespoon*
salad dressing	*2 tablespoons*
oil	*1 tablespoon*

Sugar

sugar	*1 teaspoon*
honey	*1 teaspoon*
syrup	*2 tablespoons*

Eventually, you'll know just by looking how much a serving of food is. Visual cues can be very useful portion guides.

YOU SHOULD KNOW

Seeing Is Believing

*These visual cues will help you keep
portion sizes reasonable.*

computer mouse	=	4-ounce portion of meat, chicken, seafood or 1 medium baked potato
yo-yo	=	a mini bagel or 100 calories (How many yo-yos fit into your bagel, muffin, or pastry?)
music CD	=	1 medium pancake or small waffle
tennis ball	=	medium piece of fresh fruit
ping-pong ball	=	2 ounces cheese or 2 tablespoons salad dressing, gravy, sour cream
quarter	=	1 pat butter

COUNTING CARBS

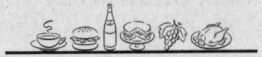

Everyone who has diabetes should know how to count carbs. Some people do it every day to check on how they are doing, some do it a few days a week, and others do it occasionally. Your Certified Diabetes Educator or Registered Dietitian will help you identify the system that is best for you.

You've got a great resource right in front of you. *The Diabetes Counter* has the carb counts for over 12,000 foods. You can look up any food you eat and know exactly how many carbs are in a serving.

The goals of carbohydrate counting are to:

- Learn which foods have carb
- Know how much carb is in each food
- Count up the carb in each meal
- Count up the carb in each snack
- Aim to eat the same amount of carb each day

Finding Carbohydrate Foods

You know that bread, pasta, cereal, and potatoes have carbs. Did you know that fruits, vegetables, cakes, ice cream, candy, jelly, cookies, sugar, milk, and beans have carbs, too? Some have more, some have less.

YOU SHOULD KNOW

Which Has More Carb?

Whole milk or skim milk?
White bread or whole wheat bread?
White sugar or brown sugar?
The carb count in each pair is the same.
The color of a food or the amount of fat in
it does not change the amount of carb.

People are creatures of habit, and most people eat only about 35 foods regularly. A simple way to get familiar with the carb counts in foods is to first list your favorites on the following chart, Carbs in My Favorite Foods. Then look up how much carb is in each food and check on pages 25–26 to be sure you are eating a normal portion size.

This might seem time consuming, but it is a really valuable exercise. This sheet will serve as a quick reference when you are planning meals and snacks. You may eventually make a number of these lists—one for each group of foods you eat. We've also had people tell us they make a list of possible options before going out to eat so they can make the best choices from a restaurant menu. There are many uses for a tool like this. You'll probably come up with your own interesting ways of using it.

CARBS IN MY FAVORITE FOODS		
Food I Usually Eat	Normal Serving Size	Grams of Carbohydrate

Your Daily Carb Budget

Thinking about the amount of carbs you can eat each day like a budget is an easy way to help you divide carbs into meals and snacks. If you had $30 a day and were told to buy 3 meals and 2 snacks, you would budget your money to cover all your food. It's the same idea with carbs. Your Certified Diabetes Educator or Registered Dietitian will help you set up your carb budget.

We recommend that 45% to 60% of your daily calories come from carb. But people don't think in terms of percentages—you just want to know what foods you can eat and when. First we have to determine how many carbs you can eat each day, based on the number of calories you are eating daily. On page 19, you figured out how many calories you needed each day. Find that number on the following chart, **My Daily Calories and Carbs**, and you'll find a target amount of carbs to eat. This number may vary slightly if you have already set up a carb budget with a diabetes educator, but the concept remains the same.

YOU SHOULD KNOW
Your Daily Carb Budget
Each day I can eat

Calories ____

Carbs ____

MY DAILY CALORIES AND CARBS	
Calories Each Day	**Grams of Carb Each Day**
1200	150
1300	160
1400	175
1500	190
1600	200
1700	215
1800	225
1900	240
2000	250
2100	265
2200	275
2300	290
2400	300
2500	315
2600	325
2700	340

*Carb recommendations are based on 50% of daily calories as carbohydrates.

Carbohydrate-containing foods have the greatest impact on your blood sugar. Eat too many carbs and your blood sugar goes up; eat too few and your blood sugar may drop too low. Eat the right amount and your diabetes will be well controlled.

YOU SHOULD KNOW

Counting carbs helps to manage your diabetes and keeps you healthy.

LET'S EAT—
PUTTING IT ALL TOGETHER

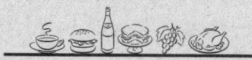

OK, you are ready to take charge. You know how many calories you need each day. You know how many carbs to eat each day. You are starting to understand how to identify foods with carbs, and why it is important to keep track of how much you eat. Now let's put all that information to use by planning meals and snacks for each day.

It's important to try to eat your meals and snacks at the same time each day. This timing helps your body use the carbs you eat and helps keep your blood sugar normal. If there is a long time between meals, your blood sugar could drop very low. If you eat fewer but larger meals, your blood sugar may go up too high.

What Is a Carb Choice?

1 carb choice = 15 grams of carbohydrate
1 slice of bread = 15 grams of carbohydrate

The easiest way to understand carb choices is to compare everything to a slice of bread, which contains

15 grams of carbs, making it a 1 carb choice. If you look up a food, such as a slice of apple pie, and you see that it has 45 grams of carbs; it equals 3 slices of bread or 3 carb choices. If that doesn't fit into your carb budget, you can eat half a slice of pie or pick something similar, like a baked apple, that is lower in carbs. Other typical carb choices, all of which have 15 grams of carb, are on the following chart titled Carb Choices.

CARB CHOICES

1 CARB CHOICE = 15 GRAMS OF CARBOHYDRATE

Breads and Cereals	Fruits	Vegetables
⅓ cup cooked rice	½ banana	⅓ cup beans
½ roll	1 small apple, orange, peach	½ cup green peas
1 (4-inch) pancake	4 fresh apricots	½ cup corn
½ cup cooked cereal	½ cup plantain melon	½ cup plantain
¾ cup ready-to-eat cereal (unsweetened)	12 cherries	½ cup boiled or mashed potato
½ cup ready-to-eat cereal (sweetened)	18 grapes	1 cup winter squash
8 animal crackers	½ papaya	
6 saltines	½ cup unsweetened canned fruit	
3 cups popcorn	¾ cup fresh berries	
½ cup pasta	1 cup fresh strawberries	
	1¼ cups cubed watermelon	
	½ cup fruit juice	
	⅓ cup prune juice	

Planning Your Day

Let's assume you can eat 1800 calories a day. A person eating 1800 calories a day can eat 225 grams of carb each day. (See chart, page 32, My Daily Calories and Carbs.) If you divide 225 by 15, you will find out how many carb choices you can eat.

$$225 \div 15 = 15 \text{ carb choices a day}$$
Daily Carbs ÷ 1 Carb Choice = Number of Carb
Choices allowed each day

The rest is simple! Here are some basic meal planning tips to help you get started.

- Divide your carb budget for the day between your meals and snacks.

- Eat some carb at every meal.
  Women: at least 2 to 3 carb choices at each meal
  Men: at least 3 to 4 carb choices at each meal

- Eat at least 1 carb at every snack; eat at least 2 snacks a day.

- Include a protein choice or a fat choice at each meal or snack.

- Do not eat carbs alone—it will make your blood sugar rise too high.

- Don't skip meals.

Religious Fast Days
Many faiths have fast days. Anyone with diabetes should get medical advice on changing medications, adjusting fluids, and monitoring blood sugar levels during fasting.
At break-the-fast meals, choose wisely and be careful not to overeat.

The following charts, Sample Day for Women and For Men, use the example we started earlier for a person eating 1800 calories a day, including 15 carb choices.

SAMPLE DAY
For Women
Dividing Your Daily Carb Budget
Between Meals and Snacks

Daily Carb Budget: 15 Carb Choices or 225 grams Carb

Breakfast	3	Carb choices	=	45 grams Carb
A.M. Snack	1	Carb choices	=	15 grams Carb
Lunch	4	Carb choices	=	60 grams Carb
P.M. Snack	1	Carb choices	=	15 grams Carb
Dinner	4	Carb choices	=	60 grams Carb
Night Snack	2	Carb choices	=	30 grams Carb
Total	**15**	**Carb choices**	=	**225** total grams Carb

The main difference between the Sample Day for Women and the Sample Day for Men is the way carbs are divided between meals and snacks. Women should eat 2 to 3 carb choices at each meal; men should eat 3 to 4 carb choices at each meal.

SAMPLE DAY
For Men
Dividing Your Daily Carb Budget
Between Meals and Snacks

Daily Carb Budget: 15 Carb Choices or 225 grams Carb

Breakfast	4	*Carb choices*	=	60 *grams Carb*
A.M. Snack	1	*Carb choices*	=	15 *grams Carb*
Lunch	4	*Carb choices*	=	60 *grams Carb*
P.M. Snack	1	*Carb choices*	=	15 *grams Carb*
Dinner	4	*Carb choices*	=	60 *grams Carb*
Night Snack	1	*Carb choices*	=	15 *grams Carb*
Total	**15**	**Carb choices**	=	**225** total grams Carb

Use the following box to divide your daily carb budget into a pattern you can follow for meals and snacks. Your diabetes educator may have you change this pattern depending on your medication and your blood sugar values. Or you may adjust the pattern if you are eating out or your activity schedule changes. The goal is to attempt to evenly divide the carbs you eat throughout the day and never go without food for long periods.

Dividing Your Daily Carb Budget
Between Meals and Snacks

Daily Carb Budget: _____ **Carb Choices or** _____ **grams Carb**

Breakfast	_____ *Carb choices*	=	_____ *grams Carb*
A.M. *Snack*	_____ *Carb choices*	=	_____ *grams Carb*
Lunch	_____ *Carb choices*	=	_____ *grams Carb*
P.M. *Snack*	_____ *Carb choices*	=	_____ *grams Carb*
Dinner	_____ *Carb choices*	=	_____ *grams Carb*
Night Snack	_____ *Carb choices*	=	_____ *grams Carb*
Total	_____ **Carb choices**	=	_____ **total grams Carb**

To take this planning one step further, here is a sample day for a woman eating 1800 calories with a carb budget of 225 grams.

SAMPLE MENU FOR A WOMAN

1800 Calories
Carb Budget: 225 grams or 15 Carb Choices

Food	Portion	Calories	Carbs
Breakfast Carb Budget			**45**
Pink grapefruit sections	½ cup	37	9
Fresh blueberries	¼ cup	20	5
Corn flakes	¾ cup	100	24
Nonfat milk	1 cup	86	12
Coffee + sugar substitute	as desired	0	0
Breakfast Subtotals		**243**	**50**

(continued)

Morning Snack Carb Budget			**15**
Apple	1 small	63	16
Cheddar cheese, lowfat	1 ounce	49	1
Morning Snack Subtotals		**112**	**17**
Lunch Carb Budget			**60**
Tuna salad	½ cup	192	10
Rye bread	2 slices	130	24
Swiss cheese	1 oz	107	1
Tossed salad	1½ cups	32	7
Low cal Italian dressing	2 tbsp	32	2
Diet cola	1 can	0	0
Light flavored yogurt	1 pkg	100	16
Lunch Subtotals		**593**	**60**
Afternoon Snack Carb Budget			**15**
Graham crackers	2 squares	60	10
Lowfat cream cheese	1 tbsp	60	2
Tea + sugar substitute	as desired	0	0
Afternoon Snack Subtotals		**120**	**12**
Dinner Carb Budget			**60**
Roast chicken w/skin	½ breast	142	0
Rice	⅔ cup	137	30
Cracked pepper	sprinkle	0	0
Butter	1 tablespoon	108	tr
Broccoli, cooked	1 cup	46	8
Vanilla ice cream (no sugar added)	¾ cup	165	21
Sparkling water	as desired	0	0
Dinner Subtotals		**598**	**59**
Evening Snack Carb Budget			**30**
Popcorn	2 cups	62	12
Nonfat milk	1 cup	86	12
Sugar free chocolate syrup	2 tbsp	15	5
Evening Snack Subtotals		**163**	**29**
Day's Totals		**1829**	**227**

If the sample day was being planned for a man, the food choices would be very similar. Simply adjust the carb choices to reflect the way your individual carb budget is set up for the day. When you are first getting used to counting carbs and learning to manage your condition, it is helpful to keep daily food records. Your diabetes educator may have already suggested this. It's also smart to check yourself regularly to see if you are eating the calories and carbs that meet your treatment goals. The following Sample Daily Menu planning sheet will be a useful tool. Share the days you record with your diabetes educator to get feedback and fine-tune the management of your condition.

SAMPLE DAILY MENU

Date _____

_____ Calories Per Day

Daily Carb Budget: _____ grams Carbs or _____ Carb Choices

Food	Portion	Calories	Carbs
Breakfast Carb Budget			_____
Breakfast Subtotals		_____	_____
Morning Snack Carb Budget			_____
Morning Snack Subtotals		_____	_____
Lunch Carb Budget			_____
Lunch Subtotals		_____	_____
Afternoon Snack Carb Budget			_____
Afternoon Snack Subtotals		_____	_____
Dinner Carb Budget			_____
Dinner Subtotals		_____	_____
Evening Snack Carb Budget			_____
Evening Snack Subtotals		_____	_____
Day's Totals		_____	_____

EATING OUT

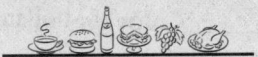

Whether it's a business lunch with clients, takeout on the way home from work, or a quick burger with your kids, eating out is part of the way we live. It's easy, quick, and fun, and it can be healthy. Eating out, even regularly, can definitely fit into your diabetic meal plan.

You walk into a restaurant, you're shown to a table, and handed a menu. Believe it or not, your key to successful eating out is right there in your hands. Read the menu carefully. Don't be afraid to ask for special options or substitutions. Many restaurants cater to diners' health needs. Some regularly offer "healthy" choices.

Menu selections that tend to have fewer calories and less fat are:

au jus (in its own juice)	grilled
baked	julienne
boiled	lean
broiled	marinara
cooked with lemon juice	poached
cooked with wine	roasted
deviled	steamed
fresh	stir fry
garden fresh	without skin

Menu choices that have more calories or fat are:

au gratin	gravy
battered	hollandaise
buttered	kiev
breaded	parmesan
casserole	parmigiana
cheese sauce (mornay)	pastry
cream sauce (à la king)	pot pie
creamy (béchamel)	prime
creamed	remoulade
crispy	rich
deep fried	scalloped
escalloped	thermidor
fried	

Simply apply the meal planning skills and carb counting strategies you use every day when you eat out. All restaurants have low calorie and no calorie sweeteners. Most carry sugar-free syrups and jelly, lowfat or nonfat salad dressings, nonfat milk, and diet drinks. Menu choices such as salads, fish, broiled lean meats, vegetables, fresh fruit, and whole grain breads are readily available. Do not be afraid to take control: ask questions, suggest substitutions, and be creative in putting together a meal you'll enjoy that fits into your daily carb and calorie budget.

Let's Order

- *Don't be afraid to ask:*
  Can I split a dinner between two?
  Can my choice be broiled instead of fried?
  Can I skip the potato and order double vegetables?
  Can I swap French fries for salad or sliced tomato?
  Can the chef leave out the salt?

- *Avoid temptation.*
  Stay away from all-you-can-eat buffets; it's too temping to overeat.
  Don't supersize your choice; large portions mean more carbs and calories.
  Take one roll and ask that the bread basket be removed from the table.
  Request no butter for the bread.
  Keep the vegetable tray and give back the chips and dip.

- *"Something to drink?"—"Water, thank you."*
  Choose calorie-free drinks—water, mineral water, club soda, unsweetened iced tea.
  Choose lower calorie drinks—wine, wine spritzers, fruit juice with club soda, diet soda.
  Limit alcohol; many drinks are packed with calories and carbs.

- *Make an "appetizer" a meal.*
  Order an appetizer or starter portion as an entrée.
  Ask if a lunch portion can be ordered at dinner.
  Share a main dish and order extra vegetables.

- *Play with your food.*
  Trim away excess fat.
  Remove skin from poultry.

- *Put toppings on the side.*
  Butter, gravy, salad dressing, sauce, sour cream, syrup, guacamole, grated cheese.
  Use very small portions to enhance flavor and avoid piling on calories.
  To get the flavor with fewer calories, try dipping your fork into the "extra" and then spear a piece of food, rather than dunking each bite.

- *Eat slowly.*
  Enjoy the company—talk more, eat less.
  Enjoy the ambiance of the restaurant.

- *Eat until you feel fine, not full—be mindful of how your body feels.*
  You don't have to clean your plate.
  Ask for a "doggie bag" to take home.

- *Be smart about dessert.*
  Share with another person—or better yet with the whole table.
  Order fresh fruit.
  End the meal with a richly flavored coffee or interesting tea instead of dessert.

YOU SHOULD KNOW

The Diabetes Counter *is a great
eating out resource. In addition to 71
restaurant chains in Part Two, there are
over 800 take-out choices listed.*

Think Before You Drink

As with many issues we have discussed, when it comes
to alcohol, there is good news and bad news. The good
news is that light to moderate use of alcohol lowers the
risk for diabetes and raises your HDL (good) cholesterol. The bad news is that heavy drinking increases
the risk for prediabetes and diabetes. Here are some
things to consider when adding alcohol to your diabetic meal plans.

- Limit alcoholic drinks to 1 a day for women and
  2 for men.

- Always drink alcohol with food, because drinking
  on an empty stomach can make your blood sugar
  drop too low.

- Alcohol by itself (gin, vodka, whiskey, rum) does
  not require insulin to be used for energy, so it does
  not cause blood sugar to go up.

- Mixed drinks, beer, and wine contain carbs and
  may raise your blood sugar.

- Light beer is very low in carbs and does not need
  to be counted into your daily carb budget.

- Regular beer has more carbs. One 12-ounce bottle should be counted as 1 carb choice in your daily carb budget.

- If you drink daily, the calories need to be added to your daily calorie intake. Alcohol calories do not need to be counted if you drink very infrequently.

YOU SHOULD KNOW

1 Alcoholic Drink Equals

12 ounces light beer—1 bottle or can
1.5 ounces 80-proof distilled spirits—1 shot glass
5 ounces wine—1 moderate-size wineglass

A Word About Tobacco

Many people use chewing tobacco and, surprisingly, the sugar content can affect blood sugar control. Pouch tobaccos contain between 24% and 65% sugar; plug tobaccos have 13% to 50% sugar. A 1.2-ounce can contains 10 or more grams of sugar. If you use smokeless tobacco regularly, it could affect your blood sugar.

All ABOUT SUGAR

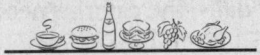

You are probably wondering why we haven't talked much about sugar up to now. In the past, people with diabetes were told they could not eat sugar because it would make their blood sugar go up too high. There is even a long-standing myth that eating too much sugar causes diabetes. It's not true.

Research has shown that sugar has the same effect on blood sugar as any other carbs you eat. Calorie for calorie, sugar raises blood sugar about the same amount as bread, pasta, or potatoes. You can eat sugar, and foods with sugar, as long as you count them in your total carb budget for the day.

Counting Sweets

As you chose different sweets, you need to know how each affects your carb budget for the day.

Let's start with the simplest sugars and sweeteners.

Sugars include table sugar, honey, brown sugar, molasses, fructose, corn syrup, maple syrup, raw sugar, powdered sugar, and agave syrup. Each contains carbs and you need to count the carb in your daily carb budget.

YOU SHOULD KNOW
Sugar Counts
1 teaspoon sugar = 4 grams carb

Reduced calorie sweeteners are often found in low calorie and low sugar foods like chewing gum, candy, cookies, and desserts. They appear on labels as *sorbitol, mannitol, xylitol, isomalt, lactitol, maltitol,* and *trehalose.* These sugar substitutes, called sugar alcohols, are absorbed slowly by the body, so they have less impact on blood sugar levels. But they still contain carbs and calories—about half the calories in sugar. If you regularly eat foods with sugar alcohols, you need to count them in your carb budget for the day.

YOU SHOULD KNOW

How to Count Sugar Alcohol as Part of Your Daily Carb Intake

Sugar alcohol is listed on the nutrition label. Subtract half the sugar alcohol from the total carbohydrate. Count the answer in your carb budget for the day.

For example:

1 energy bar = 15 grams of carb and 6 grams of sugar alcohol

Half the sugar alcohol = 3 grams

15 – 3 = 12

Count 12 grams of carb in your daily carb budget when you eat this energy bar for a snack.

No calorie sweeteners or artificial sweeteners don't contain calories or carbs and they don't affect your blood sugar. They are often referred to as "free foods" and you can eat them as often as you wish.

Artificial and Zero Calorie Natural Sweeteners	
Generic name	**Brand name**
Saccharin	*Sweet'N Low*
	Sweet Twin
	Necta Sweet
Aspartame	*NutraSweet*
	Equal
	SugarTwin
	AminoSweet
Acesulfame-K	*Sunette*
	Sweet & Safe
	Sweet One
Sucralose	*Splenda*
Stevia	*Truvia*
	PureVia
	SweetLeaf
	Only Sweet
	Stevia Extract In The Raw

Desserts

Having diabetes does not mean you have to give up desserts. Instead of "give it up," think "down-size and negotiate." Eat a smaller portion or trade dessert for a meal carb. Many desserts, like custard, rice pudding, or fruit-based sweets, are good for you and can be part of a healthy meal. Purely indulgent choices are not off-limits, either—in those cases just think small. Instead of a large candy bar, have a snack size. Try mini-cupcakes. With a little creative planning, there is a way to fit in your favorites.

- Small amounts of dried fruit can satisfy a sweet tooth.

- Eat smaller amounts of your favorites—½ cup of ice cream instead of a soup bowl full.

- When you eat out, split dessert with someone, or better yet share with the whole table.

- Try lower calorie, lower sugar recipes.

- Buy lower sugar versions of favorites, but remember that low sugar doesn't always equal low calorie.

- Drink diet soda, sugar free drinks, and use no calorie sweeteners in coffee and tea.

Instead of Apple Pie, Try . . .
In a microwave-safe serving dish, place:
1 small apple, peeled and sliced
1 tablespoon raisins
1 teaspoon chopped walnuts
Pinch of cinnamon
1 pkg artificial sweetener
Cover with plastic wrap or wax paper and
microwave on high for 1 minute 45 seconds.
Calories: 106   *Carb: 23*
À la mode, with ¼ cup light vanilla ice cream:
Calories: 150   *Carb: 31*

ALL ABOUT FIBER

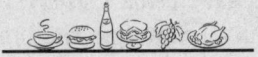

Few of us eat enough fiber, according to experts. Although nutrition guidelines recommend that we all eat at least 3 servings of whole grains a day, few of us do. Most eat less that 1 serving and we all eat too few fruits, vegetables, and beans, the other fiber-rich foods. We average about 15 grams of fiber a day, only half of what we should be eating.

Fiber is the part of carbohydrates that you can't digest, which is why it has no calories. The main sources of fiber are fruits, vegetables, beans, and whole grains—all good-for-you foods. Eating more high-fiber foods helps normalize blood sugar, reduce cholesterol, prevent colon cancer and constipation, and can even slightly lower blood pressure. Not bad for something that has no calories!

FIBER TIP

One easy way to add more fiber to your diet is to simply switch from white bread to whole wheat bread—the same amount of carbs per portion but with more fiber.

Figuring out how much fiber to eat each day is easy. Simply select your sex and age range on the following table and use that recommendation as your daily target fiber intake.

DAILY FIBER RECOMMENDATIONS

Men	
19-50 years	38 grams of fiber
50 and older	30 grams of fiber
Women	
19-50 years	25 grams of fiber
50 and older	21 grams of fiber
pregnant	28 grams of fiber

You don't need to track your fiber intake daily, but you should be aware of which foods contain fiber. *The Diabetes Counter* lists fiber so you can see which are the best sources. Every so often, as you are adding up your daily carb intake, add up fiber as well to see if you are getting the recommended amount.

If you normally eat little fiber—and that's the case for most of us—add foods rich in fiber slowly. Fiber-rich foods include beans, berries, bran, fruits, oatmeal, vegetables, popcorn, and whole grains. Don't go overboard, because it takes your body a little time to adjust to the extra bulk passing through your digestive tract. At first you may find you are a little gassy; this will pass as you adjust to the higher fiber intake. And be sure to drink plenty of fluids. Fiber soaks up fluids like a sponge. This not only helps you feel fuller longer, but helps form soft, easily passed stools.

FIBER TIP

*High fiber foods have 5 or more
grams of fiber in a serving.
A good source of fiber has 2 or more
grams of fiber in a serving.*

Add a Little Fiber to Your Life

- Eat whole fruits and vegetables instead of drinking juices.
- Don't peel! Eat the fiber-rich skins of cucumbers, apples, pears, potatoes, and zucchini.
- Eat more berries—blueberries, blackberries, raspberries, strawberries.
- Choose whole grains—brown rice, cornmeal, barley, cracked wheat, rye, whole wheat.
- Eat whole grain or high fiber cereals—oatmeal, oat flakes, bran, shredded wheat.
- Choose whole wheat bread, bagels, pasta, pretzels, crackers, and rolls.
- Eat beans, lentils, and peas a few times a week.
- Try soybeans in every form—soynuts, tofu, tempeh, edamame.
- Snack on fig newtons, graham crackers, and popcorn.
- Eat dried fruits and raisins.
- Sprinkle ground flaxseed, bran, or whole wheat granola on cereal or yogurt for a healthy crunch.

- Experiment with higher fiber versions of old favorites, like brown rice instead of white rice, buckwheat noodles instead or regular noodles, or baked sweet potatoes instead of white potatoes.

- Have vegetarian meals a few times a week.

- Try some of the new fiber-fortified foods like high-fiber cereal bars and breads.

Mash It, Smash It, Break It Apart
*Fiber is fiber, no matter how you process
or cook it.*
*Canned pureed pumpkin is a rich source of
fiber, as is split pea soup, mashed sweet potatoes,
cream of broccoli soup, or a fruit smoothie.*

MONITORING DIABETES

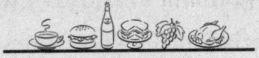

Many diabetes experts believe that self-monitoring is the key to successfully managing diabetes, reducing risks, and minimizing complications. Your diabetes educator, doctor, and dietitian will help you learn how to best monitor your condition.

Counting carbs and keeping a record of what you eat is one self-monitoring tool. Monitoring your blood sugar is another important tool you will use.

Checking Blood Sugar

Blood sugar is checked 2 ways: self-monitoring and the A1C test.

Your diabetes educator will tell you how often to check your blood sugar at home using a glucose monitor. At first, you may do it more often to be sure your medication and your diet are working together. Some people test 4 times a day, before each meal and at bedtime. If you have type 2 diabetes and your blood sugar is stable, you may test less frequently, 3 to 7 days a week before breakfast and randomly at other times during the day. At least 1 to 3 times a month, you should test before each meal and at bedtime to be sure your levels are within range.

You may be asked to keep a blood sugar log and bring these records when you get a checkup. The numbers you record will help your doctor decide which type and how much of a drug or insulin you should be taking. They also give your diabetes educator information that will help in adjusting your daily carb budget.

YOU SHOULD KNOW

Target Blood Sugar Values for People with Diabetes

Time to Check	Target Values
Upon waking, before eating	*90 to 130*
Before meals (at least 3 hours since your last meal)	*90 to 130*
2 hours after eating	*less than 160*
Bedtime (if lower, have a bedtime snack)	*110 to 150*

A1C is a blood test measuring a compound in your blood called *glycosylated hemoglobin*. The amount of this compound reveals the average blood sugar level over the last 6 to 12 weeks. The higher the A1C number, the higher your blood sugar has been. For good control the A1C value should be below 7%; a value of 6.5% means your average blood sugar is less than 155, which is very good. A1C tests should be done periodically throughout the year and are an excellent tool for monitoring long-term management of diabetes.

YOU SHOULD KNOW

*Blood sugar below 70 is too low and
above 240 is too high.
Blood sugar equal to or over 200 increases your
risk for infection and slows down wound healing.*

Low Blood Sugar—Hypoglycemia

Though your goal is to keep your blood sugar level
down, if it goes too low this can be a problem, as well.
The most common causes of low blood sugar are too
much insulin or oral medication, eating too little food,
exercising without eating extra food, or drinking alcohol on an empty stomach.

YOU SHOULD KNOW

Physical Signs of Low Blood Sugar
Sweating
Weakness
Hunger
Anxiety
Fast heartbeat
Irritability
Unable to think clearly
Headache
Drowsiness
Numbness or tingling around the lips

If you ever think that your blood sugar is too low, test
yourself with your glucose monitor. If the level is 70 or

lower, have one of these "quick fix" foods immediately to raise your blood sugar. Each equals 15 grams of carbohydrate or 1 carb choice.

- Glucose gel packet or glucose tablets equaling 15 grams of carb
- ½ cup fruit juice
- 1 cup milk
- 1 to 2 teaspoons sugar or honey
- ½ cup of regular soda
- ½ cup of regular Jell-O
- 2 tablespoons raisins
- 6 jelly beans
- 5 to 6 pieces of hard candy

Test your blood again in 15 minutes. If it is still below 70, eat another 15-gram carb choice. Wait 15 minutes and test your blood again. If it is an hour or more before your next meal, have a snack that contains both a carb and a protein. Good examples are:

- Peanut butter and crackers
- Cheese and crackers
- Half a ham or turkey sandwich
- Milk and cereal
- Hard or soft cooked egg and toast

It's a good idea to keep some of these "quick fix" choices in your house, office desk drawer, or in the car when you drive long distances, just in case.

You Should Get a Round of Applause

Good diabetes control takes discipline, effort, and commitment.

You need to monitor your diet, exercise, blood glucose, and drugs.

Keep up the good work!

A WORD ABOUT THE GLYCEMIC INDEX

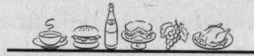

Decades ago, researcher David Jenkins at the University of Toronto coined the term *glycemic index* (GI). This index ranks carbohydrate foods by the amount they raise blood sugar after eating. Foods with a high glycemic index raise blood sugar levels quickly. Foods with a low GI produce a much smaller rise in blood sugar levels, which helps keep blood sugar within a normal range.

The theory behind the glycemic index is correct. Some foods do raise blood sugar quickly; others do not. But in practice, it's not that simple.

The glycemic index measures the ability of foods to raise blood sugar when eaten alone. Straight glucose was given a rating of 100 and individual foods were measured against it. But the gycemic index of food combinations can be very different. White bread has a very high glycemic index. If you add peanut butter to white bread, the glycemic response goes down because peanut butter, a high fat food, has a low glycemic index. The same goes for a baked potato, another high glycemic food: top it with cheese sauce and broccoli, and the glycemic index plunges.

It gets even more complicated. Ripe fruits have a lower glycemic index than unripe fruits. That's right, a hard peach will raise your blood sugar faster than a ripe, juicy one. Cooking pasta al dente is fine; overcook it, and its glycemic value goes up. Regular ice cream has a low glycemic index, because the fat in it slows down the absorption of sugar. Even sugars vary. Glucose is high on the index, but fructose (fruit sugar) is low.

GLYCEMIC INDEX OF COMMON FOODS	
High (greater than 70)	
White rice	126
Baked potato	121
Cornflakes	119
Rice cakes	117
Jellybeans	114
Carrots	101
White bread	101
Glucose	**100**
Wheat bread	99
Soda	97
Sucrose	92
Cheese pizza	86
Spaghetti	83
Popcorn	79
Corn	78
Banana	76
Orange juice	74

(continued)

Moderate (between 56 and 69)

Peas	*68*
Orange	*62*
Bran cereal	*60*
Apple juice	*58*
Pumpernickel bread	*58*

Low (55 and below)

Apple	*52*
Nonfat milk	*46*
Kidney beans	*42*
Fructose (fruit sugar)	*32*

Source: *Dietary Reference Intakes for Energy, Carbohydrate, Fiber, Fat, Fatty Acids, Cholesterol, Protein and Amino Acids, Part 1,* Institute of Medicine of the National Academies, The National Academies Press, 2002.

Bottom Line

Research into the health effects of the glycemic index is still evolving. Most experts agree that eating more high-fiber foods and fewer processed foods is good. Low GI foods include nonstarchy vegetables, most fruits, and dairy products—all good choices for someone with diabetes. Using the index might help you fine-tune some of your carb choices, but exclusively eating-by-the-numbers could steer you away from otherwise healthy foods.

If you want to incorporate glycemic index choices into your carb budget for the day, that's fine. Some research has shown that this approach can give you a better blood sugar response.

YOU SHOULD KNOW

If you are considering using the glycemic index to help manage your diabetes, discuss the benefits with your diabetes educator, who can help you tailor this approach to your treatment goals.

WHERE TO GO FOR MORE INFORMATION

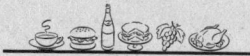

There are many resources available to help you learn more about diabetes, its treatment, and the newest research findings. Many food companies and pharmaceutical firms offer publications, newsletters, and recipes. Take advantage of all these resources because they provide interesting and worthwhile information. You can start with the following well-known and reliable resources.

American Diabetes Association
National Service Center
1701 North Beauregard Street
Alexandria, VA 22311
800-DIABETES (1-800-342-2383)
www.diabetes.org

Canadian Diabetes Association (CDA)
National Life Building
1400-522 University Avenue
Toronto, ON M5G 2R5
Canada
800-226-8464
www.diabetes.ca

Centers for Disease Control and Prevention
CDC-INFO
National Center for Chronic Disease Prevention and
Health Promotion
1600 Clifton Road
Atlanta, GA 30333
800-CDC-INFO (800-232-4636)
www.cdc.gov/diabetes

Diabetes Action Resource and Education Foundation
426 C Street, NE
Washington, DC 20002
202-333-4520
www.diabetesaction.org

Diabetes Exercise and Sports Association (DESA)
8001 Montcastle Drive
Nashville, TN 37221
800-898-4322
www.diabetes-exercise.org

Indian Health Service National Diabetes Program
5300 Homestead Road, NE
Albuquerque, NM 87110
505-246-4182
www.ihs.gov/MedicalPrograms/Diabetes/index.asp

International Diabetes Institute (IDI)
250 Kooyoung Road
Caulfield, Victoria 3162
Australia
061-03-9258-5050
www.diabetes.com.au or www.diabetes.org.au

National Diabetes Education Program (NDEP)
One Diabetes Way
Bethesda, MD 20814-9692
800-438-5383
www.ndep.nih.gov

National Diabetes Information Clearing House (NDIC)
1 Information Way
Bethesda, MD 20892-3560
800-860-8747
www.diabetes.niddk.nih.gov

USING YOUR DIABETES COUNTER

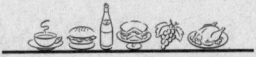

The Diabetes Counter lists the portion size, calories, fat, carbohydrate, fiber, and sugar values for more than 12,000 foods. Now you can compare the values in your favorite foods and, when necessary, choose substitutes before you go out to shop or eat. This will save you time and help you decide what to buy.

The carbohydrate and calorie values will help you stay within your carb and calorie budget for the day. Fat values have been included to help you plan lower fat meals to reduce your risk for heart disease. Sugar values are included to make you aware of which foods are high in sugar. Sugar is not counted separately, but is part of your total carb budget for the day. Fiber values are included to make you aware of which foods are high in fiber. Fiber, like sugar, is found in foods that contain carbohydrates. It is a good idea to occasionally track your fiber intake for a day or two to see if you are meeting the requirements for your age and sex. (See page 53.)

The counter section of the book is divided into two parts: Part One: Brand Name, Nonbranded (Generic), and Take-out Foods (page 75); and Part Two: Restaurant Chains (page 483). Each part lists foods or restaurant chains alphabetically.

In Part One, for each category, you will find non-branded (generic) foods listed first, in alphabetical order, followed by an alphabetical listing of brand name foods. The nonbranded listings will help you estimate calorie, fat, carbohydrate, fiber, and sugar values when you don't see your favorite brands. They can also help you evaluate store brands. Large categories are divided into subcategories, such as canned, fresh, frozen, and ready-to-eat, to make it easier to find what you're looking for. Some categories have "see" and "see also" references to help you find related items.

Because we eat out so often, more than 800 take-out foods are listed in Part One. These are found in the take-out subcategory in many categories throughout Part One. Foods you take out or order in are rarely nutrition labeled.

Most foods are listed alphabetically. In some cases, though, foods are grouped by category. For example, a tuna sandwich is found in the SANDWICH category. Other group categories include:

Asian Food: **Page 83**
Includes all types of Asian foods except egg rolls and sushi, which are found in the egg rolls and sushi categories.

Deli Meats/Cold Cuts: **Page 219**
Includes all sandwich meats
except chicken, ham and turkey,
which have their own separate
categories.

Dinner: **Page 221**
Includes all prepared dinners listed
by brand name, except pasta dinners,
which are found in the pasta dinner
category.

Liquor/Liqueur: **Page 296**
Includes all alcoholic beverages and
mixed drinks except beer, champagne,
and wine, which have their own
separate categories.

Nutrition Supplements: **Page 320**
Includes all dieting aids, meal
replacements, and drinks, except
energy bars and energy drinks,
which have their own separate
categories.

Sandwiches: **Page 393**
Includes popular sandwich, calzone,
and panini choices.

Snacks: **Page 412**
Includes a variety of snack items, such
as pork rinds and cheese puffs.

Spanish Food: **Page 432**
> Includes all types of Spanish and
> Mexican foods except salsa and
> tortillas, which have their own
> separate categories

In Part Two, Restaurant Chains, 71 national and regional restaurant, coffee, doughnut, frozen yogurt, ice cream, pizza, sandwich, soup, and sushi chains are listed. Brand-name foods are required by federal law to have nutrition information on labels, but restaurants are different. In most areas of the country, restaurants provide this information voluntarily.

With *The Diabetes Counter* as your guide, you will never again wonder how much carbohydrate is in the foods you eat.

DEFINITIONS

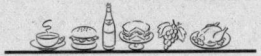

as prep (as prepared): refers to food that has been prepared according to package directions

lean and fat: describes meat with some fat on its edges that is not cut away before cooking, or poultry prepared with skin and fat as purchased

lean only: refers to lean meat that is trimmed of all visible fat, or poultry without skin

not prep (not prepared): refers to food that has not been cooked and may require the addition of other ingredients to prepare

shelf stable: refers to prepared products found on the supermarket shelf that are not canned or frozen but are packaged and ready-to-eat, or are ready to be heated and do not require refrigeration

take-out: describes prepared dishes that you purchase ready-to-eat; those included serve as a guide to the calories, fat, carbohydrate, fiber, and sugar in products you may buy

ABBREVIATIONS

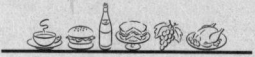

avg	=	average
diam	=	diameter
fl	=	fluid
frzn	=	frozen
g	=	gram
in	=	inch
lb	=	pound
lg	=	large
med	=	medium
mg	=	milligram
oz	=	ounce
pkg	=	package
pt	=	pint
prep	=	prepared
qt	=	quart
reg	=	regular
sec	=	second
serv	=	serving
sm	=	small
sq	=	square
tbsp	=	tablespoon
tr	=	trace
tsp	=	teaspoon
w/	=	with
w/o	=	without
<	=	less than

NOTES

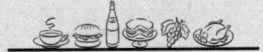

cal = calories
fat = fat
carb = carbohydrates
fiber = fiber
sugar = sugar
All fat, carbohydrate, fiber and sugar values are given
    in grams.
− (dash) indicates that values are not available
tr (trace) = less than 1 gram of fat, carbohydrate, fiber,
    or sugar
0 (zero) indicates there are no calories, fat,
    carbohydrate, fiber, or sugar in that food

Discrepancies in figures are due to rounding of values, product reformulation, and reevaluation. The current labeling law allows rounding. Some of the data listed are analysis data, obtained directly from manufacturers, not from labels; therefore, some values may differ slightly from the labels because the values have not been rounded.

PART ONE

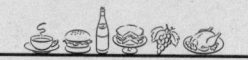

Brand Name, Nonbranded (Generic), and Take-out Foods

YOU SHOULD KNOW

*Naturally occurring compounds
in certain healthy foods may help
you manage your diabetes.*
*Green and black tea help boost insulin
activity and protect the eyes from damage.*
Cinnamon lowers blood sugar.
Buckwheat lowers blood sugar.
*Cherries lower blood sugar and help
increase insulin production.*
*Foods high in vitamin C, like citrus
fruits, strawberries, watermelon,
and orange juice, help prevent some
complications from diabetes.*

FOOD	PORTION	CAL	FAT	CARB	SUGAR	FIBER
ABALONE						
breaded & fried	1 serv (3 oz)	162	6	9	tr	tr
steamed	1 serv (3 oz)	127	3	6	tr	0
ACAI JUICE						
Arthur's						
Acai Plus	1 bottle (11 oz)	230	5	45	25	5
Bossa Nova						
Acai Juice Blueberry	8 oz	89	0	21	18	0
Acai Juice Mango	8 oz	89	0	23	16	0
Acai Juice Original	8 oz	94	0	21	18	0
Acai Juice Passion Fruit	8 oz	89	0	23	18	0
Acai Juice Raspberry	8 oz	89	0	23	18	0
O.N.E.						
Amazon Acai	1 bottle (11 oz)	157	3	32	29	3
ACEROLA						
fresh	1 (5 g)	2	tr	tr	–	tr
ACEROLA JUICE						
juice	1 cup	56	1	12	11	1
ADZUKI BEANS						
canned sweetened	½ cup	351	tr	81	–	–
dried cooked w/o salt	½ cup	147	tr	28	–	8
AKEE						
fresh	3.5 oz	223	20	5	–	–

ALE (see BEER AND ALE)

ALCOHOL (see BEER AND ALE, CHAMPAGNE, LIQUOR/LIQUEUR, MALT, WINE)

FOOD	PORTION	CAL	FAT	CARB	SUGAR	FIBER
ALFALFA						
sprouts	½ cup	40	tr	1	tr	tr

FOOD	PORTION	CAL	FAT	CARB	SUGAR	FIBER
ALLIGATOR						
cooked	3 oz	126	2	0	0	0
ALLSPICE						
ground	1 tsp	5	tr	1	–	tr
ALMONDS						
almond butter w/ salt	2 tbsp	203	19	7	2	1
almond butter w/o salt	2 tbsp	203	19	7	–	1
almond paste	¼ cup	260	16	27	21	3
chocolate covered	6 pieces (0.6 oz)	102	8	6	3	2
dry roasted w/ salt	¼ cup	206	18	7	2	4
dry roasted w/o salt	¼ cup	206	18	7	2	4
honey roasted	¼ cup	214	18	10	–	5
jordan almonds	6 (0.7 oz)	99	4	14	13	1
oil roasted w/ salt	¼ cup	238	22	7	2	4
oil roasted w/o salt	¼ cup	238	22	7	2	4
praline	17 pieces (1.4 oz)	210	12	21	17	3
yogurt covered	6 pieces (0.8 oz)	122	8	10	8	1
Back To Nature						
California Sea Salt Roasted	1 oz	160	14	6	1	3
Diamond						
Slivered	¼ cup (1 oz)	170	15	6	1	3
Fisher						
Roasted & Salted	¼ cup (1 oz)	170	15	5	1	3
Godiva						
Dark Chocolate Almonds	1 pkg (2 oz)	310	24	23	14	5
Justin's						
Almond Butter Classic	2 tbsp (1.1 oz)	200	18	6	1	4
Almond Butter Maple	2 tbsp (1.1 oz)	190	16	8	4	3

FOOD	PORTION	CAL	FAT	CARB	SUGAR	FIBER
Mrs. May's						
Almond Crunch	1 oz	156	13	8	3	3
Naturally More						
Almond Butter	2 tbsp	190	16	8	2	4
AMARANTH						
leaves cooked	½ cup	14	tr	3	–	–
uncooked	½ cup (3.4 oz)	365	6	65	–	15
ANCHOVY						
boneless	1 oz	60	3	0	0	0
canned in oil drained	1 can (2 oz)	94	4	0	0	0
fresh	1 (4 g)	8	tr	0	0	0
fresh fillets	3 (0.4 oz)	21	1	tr	–	–
Polar						
Rolled Fillets w/ Capers In Olive Oil	7 pieces (0.6 oz)	40	3	0	0	0
ANGLERFISH						
raw	3.5 oz	72	1	0	0	0
ANISE						
seed	1 tsp	7	tr	1	–	tr
ANTELOPE						
roasted	4 oz	215	4	0	0	0
APPLE						
CANNED						
sliced sweetened	½ cup	68	1	17	15	2
Polar						
Fuji	½ cup	50	0	12	11	2
DRIED						
chopped	½ cup	104	tr	28	24	4
cooked w/o sugar	½ cup	73	tr	20	17	3
rings	5	78	tr	21	18	3

FOOD	PORTION	CAL	FAT	CARB	SUGAR	FIBER
Chukar Cherries						
Cherry Apple Slices	10 (1 oz)	110	0	28	24	4
Crispy Green						
Freeze-Dried	1 pkg (0.35 oz)	40	0	8	7	1
Mrs. May's						
Fruit Chips	1 pkg	35	0	8	7	1
Nature's Envy						
Apple Chips Original	1 pkg (0.8 oz)	80	0	20	17	tr
Stoneridge Orchards						
Green Wedges	⅓ cup (1.4 oz)	140	0	32	27	1
Sun-Maid						
Apples	¼ cup (1.4 oz)	120	0	29	22	2
FRESH						
apple	1 sm	55	tr	15	11	3
apple	1 med	72	tr	19	14	3
apple	1 lg	110	tr	29	22	5
candied	1 sm (4.9 oz)	79	3	40	32	3
candied	1 med (6.5 oz)	234	4	52	42	4
candied	1 lg (9.8 oz)	357	6	79	64	6
w/ skin sliced	1 cup	57	tr	15	11	3
w/o skin sliced	1 cup	53	tr	14	11	1
Chiquita						
Apple	1 (6.4 oz)	95	0	25	19	4
Apple Bites	1 pkg (2.5 oz)	30	0	8	5	2
Apple Bites w/ Caramel	1 pkg (2.5 oz)	70	0	17	13	2
Eastern Select						
Gala	1 (5.5 oz)	80	0	22	16	5
FROZEN						
sliced w/o sugar	½ cup	42	tr	11	–	2
REFRIGERATED						
Country Crock						
Cinnamon Apples	½ cup (4.4 oz)	130	3	26	22	1

FOOD	PORTION	CAL	FAT	CARB	SUGAR	FIBER
TAKE-OUT						
baked	1 (6 oz)	128	tr	42	37	4
baked no sugar	1 (5.6 oz)	136	tr	24	18	4
fried apple rings	1 serv (2.7 oz)	91	4	15	12	2
APPLE JUICE						
cider	1 cup	117	tr	29	27	tr
juice + vitamin C & calcium	1 cup	117	tr	29	27	tr
mulled cider	1 serv	265	1	42	–	6
unsweetened w/o vitamin C	1 cup	117	tr	29	27	tr
Back To Nature						
100% Juice	1 pkg (6 oz)	80	0	21	20	–
Izze						
Sparkling Fortified Apple	1 can (8.4 oz)	90	0	23	21	–
Land O Lakes						
Juice	1 cup (8 oz)	120	0	29	26	0
Mott's						
100% Natural	1 bottle (14 oz)	200	0	48	48	0
Nantucket Nectars						
100% Juice Pressed Apple	8 oz	120	0	30	26	tr
Organic Cloudy Apple	8 oz	120	0	29	28	0
Santa Cruz						
Organic	8 oz	120	0	30	30	0
Snapple						
100% Juice Green Apple	8 oz	160	0	41	39	–
Juice Drink Apple	8 oz	110	0	27	27	–
APPLESAUCE						
sweetened	½ cup	97	tr	25	21	2

FOOD	PORTION	CAL	FAT	CARB	SUGAR	FIBER
unsweetened	½ cup	52	tr	14	12	2
GoGo Squeez						
Apple	1 pkg (3 oz)	60	1	14	13	1
Apple Banana	1 pkg (3 oz)	60	tr	14	11	1
Apple Cinnamon	1 pkg (3 oz)	50	tr	10	9	1
Apple Peach	1 pkg (3 oz)	60	tr	13	12	1
Mott's						
Healthy Harvest Granny Smith No Sugar Added	1 pkg (3.9 oz)	50	0	13	11	1
Organic Original	½ cup (4.5 oz)	110	0	27	25	1
Organic Unsweetened	½ cup (4.3 oz)	50	0	14	–	1
Musselman's						
Unsweetened	1 pkg (4 oz)	50	0	12	8	2
Revolution Foods						
Organic Unsweetened	1 pkg (4 oz)	50	0	13	10	2
Santa Cruz						
Organic	½ cup (4.5 oz)	60	0	13	11	2
Organic Apple Apricot	1 pkg (4 oz)	60	0	14	11	2
Organic Apple Blueberry	1 pkg (4 oz)	60	0	14	11	2
Organic Apple Cherry	½ cup (4.5 oz)	60	0	15	12	2

APRICOT JUICE

FOOD	PORTION	CAL	FAT	CARB	SUGAR	FIBER
nectar	6 oz	106	tr	27	26	1
Santa Cruz						
Organic Nectar	8 oz	120	0	29	27	tr

APRICOTS

FOOD	PORTION	CAL	FAT	CARB	SUGAR	FIBER
canned heavy syrup	½ cup	91	tr	23	20	3
canned in juice	½ cup	59	tr	15	13	2
canned in water	½ cup	33	tr	8	6	2
canned light syrup	½ cup	80	tr	21	19	2
dried halves	6	51	tr	13	11	2
dried halves cooked w/o sugar	½ cup	106	tr	28	24	3

FOOD	PORTION	CAL	FAT	CARB	SUGAR	FIBER
fresh	1	17	tr	4	3	1
fresh sliced	½ cup	40	tr	9	8	2
frozen sweetened	½ cup	119	tr	30	–	3
Elizabeth's Natural						
Turkish Dried	5 (1.8 oz)	90	0	22	19	3
Harvest Bay						
Dried	5 (1.4 oz)	60	0	15	15	3
S&W						
Whole In Heavy Syrup	½ cup (4.5 oz)	120	0	29	28	1
ARROWHEAD						
corm boiled	1 med	9	tr	2	–	–
ARROWROOT						
raw	1 root (1.2 oz)	21	tr	4	–	tr
raw root sliced	1 cup	78	tr	16	–	2
ARTICHOKE						
CANNED						
hearts in oil	1 serv (3 oz)	100	7	9	1	4
Cento						
Hearts Quartered Marinated	2 pieces	20	2	2	–	–
Polar						
Hearts	2	18	0	3	0	2
Hearts Quartered Marinated	1 oz	25	2	5	0	1
Progresso						
Hearts	2 (4.6 oz)	30	0	7	2	2
Hearts Marinated	2 (1.1 oz)	60	5	2	7	0
Roland						
Hearts	½ cup (4.6 oz)	50	0	9	1	4
The Gracious Gourmet						
Artichoke Parmesan Tapenade	2 tbsp (1 oz)	30	2	3	0	tr

FOOD	PORTION	CAL	FAT	CARB	SUGAR	FIBER
FRESH						
cooked	1 med	60	tr	13	1	7
hearts cooked	½ cup	42	tr	9	1	5
Ocean Mist						
Lemon	1 (4.2 oz)	60	0	13	1	6
FROZEN						
cooked	1 cup	42	tr	9	1	5
cooked w/o salt	1 pkg (9 oz)	108	1	22	2	11
TAKE-OUT						
stuffed	1 (8.8 oz)	397	14	54	6	10

ASIAN FOOD (see also CURRY, DINNER, EGG ROLLS, SAUCES, SOY SAUCE, SUSHI)

FOOD	PORTION	CAL	FAT	CARB	SUGAR	FIBER
CANNED						
chow mein chicken w/o noodles	1 cup	194	8	10	6	2
La Choy						
Chow Mein Beef	1 cup	90	2	11	2	2
Chow Mein Chicken	1 cup (9.3 oz)	100	3	10	3	2
Sweet & Sour Noodles	1 cup	150	2	29	23	5
Teriyaki Chicken	1 cup (8.6 oz)	120	4	16	7	3
FRESH						
wonton wrapper	1 (0.3 oz)	23	tr	5	–	tr
FROZEN						
Amy's						
Asian Noodle Stir Fry	1 pkg	290	7	50	16	4
Indian Mattar Paneer	1 pkg (10 oz)	320	8	54	8	6
Indian Palak Paneer	1 pkg (9.9 oz)	270	9	38	5	5
Indian Paneer Tikka	1 pkg (9.4 oz)	320	18	36	6	5
Indian Vegetable Korma	1 pkg (9.4 oz)	310	12	41	7	7
Thai Stir Fry	1 pkg (9.4 oz)	310	11	45	2	5
Ethnic Gourmet						
Bhartha Eggplant	1 pkg (11 oz)	300	9	47	2	10
Dal Bahaar	1 pkg (11 oz)	360	8	61	5	8
Kaeng Kari Kai	1 pkg (10 oz)	390	11	54	13	2

FOOD	PORTION	CAL	FAT	CARB	SUGAR	FIBER
Korma Chicken	1 pkg (10 oz)	340	9	44	4	3
Korma Vegetable	1 pkg (11 oz)	300	6	52	5	4
Kotopoulo Domato Ke Feta	1 pkg (10 oz)	340	11	41	1	5
Pad Thai Chicken	1 pkg (10 oz)	410	7	66	22	3
Pad Thai Shrimp	1 pkg (10 oz)	410	7	70	24	3
Tandoori Chicken w/ Spinach	1 pkg (10 oz)	170	5	19	4	3
French Meadow Bakery						
Vegetarian Dal Makhani	1 pkg (12 oz)	370	19	39	2	5
Healthy Choice						
Five Spice Beef & Vegetables	1 pkg (10 oz)	310	5	49	17	7
General Tso's Spicy Chicken	1 pkg (10.7 oz)	310	4	50	10	5
Joy Of Cooking						
Lo Mein Vegetable	1 cup (7.7 oz)	220	3	40	6	11
Organic Classics						
Thai Chicken Curry	1 pkg (10 oz)	420	17	50	4	3
SHELF-STABLE						
Healthy Choice						
Fresh Mixers Sesame Teriyaki Chicken	1 pkg (7.9 oz)	380	6	69	16	3
Fresh Mixers Sweet & Sour Chicken	1 pkg (7.9 oz)	390	3	78	22	5
Fresh Mixers Szechwan Beef w/ Asian Noodles	1 pkg (6.9 oz)	370	6	65	18	4
TAKE-OUT						
beef & broccoli	1 cup	221	12	10	3	3
beef w/ black bean sauce	1 serv (7 oz)	288	14	6	5	1

FOOD	PORTION	CAL	FAT	CARB	SUGAR	FIBER
buddha's delight w/ cellophane noodles fat choi jai	1 serv (7.6 oz)	211	4	44	3	2
bun baked red bean	1 (1.1 oz)	102	3	16	–	1
cha siu bao steamed buns w/ chicken filling	1 (2.3 oz)	160	3	26	4	tr
chicken masala	1 serv (8 oz)	430	25	8	–	0
chicken tandoori	1 serv (4 oz)	156	8	2	–	0
chicken tikka	1 serv (2.5 oz)	173	8	1	–	1
chinese garlic chicken	1 cup (5.7 oz)	290	19	8	3	1
chinese style fried egg noodles w/ seafood & lettuce	1 serv (14 oz)	694	37	63	1	8
chow mein beef w/o noodles	1 cup	271	15	12	4	3
chow mein chicken w/ noodles	1 cup (7.7 oz)	273	14	20	5	2
chow mein noodles	1 cup	237	14	26	tr	2
chow mein pork w/o noodles	1 cup	284	16	12	4	3
chow mein shrimp w/o noodles	1 cup	154	5	11	6	2
chow mein vegetable w/o noodles	1 cup	224	15	16	8	4
dim sum deep fried beancurd w/ shrimp	1 (1.1 oz)	77	6	2	–	1
dim sum deep fried yam	1 (2.4 oz)	201	12	23	–	2
dim sum meat filled	3 pieces (4 oz)	124	3	11	1	1
dim sum steamed chives & prawns	1 (1.2 oz)	48	2	5	–	1
egg foo yung beef	1 patty (6 oz)	243	16	7	3	1
egg foo yung chicken	1 patty (3 oz)	121	8	4	2	1
egg foo yung pork	1 patty (3 oz)	125	8	4	2	1

FOOD	PORTION	CAL	FAT	CARB	SUGAR	FIBER
egg foo yung shrimp	1 patty (3 oz)	153	12	3	2	1
filipino chicken adobo	1 serv (15 oz)	555	26	45	tr	1
foochow fish ball	1 (1 oz)	36	2	3	0	1
fried rice	1 cup	333	12	42	2	1
fried rice beef	1 cup	346	14	42	1	1
fried rice chicken	1 cup	329	12	42	1	1
fried rice pork	1 cup	335	13	42	1	1
fried rice shrimp	1 cup	323	12	42	2	1
general tso's chicken	1 cup (5 oz)	296	17	16	5	1
green beans szechuan style	1 cup	176	12	16	3	6
indian style fried egg noodles w/ eggs, tomato sauce, & lime	1 serv (15 oz)	721	31	80	2	8
korean spicy shredded chicken	1 serv (5 oz)	258	16	5	5	2
kung pao beef	1 cup	410	30	9	2	2
kung pao chicken	1 cup (5.7 oz)	434	31	12	4	2
kung pao pork	1 cup	460	34	12	4	2
kung pao shrimp	1 cup	345	20	11	3	2
lemon chicken w/o vegetables	1 serv (6.6 oz)	503	28	26	3	1
lo mein beef	1 cup	286	11	31	3	3
lo mein chicken	1 cup (7 oz)	280	9	33	3	3
lo mein meatless	1 cup	234	6	38	3	3
lo mein pork	1 cup	314	14	34	3	3
lo mein shrimp	1 cup	236	7	33	2	4
moo goo gai pan chicken	1 cup (7.6 oz)	272	19	12	5	3
moo shu pork w/o pancake	1 cup	512	46	5	2	1
pakhoras	1 (2.5 oz)	163	8	16	–	4
paneer pakhora	1 (2.2 oz)	183	13	8	–	2

FOOD	PORTION	CAL	FAT	CARB	SUGAR	FIBER
peking duck w/ pancakes & seafood sauce	1 serv (14 oz)	1871	121	157	39	5
phad thai w/ chicken	1 cup (7 oz)	358	15	39	5	2
pork w/ chinese cabbage	1 serv (4 oz)	120	8	1	0	1
sesame seed paste bun	1 (2.5 oz)	220	6	39	12	2
shrimp chips banh phong tom	6 med	214	14	20	1	tr
shrimp w/ lobster sauce	1 cup	298	12	8	2	1
shu mai chicken & vegetable dumplings	6 (3.6 oz)	160	5	18	6	1
sukiyaki beef	1 cup	165	7	6	4	1
sukiyaki chicken	1 serv (18 oz)	436	8	19	7	4
sweet & sour chicken w/o rice	1 cup	670	37	36	4	2
sweet & sour pork w/ rice	1 cup	268	6	40	10	2
sweet & sour pork w/o rice	1 cup	231	8	25	15	2
sweet & sour shrimp	1 cup	480	30	46	40	1
szechuan chicken	1 cup (5.7 oz)	180	9	9	2	2
szechuan shrimp & vegetables	1 cup	159	7	10	3	2
tempura vegetable	8 pieces	90	6	8	1	1
tempura hawaiian fish tofu vegetable	2 cups	285	22	13	9	2
teriyaki beef	1 cup	454	19	13	9	tr
teriyaki chicken	¾ cup	399	27	7	–	–
teriyaki chicken w/ rice	1 serv (11 oz)	430	6	77	10	1
teriyaki shrimp	1 cup	271	3	14	6	1
thai style pineapple rice w/ ham & pork floss	1 serv (7.7 oz)	408	14	60	22	6
wonton fried meat filled	1 (0.7 oz)	54	3	5	tr	tr

FOOD	PORTION	CAL	FAT	CARB	SUGAR	FIBER
wonton meat & shrimp boiled	1 (0.5 oz)	19	1	2	–	tr

ASPARAGUS
CANNED

FOOD	PORTION	CAL	FAT	CARB	SUGAR	FIBER
spears	1	3	tr	tr	tr	tr
spears	1 cup	46	2	6	3	4
Del Monte						
Spears Extra Long	½ cup	20	0	3	0	1
Green Giant						
Spears Extra Long	5	20	0	3	1	1
McSweet						
Pickled Spears	6 (1 oz)	25	0	6	6	0
S&W						
Spears	½ cup (4.4 oz)	20	0	3	0	1
FRESH						
cooked	½ cup	20	tr	4	1	2
cooked	4 spears	13	tr	2	1	1
spears raw	4	10	tr	2	1	1
Ocean Mist						
Spears	5 (3.3 oz)	25	0	4	2	2
FROZEN						
cooked	1 pkg (10 oz)	53	1	6	1	5
cooked	4 spears	11	tr	1	tr	1
Joy Of Cooking						
Tender	½ cup (3.3 oz)	70	5	4	1	1

ATEMOYA

FOOD	PORTION	CAL	FAT	CARB	SUGAR	FIBER
fresh	½ cup	94	1	24	–	–

AVOCADO

FOOD	PORTION	CAL	FAT	CARB	SUGAR	FIBER
california mashed	¼ cup	96	9	5	tr	4
california peeled & pitted	1	289	27	15	1	12

FOOD	PORTION	CAL	FAT	CARB	SUGAR	FIBER
florida mashed	¼ cup	69	6	5	0	1
florida peeled & pitted	1	365	31	24	7	17
Cabilfrut						
Hass fresh	⅕ med (1.1 oz)	55	3	3	0	3
Chiquita						
fresh	1 (7 oz)	322	29	17	1	13
Simply Avo						
Hass Avocado Pulp	2 tbsp	50	5	3	1	2
Hass Halves	⅙ pkg (1.1 oz)	50	5	3	0	2
Wholly Guacamole						
Classic	2 tbsp	50	4	2	0	2
Organic	2 tbsp	50	5	2	0	2
Pico De Gallo Style	2 tbsp	40	3	2	0	2
TAKE-OUT						
guacamole	1 serv (2.2 oz)	105	10	5	1	2
BACON						
bacon grease	1 tbsp	116	13	0	0	0
beef breakfast strips cooked	3 strips	153	12	tr	0	0
gammon lean & fat grilled	4.2 oz	274	15	0	–	0
pan fried	3 strips	109	9	tr	–	0
turkey	2 (0.8 oz)	84	6	1	0	0
Applegate Farms						
Natural Dry Cured Cooked	2 slices (0.5 oz)	60	5	0	0	0
Organic Turkey	1 slice (1 oz)	35	2	0	0	0
Boar's Head						
Fully Cooked Slices	3 (0.5 oz)	70	6	0	0	0
Butterball						
Turkey Bacon	1 slice (0.5 oz)	25	2	0	0	0

FOOD	PORTION	CAL	FAT	CARB	SUGAR	FIBER
Hormel						
Microwave Ready	2 slices (0.5 oz)	80	7	0	0	0
Real Bits	1 tbsp (7 g)	25	2	0	0	0
Jimmy Dean						
Lower Sodium	1 slice (0.3 oz)	50	4	0	0	0
Original	1 slice (0.3 oz)	50	4	0	0	0
Thick Slice	1 slice (0.5 oz)	80	6	0	0	0
Oscar Mayer						
Bacon Bits	1 tbsp (7 g)	25	2	0	0	0
Hardwood Smoked	2 slices (0.5 oz)	70	6	0	0	0
Lower Sodium	3 slices (0.5 oz)	70	6	0	0	0
Ready To Serve	3 slices	70	5	0	0	0
Uncured	3 slices (0.5 oz)	60	5	1	1	0
BACON SUBSTITUTES						
bacon bits meatless	1 tbsp	33	2	2	0	1
meatless	1 strip	16	1	tr	0	tr
BAGEL						
cinnamon raisin	1 mini	71	tr	14	2	1
cinnamon raisin	1 lg (4 in)	244	2	49	5	2
egg	1 lg (4.5 in)	364	3	69	–	3
low carb	1 (4 oz)	216	0	42	0	14
mini onion	1 (1.4 oz)	100	0	20	1	1
oat bran	1 lg (4 in)	227	1	47	1	3
plain	1 sm (3 in)	190	1	37	–	2
plain	1 med (3.5 in)	289	2	56	–	2
plain	1 lg (4.5 in)	360	2	70	–	3

FOOD	PORTION	CAL	FAT	CARB	SUGAR	FIBER
Finagle A Bagel						
Cinnamon Raisin	1 (4 oz)	300	1	67	18	5
Everything	1 (4 oz)	310	3	62	8	5
Onion	1 (4 oz)	300	1	65	8	4
Plain	1 (4 oz)	290	1	63	8	4
Poppy Seed	1 (4 oz)	310	4	60	9	4
Sesame	1 (4 oz)	310	5	60	8	5
French Meadow Bakery						
100% Spelt	1 (3.4 oz)	270	2	52	1	8
Hemp	1 (3.4 oz)	280	8	35	3	13
Sprouted Cinnamon Raisin	1 (3.5 oz)	270	2	50	11	7
Natural Ovens						
Blueberry	1 (3 oz)	250	2	47	13	5
Brainy	1 (3 oz)	230	3	40	7	8
Whole Wheat	1 (3 oz)	230	3	40	7	8
Pepperidge Farm						
100% Whole Wheat Mini	1 (1.4 oz)	100	1	20	3	3
Thomas'						
100% Whole Wheat Mini	1 (1.5 oz)	110	1	22	3	3
Bagel Holes Plain	3 (1.6 oz)	120	1	24	3	1
BAKING POWDER						
baking powder	1 tsp	2	0	1	0	0
low sodium	1 tsp	5	tr	2	0	tr
Davis						
Baking Powder	1 tsp	0	0	tr	0	0
BAKING SODA						
baking soda	1 tsp	0	0	0	0	0

FOOD	PORTION	CAL	FAT	CARB	SUGAR	FIBER
BALSAM PEAR (BITTER GOURD)						
leafy tips cooked w/o salt	1 cup	20	tr	4	1	1
leafy tips raw	1 cup	14	tr	2	–	–
pods raw sliced	1 cup	16	tr	3	–	3
pods sliced cooked w/ salt	1 cup	24	tr	5	2	3
BAMBOO SHOOTS						
canned sliced	½ cup	12	tr	2	1	1
fresh sliced cooked w/ salt	½ cup	7	tr	1	–	1
raw sliced	½ cup	20	tr	4	2	2
La Choy						
Bamboo Shoots	½ cup	10	0	2	0	tr
Polar						
Sliced	½ cup	25	0	3	1	2
BANANA						
baked	1 (4.5 oz)	163	tr	42	26	4
banana chips	1 oz	147	10	17	–	2
fresh	1 sm (6 in)	90	tr	23	12	3
fresh	1 lg (8 in)	121	tr	31	17	4
fresh	1 med (7 in)	105	tr	27	14	3
fresh baby	1 extra sm (<6 in)	72	tr	19	10	2
fresh mashed	½ cup	100	tr	26	14	3
fresh sliced	1 cup	134	1	34	18	4
green fried	1 (3.1 oz)	152	8	21	11	2
green pickled	½ cup	240	22	11	6	1
green sliced fried	1 cup	323	18	45	24	5
powder	1 tbsp	21	tr	5	3	1
red ripe	1 (7 in)	93	tr	24	13	3
red ripe sliced	1 cup	134	1	34	18	4

FOOD	PORTION	CAL	FAT	CARB	SUGAR	FIBER
whole dried	1 piece (1.2 oz)	130	1	33	22	2
Brothers-All-Natural						
Crisps	1 pkg (0.58 oz)	66	0	16	8	2
Chiquita						
fresh	1 med (4.1 oz)	105	0	27	14	3
Crispy Green						
Freeze-Dried	1 pkg (0.5 oz)	55	0	13	8	2
Kopali						
Organic Dark Chocolate Covered	½ pkg (1 oz)	120	6	19	17	2
Nana Flakes						
100% Natural	1 tbsp (0.2 oz)	22	0	6	3	1
Tree Of Life						
Dried Sweetened	½ cup (1.6 oz)	240	15	27	18	4
TAKE-OUT						
batter dipped fried	1 sm (4 oz)	266	15	32	9	3
batter dipped fried sliced	1 cup	335	19	40	12	3
fried dwarf w/ cheese	1 (1.4 oz)	84	5	10	5	1
fritter	1 (2.3 oz)	197	5	36	14	2

BANANA JUICE
Snapple

Juice Drink Go Bananas	8 oz	110	0	28	28	–

BARBECUE SAUCE

barbecue	2 tbsp	52	tr	13	9	tr
low sodium	2 tbsp	52	tr	13	9	tr
Bear-Man						
Black Bear Boogie	2 tbsp	40	1	8	5	0
Growlin' Grizzly	2 tbsp	60	1	12	8	tr

FOOD	PORTION	CAL	FAT	CARB	SUGAR	FIBER
Chef Hymie Grande						
Cascabel Express Barbecue Glaze	2 tbsp (1.2 oz)	30	0	7	5	1
Polapote Barbecue Glaze	2 tbsp (1.2 oz)	30	0	7	4	2
Dave's Gourmet						
Badlands BBQ	2 tbsp (1.1 oz)	40	1	8	7	–
Naturally Fresh						
BBQ	2 tbsp	40	0	10	8	0
OrganicVille						
Original No Added Sugar	2 tbsp (1 oz)	50	0	13	11	tr
Ribber City						
Kansas City	2 tbsp (1.1 oz)	40	0	11	9	0
The Gracious Gourmet						
Spicy Barbeque Glaze	2 tbsp (1 oz)	35	1	7	6	0
World Harbors						
Bar-B	2 tbsp (1.2 oz)	70	0	16	14	0
Buccaneer Blends Fra Diavlo	2 tbsp (1.2 oz)	45	0	11	10	0
Buccaneer Blends Honey Mango	2 tbsp (1.3 oz)	60	0	13	12	0
Buccaneer Blends Sticky Rum	2 tbsp (1.2 oz)	50	0	13	12	0
BARLEY						
flour	1 cup	511	2	110	1	15
pearled cooked	1 cup (5.5 oz)	193	1	44	tr	6
pearled uncooked	¼ cup	176	1	39	tr	8
BARRACUDA						
broiled	4 oz	239	14	tr	tr	0
cooked flaked	1 cup	287	16	1	tr	0
poached	4 oz	227	11	0	0	0

FOOD	PORTION	CAL	FAT	CARB	SUGAR	FIBER
TAKE-OUT						
breaded & fried	4 oz	282	17	5	tr	tr
BASIL						
fresh chopped	2 tbsp	1	tr	tr	tr	tr
ground	1 tsp	4	tr	1	tr	1
leaves fresh	5	1	tr	tr	tr	tr
BASS						
breaded baked	4 oz	205	7	10	1	1
pickled mero en escabeche	2 oz	156	14	tr	tr	tr
striped baked	3 oz	105	3	0	0	0
striped bass farm raised	4 oz	110	3	0	0	0
BAY LEAF						
crumbled	1 tsp	2	tr	tr	tr	tr

BEAN SPROUTS (see ALFALFA, SPROUTS)

BEANS (see also individual names)

FOOD	PORTION	CAL	FAT	CARB	SUGAR	FIBER
CANNED						
baked beans plain	½ cup	119	tr	27	–	5
baked beans vegetarian	½ cup	119	tr	27	–	5
baked beans w/ franks	½ cup	184	9	20	–	9
baked beans w/ pork	½ cup	134	2	25	–	7
baked beans w/ pork & tomato sauce	½ cup	119	1	24	7	5
refried beans	½ cup	134	1	23	–	–
Allens						
Original Baked	½ cup	150	1	29	10	8
Refried Black Beans No Fat Added	½ cup	120	0	23	1	8
Amy's						
Organic Refried	½ cup	140	3	21	1	6

FOOD	PORTION	CAL	FAT	CARB	SUGAR	FIBER
Organic Refried Light In Sodium	½ cup (4.6 oz)	140	3	21	1	6
B&M						
Baked Original	½ cup (4.6 oz)	180	3	31	10	8
Barbeque Baked	½ cup (4.6 oz)	190	1	39	19	9
Country Style	½ cup (4.6 oz)	170	1	35	15	7
Vegetarian	½ cup (4.6 oz)	160	1	31	12	8
Bush's						
Honey	½ cup	160	1	32	14	6
Gebhardt						
Refried	½ cup	90	2	16	0	4
Refried Fat Free	½ cup	80	0	17	tr	5
Refried Jalapeno	½ cup	100	2	17	1	5
Green Giant						
Three Bean Salad	½ cup	80	0	18	10	3
Hormel						
Kid's Kitchen Microwave Meals Beans & Wieners	1 pkg (7.7 oz)	310	13	37	14	7
Read						
3 Bean Salad	⅓ cup	60	0	13	8	2
Rosarita						
Refried	½ cup	120	2	18	tr	6
Refried Black Beans No Fat	½ cup	110	0	19	0	8
Refried Fat Free	½ cup	100	0	19	tr	6
Refried Vegetarian	½ cup	120	2	19	0	7
Van Camp's						
Baked Beans Homestyle	½ cup	170	1	33	15	6
Beanee Weenee BBQ	1 can	260	8	35	12	9
Beanee Weenee Original	1 can	240	8	29	8	8
Beanee Weenee w/ Chili	1 can	240	9	26	2	6
Pork And Beans	½ cup	110	1	23	7	6

FOOD	PORTION	CAL	FAT	CARB	SUGAR	FIBER
Wagon Master						
Pork & Beans	½ cup	130	1	23	4	9
TAKE-OUT						
baked beans	½ cup	191	7	27	–	7
barbecue beans	3.5 oz	120	tr	26	–	–
frijoles a la charra w/ pork tomatoes & chili peppers	1 cup	341	22	23	2	5
refried beans	½ cup	43	2	5	–	–
three bean salad	1 cup	114	5	15	2	5
BEAR						
simmered	3 oz	220	11	0	0	0
BEAVER						
roasted	4 oz	240	8	0	0	0
BEE POLLEN						
bee pollen	1 tsp (5 g)	16	tr	2	2	tr
Tree Of Life						
Bee Pollen	1 tsp (7 g)	30	1	3	0	0
BEECHNUTS						
dried	1 oz	163	14	10	–	–
BEEF (see also BEEF DISHES, JERKY, MEATBALLS, VEAL)						
CANNED						
corned beef	1 oz	71	4	0	0	0
Hormel						
Corned Beef	1 serv (2 oz)	120	6	0	0	0
Dried Beef	1 oz	50	2	1	1	0
Libby's						
Corned Beef	2 oz	120	7	0	0	0
Potted Meat	¼ cup	120	9	0	0	0
Roast Beef w/ Gravy	⅔ cup	140	4	3	0	0

FOOD	PORTION	CAL	FAT	CARB	SUGAR	FIBER
FRESH						
arm pot roast trim 0 fat braised	3.5 oz	297	19	0	0	0
arm pot roast trim 1/8 in fat braised	3.5 oz	302	19	0	0	0
beef crumbles 70% lean pan browned	3 oz	230	15	0	0	0
bottom round roast trim 0 fat braised	4 oz	253	10	0	0	0
bottom round roast trim 0 fat roasted	3.5 oz	187	8	0	0	0
bottom round roast trim 1/2 in fat braised	4 oz	337	22	0	0	0
bottom round roast trim 1/8 in fat braised	4 oz	280	13	0	0	0
bottom round roast trim 1/8 in fat roasted	4 oz	247	13	0	0	0
bottom sirloin butt roast trim 0 fat roasted	3.5 oz	182	8	0	0	0
brisket flat half trim 1/8 in fat braised	3.5 oz	298	19	0	0	0
brisket flat trim 0 fat braised	3.5 oz	221	9	0	0	0
brisket point half trim 0 fat braised	3.5 oz	358	29	0	0	0
brisket point half trim 1/4 in fat braised	3.5 oz	404	22	0	0	0
brisket point half trim 1/8 in fat braised	3.5 oz	349	27	0	0	0
chuck boston cut roast trim 0 fat roasted	3.5 oz	207	11	0	0	0
chuck boston cut roast trim 1/4 in fat roasted	3.5 oz	242	15	0	0	0

FOOD	PORTION	CAL	FAT	CARB	SUGAR	FIBER
chuck bottom roast trim 0 fat braised	3.5 oz	334	24	0	0	0
chuck bottom roast trim ¼ in fat braised	3.5 oz	345	26	0	0	0
chuck fillet steak trim 0 fat broiled	4 oz	181	6	0	0	0
chuck top roast trim 0 fat broiled	4 oz	245	13	0	0	0
club steak trim ½ in fat broiled	4 oz	384	29	0	0	0
corned beef brisket cooked	3 oz	213	16	tr	0	0
crosscut shank trim ¼ in fat stewed	1 serv (6.8 oz)	510	28	0	0	0
delmonico steak trim ¼ in fat broiled	4 oz	409	33	0	0	0
entrecote steak trim ½ in fat broiled	4 oz	413	33	0	0	0
eye round roast trim 0 fat roasted	4 oz	190	5	0	0	0
eye round roast trim ¼ in fat roasted	4 oz	283	17	0	0	0
filet mignon roast trim ¼ in fat roasted	4 oz	376	29	0	0	0
filet mignon roast trim ⅛ in fat roasted	4 oz	367	28	0	0	0
filet mignon trim 0 fat broiled	4 oz	247	13	0	0	0
filet mignon trim ⅛ in fat broiled	4 oz	303	19	0	0	0
ground 70% lean broiled	3.5 oz	273	18	0	0	0

FOOD	PORTION	CAL	FAT	CARB	SUGAR	FIBER
ground 75% lean broiled	2.5 oz	195	13	0	0	0
ground 80% lean broiled	3 oz	234	15	0	0	0
ground 85% lean pan fried	3 oz	197	12	0	0	0
ground 90% lean pan fried	3 oz	173	9	0	0	0
ground 95% lean pan fried	3 oz	139	5	0	0	0
ground lowfat w/ carrageenan raw	4 oz	160	7	tr	–	–
london broil trim 0 fat broiled	3.5 oz	188	8	0	0	0
london broil trim ¼ in fat broiled	4 oz	260	12	0	0	0
new york strip steak trim 0 fat broiled	4 oz	219	9	0	0	0
oxtails cooked	6 pieces (6.3 oz)	472	26	0	0	0
porterhouse steak trim 0 fat broiled	1 lb	1252	87	0	0	0
porterhouse steak trim ¼ in fat broiled	1 lb	1492	117	0	0	0
porterhouse steak trim ⅛ in fat broiled	4 oz	337	25	0	0	0
porterhouse steak trim ⅛ in fat broiled	1 lb	1324	99	0	0	0
rib eye roast trim ¼ in fat roasted	3.5 oz	365	30	0	0	0
rib eye steak trim ⅛ in fat broiled	4 oz	221	9	0	0	0

FOOD	PORTION	CAL	FAT	CARB	SUGAR	FIBER
rib roast trim ¼ in fat roasted	4 oz	406	33	0	0	0
rib steak trim ¼ in fat broiled	4 oz	388	31	0	0	0
round tip roast trim 0 fat roasted	4 oz	213	9	0	0	0
sandwich steaks thinly sliced	1 serv (2 oz)	173	15	0	0	0
shell steak trim ¼ in fat broiled	4 oz	366	27	0	0	0
shortribs lean & fat braised	1 serv (7.8 oz)	1060	94	0	0	0
skirt steak trim 0 fat broiled	4 oz	289	19	0	0	0
t-bone steak trim 0 fat broiled	4 oz	280	18	0	0	0
t-bone steak trim ¼ in fat broiled	1 lb	1388	103	0	0	0
t-bone steak trim ⅛ in fat broiled	1 lb	804	56	0	0	0
tip round roast trim ⅛ in fat roasted	4 oz	248	13	0	0	0
top loin steak boneless trim ⅛ in fat broiled	4 oz	299	19	0	0	0
top round roast trim 0 fat braised	4 oz	237	7	0	0	0
top round roast trim ¼ in fat braised	4 oz	281	13	0	0	0
top round roast trim ¼ in fat roasted	4 oz	265	15	0	0	0
top round steak trim ¼ in fat pan fried	4 oz	314	17	0	0	0

FOOD	PORTION	CAL	FAT	CARB	SUGAR	FIBER
top sirloin steak trim ⅛ in fat broiled	4 oz	275	16	0	0	0
top sirloin steak trim ⅛ in fat pan fried	4 oz	355	24	0	0	0
tri-tip roast trim 0 fat roasted	3.5 oz	218	12	0	0	0
tri-tip steak trim 0 fat broiled	4 oz	300	17	0	0	0
Rumba						
Cheekmeat	4 oz	300	25	0	0	0
Crosscut Hind Shank	4 oz	190	10	0	0	0
Marrow Bones	4 oz	290	22	0	0	0
Oxtail	4 oz	260	21	0	0	0
Short Ribs	4 oz	400	36	0	0	0
FROZEN						
patty broiled medium	3 oz	240	17	0	0	0
READY-TO-EAT						
dried beef smoked chopped	1 oz	37	1	1	–	0
roast beef spread	¼ cup	127	9	2	tr	tr
Applegate Farms						
Organic Roast Beef	2 oz	80	3	0	0	0
Healthy Ones						
Deli Roast Beef	2 oz	70	2	1	1	0
Oscar Mayer						
Slow Roasted Shaved	¼ pkg (1.8 oz)	60	3	0	0	0
TAKE-OUT						
roast beef rare	2 oz	70	2	0	0	0

BEEF DISHES

FOOD	PORTION	CAL	FAT	CARB	SUGAR	FIBER
CANNED						
corned beef hash	3 oz	155	10	9	–	–
Hormel						
Beef Stew	1 pkg (7.5 oz)	150	6	15	2	2

FOOD	PORTION	CAL	FAT	CARB	SUGAR	FIBER
Corned Beef Hash	1 cup (8.3 oz)	390	24	22	1	2
Corned Beef Hash 50% Reduced Fat	1 cup (8.3 oz)	290	12	24	2	2
Roast Beef Hash	1 cup (8.3 oz)	390	24	22	1	2
Roast Beef In Gravy	1 serv (5.8 oz)	130	3	8	1	0
Libby's						
Corned Beef Hash	1 cup	420	24	33	1	3
Hawaiian Corned Beef	2 oz	120	7	0	0	0
MIX						
Hamburger Helper						
Beef Pasta as prep	1 cup	270	10	24	1	1
Cheddar Cheese Melt as prep	1 cup	310	12	30	2	tr
Cheesy Baked Potato as prep	1 cup	310	11	30	2	2
Chili Cheese as prep	1 cup	340	13	33	4	1
Double Cheesy Quesadilla as prep	1 cup	350	11	36	2	tr
Italian Sausage as prep	1 cup	290	10	29	5	1
Microwave Singles Cheesy Lasagna	1 pkg	210	5	33	6	1
Philly Cheesesteak as prep	1 cup	320	13	27	2	1
Salisbury as prep	1 cup	260	10	27	1	1
Tomato Basil Penne as prep	1 cup	300	10	31	6	1
REFRIGERATED						
Hormel						
Beef Tips & Gravy	1 serv (4 oz)	170	8	4	3	1
TAKE-OUT						
beef bourguignonne	1 cup	339	12	10	3	1
beef satay + peanut sauce	2 skewers	253	16	6	4	1

FOOD	PORTION	CAL	FAT	CARB	SUGAR	FIBER
bool kogi korean marinated beef ribs	4 oz	190	10	6	4	0
bracciola	1 roll (4.7 oz)	276	14	8	1	1
bubble & squeak	5 oz	186	13	16	–	3
bulgoghi korean grilled beef	1 serv (5.2 oz)	256	15	5	3	tr
chipped beef on toast	1 slice (5 oz)	226	10	22	7	1
cornish pasty	1 (8 oz)	847	52	79	–	3
goulash w/ potatoes	1 cup	298	12	19	3	2
greek moussaka	1 serv (8.5 oz)	450	33	12	4	1
irish stew	1 cup (7 oz)	280	16	10	–	–
kebab indian	1 (5.4 oz)	553	40	2	–	–
kheena	6.7 oz	781	71	1	–	tr
koftas	5	280	22	3	–	tr
meatloaf	1 lg slice (5 oz)	294	17	9	2	1
pepper steak	1 cup	317	20	5	2	1
pot roast w/ gravy	1 serv (6 oz)	320	10	4	0	0
samosa	2 (4 oz)	652	62	20	–	2
shepherds pie	1 serv (7 oz)	282	16	20	–	2
sloppy joes	1 serv (9 oz)	398	6	48	5	12
steak & kidney pie w/ top crust	1 slice (5 oz)	400	26	23	–	1
stew w/ potatoes & vegetables	1 cup	199	5	22	3	3
stroganoff	1 cup	394	25	15	2	1
swiss steak w/ sauce	1 serv (8 oz)	234	10	8	3	1
toad in the hole	1 (4.7 oz)	383	29	23	–	1

BEEFALO

FOOD	PORTION	CAL	FAT	CARB	SUGAR	FIBER
roasted	4 oz	213	7	0	0	0

FOOD	PORTION	CAL	FAT	CARB	SUGAR	FIBER
BEER AND ALE						
alcohol free beer	7 fl oz	50	tr	11	5	–
ale brown	10 oz	77	0	8	–	0
ale pale	10 oz	88	0	12	–	0
beer cooler	1 (16 oz)	194	0	34	–	1
beer light	12 oz can	103	0	6	tr	0
beer regular	12 oz can	153	0	13	0	0
black & tan	1 serv (12 oz)	146	0	13	–	1
black velvet	1 (10 oz)	160	0	8	–	1
boilermaker	1 serv	216	0	13	–	1
lager	10 oz	80	0	4	–	0
lager & black	1 (14 oz)	241	0	39	–	–
mead	1 serv	250	0	13	–	1
pilsener lager	7 oz	85	tr	13	2	–
shandy	1 serv	125	0	12	–	1
stout	10 oz	102	0	6	–	0
trojan horse	1 (16 oz)	189	0	35	–	–
Amstel						
Light	1 bottle (12 oz)	95	0	5	–	–
Bard's						
Gluten Free	1 bottle (12 oz)	155	0	14	–	–
Beck's						
Pilsner	1 bottle (12 oz)	138	0	12	–	–
Bud						
Dry	1 bottle (12 oz)	130	0	8	–	–
Budweiser						
Beer	1 bottle (12 oz)	145	0	11	–	–
Bud Light	1 bottle (12 oz)	110	0	7	–	–

FOOD	PORTION	CAL	FAT	CARB	SUGAR	FIBER
Coors						
Lite	1 bottle (12 oz)	104	0	5	–	–
Non-Alcohol	1 bottle (12 oz)	66	0	15	–	–
Original	1 bottle (12 oz)	149	0	12	–	–
Super Dry	1 bottle (12 oz)	149	0	11	–	–
Corona						
Extra	1 bottle (12 oz)	149	0	14	–	–
Guiness						
Draft In A Bottle	1 bottle (12 oz)	128	0	11	–	–
Extra Stout	1 bottle (12 oz)	174	0	12	–	–
Heineken						
Beer	1 bottle (12 oz)	150	0	12	–	–
LaBatt						
Blue	1 bottle (12 oz)	127	0	9	–	–
Michelob						
Porter	1 bottle (12 oz)	196	0	17	–	–
Ultra	1 bottle (12 oz)	95	0	3	–	–
Miller						
Genuine Draft	1 bottle (12 oz)	143	0	13	–	–
Lite	1 bottle (12 oz)	96	0	3	–	–
MDG 64	1 bottle (12 oz)	64	0	2	–	–

FOOD	PORTION	CAL	FAT	CARB	SUGAR	FIBER
O'Douls						
Non-Alcoholic	1 bottle (12 oz)	65	0	13	–	–
RedBridge						
Gluten Free	1 bottle (12 oz)	160	0	16	–	–
Sierra Nevada						
Porter	1 bottle (12 oz)	194	0	12	–	–
Smirnoff						
Ice	1 bottle (12 oz)	241	0	38	–	–
BEET JUICE						
juice	7 oz	72	0	16	–	–
BEETS						
CANNED						
harvard	½ cup	90	tr	22	–	3
pickled	½ cup	74	tr	18	–	3
sliced	½ cup	37	tr	9	8	2
Freshlike						
Pickled Sliced	4 slices (1 oz)	20	0	4	4	0
S&W						
Sliced	½ cup (4.3 oz)	35	0	8	5	2
Sliced Pickled	1 oz	15	0	4	4	1
FRESH						
greens cooked w/o salt	½ cup	19	tr	4	tr	2
sliced cooked	½ cup	37	tr	8	7	2
whole cooked	2 med (3.5 oz)	44	tr	10	8	2

BEVERAGES (*see* BEER AND ALE, CHAMPAGNE, COFFEE, DRINK MIXERS, ENERGY DRINKS, FRUIT DRINKS, ICED TEA, LIQUOR/LIQUEUR, MALT, MILKSHAKE, SMOOTHIES, SODA, TEA/HERBAL TEA, WATER, WINE, YOGURT DRINKS)

FOOD	PORTION	CAL	FAT	CARB	SUGAR	FIBER
BISCUIT						
FROZEN						
Jimmy Dean						
Snack Size Sausage On A Biscuit	2	400	30	24	4	1
MIX						
plain as prep	1 (2 oz)	190	7	27	–	1
Bisquick						
Heart Smart	1/3 cup	140	3	27	3	1
REFRIGERATED						
plain baked	1 (1 oz)	93	4	13	tr	tr
Pillsbury						
Buttermilk	3 (2.2 oz)	150	2	29	4	1
Flaky Layers	3 (2.2 oz)	160	4	28	4	1
Grands! Butter Tastin'	1 (2 oz)	190	9	24	5	tr
Grands! Buttermilk Reduced Fat	1 (2 oz)	170	6	26	4	tr
Grands! Golden Wheat Reduced Fat	1 (2.1 oz)	180	7	27	6	2
Grands! Original	1 (2 oz)	190	9	24	5	tr
Grands! Original Reduced Fat	1 (2 oz)	170	6	26	5	tr
Perfect Portions Butter Tastin'	1 (1.9 oz)	190	9	23	4	tr
TAKE-OUT						
buttermilk	1 lg (2.7 oz)	280	13	37	1	1
oatcakes	2 (4 oz)	115	5	16	–	1
plain	1 sm (1.2 oz)	127	6	17	tr	1
tea biscuit	1 (3 oz)	210	3	30	12	1
w/ egg	1 (4.8 oz)	373	22	32	–	1
w/ egg & bacon	1 (5.3 oz)	458	31	29	1	1
w/ egg & ham	1 (6.7 oz)	442	27	30	2	1
w/ egg & sausage	1 (6.3 oz)	581	39	11	1	1

FOOD	PORTION	CAL	FAT	CARB	SUGAR	FIBER
w/ egg & steak	1 (5.2 oz)	410	28	21	–	–
w/ egg cheese & bacon	1 (5.1 oz)	477	31	33	–	–
w/ ham	1 (4 oz)	386	18	44	1	1
w/ sausage	1 (4.4 oz)	485	32	40	1	1
BLACK BEANS						
dried cooked	1 cup	227	1	41	–	15
Allens						
Black Beans	½ cup	100	1	19	1	8
Goya						
Black Beans	½ cup (4.3 oz)	90	1	19	tr	6
Tree Of Life						
Organic	½ cup (4.6 oz)	130	1	24	1	<6
BLACKBERRIES						
canned in heavy syrup	½ cup	118	tr	30	25	4
fresh	½ cup	31	tr	7	4	4
unsweetened frzn	½ cup	48	tr	12	8	4
Cascadian Farm						
Organic frzn	1 cup	80	1	22	15	7
BLACKBERRY JUICE						
canned	6 oz	65	1	13	13	tr
Izze						
Sparkling Esque Blackberry	1 bottle (12 oz)	50	0	12	11	–
BLACKEYE PEAS						
CANNED						
cowpeas	1 cup	184	1	33	–	–
w/pork	½ cup	199	4	40	–	–
DRIED						
catjang cooked	1 cup (2.9 oz)	200	1	35	–	–
peas cooked	1 cup	198	1	36	–	16

FOOD	PORTION	CAL	FAT	CARB	SUGAR	FIBER
FRESH						
cowpeas leafy tips chopped cooked	1 cup	12	tr	1	–	–
cowpeas leafy tips raw chopped	1 cup	10	tr	2	–	–
FROZEN						
cowpeas cooked	½ cup	112	tr	20	–	–
TAKE-OUT						
blackeye peas & pork	1 cup	236	5	25	4	8
BLINTZE						
TAKE-OUT						
cheese	1 (2.7 oz)	160	9	15	4	tr
BLUEBERRIES						
canned in heavy syrup	½ cup	113	tr	28	26	2
fresh	1 pt	229	1	58	40	10
fresh	½ cup	41	tr	11	7	2
frzn unsweetened	½ cup	40	1	9	7	2
Chukar Cherries						
Puget Sound Dried	¼ cup	160	0	38	20	5
White Chocolate Covered	3 tbsp (1.4 oz)	223	12	26	24	tr
Emily's						
Dark Chocolate Covered	¼ cup (1.4 oz)	170	8	27	22	2
LiteHouse						
Glaze	3 tbsp	70	0	17	15	0
Stoneridge Orchards						
Organic Dried Wild Whole	⅓ cup (1.4 oz)	130	0	33	29	2
Whole Dried	⅓ cup (1.4 oz)	130	0	33	31	1
Tree Of Life						
Dried	¼ cup (1.5 oz)	150	0	38	27	4

FOOD	PORTION	CAL	FAT	CARB	SUGAR	FIBER
BLUEBERRY JUICE						
Izze						
Sparkling Blueberry	1 bottle (12 oz)	120	0	33	31	–
Tart Is Smart						
Wild Blueberry Concentrate	0.5 oz	35	0	9	7	1
BLUEFIN						
fillet baked	4.1 oz	186	6	0	0	0
BLUEFISH						
fresh baked	3 oz	135	5	0	0	0
BOAR						
wild roasted	3 oz	136	4	0	0	0
Natural Frontier Foods						
Wild Boar Steaks	1 (4 oz)	170	8	0	0	0
BOK CHOY (*see* CABBAGE)						
BONITO						
dried	1 oz	50	2	0	0	0
fresh	3 oz	117	4	0	0	0
BORAGE						
fresh chopped	1 cup	19	tr	3	–	–
BOTTLED WATER (*see* WATER)						
BOYSENBERRIES						
frzn unsweetened	½ cup	33	tr	8	5	4
in heavy syrup	½ cup	113	tr	29	–	3
BRAINS						
beef pan fried	3 oz	167	13	0	0	0
beef simmered	3 oz	123	9	0	0	0
lamb braised	3 oz	123	9	0	0	0

FOOD	PORTION	CAL	FAT	CARB	SUGAR	FIBER
lamb fried	3 oz	232	19	0	0	0
pork braised	3 oz	117	8	0	0	0
veal braised	3 oz	116	8	0	0	0
veal fried	3 oz	181	14	0	0	0
BRAN						
corn	1 cup (2.7 oz)	170	1	65	–	65
oat	½ cup (1.6 oz)	116	3	31	–	7
oat cooked	½ cup (3.8 oz)	44	1	13	–	3
rice	½ cup (2.1 oz)	187	12	29	–	12
wheat	½ cup (2 oz)	63	1	19	–	12
Quaker						
Unprocessed	⅓ cup (0.6 oz)	35	1	11	1	8
Tree Of Life						
Oat Bran	½ cup (1.6 oz)	120	4	31	1	7
Organic Wheat Bran	¼ cup (1.1 oz)	190	18	4	1	2
BRAZIL NUTS						
dried unblanched	1 oz	186	19	4	–	–
BREAD						
CANNED						
boston brown	1 slice (1.6 oz)	88	1	19	5	2
B&M						
Raisin Brown Bread	½ in slice (2 oz)	130	1	29	16	2
FROZEN						
Cedarlane						
Organic Mediterranean Stuffed Focaccia	1 piece (4 oz)	295	10	37	4	1
MIX						
cornbread	1 piece (2 oz)	188	6	29	–	1
READY-TO-EAT						
anadama	1 piece (1.1 oz)	87	1	16	3	1
baguette whole wheat	2 oz	140	0	29	tr	1

FOOD	PORTION	CAL	FAT	CARB	SUGAR	FIBER
cassava	1 piece (3.5 oz)	299	1	71	3	3
challah	1 slice (1.4 oz)	115	2	19	1	1
cinnamon	1 slice (0.9 oz)	69	1	13	1	1
cracked wheat	1 slice (1.1 oz)	78	1	15	–	2
cuban bread	1 slice (1.1 oz)	83	1	16	1	1
french	1 slice (1.1 oz)	88	1	17	tr	1
italian	1 loaf (1 lb)	1255	4	256	–	–
navajo fry	1 piece	281	10	41	2	–
oat bran	1 slice (1.1 oz)	71	1	12	2	1
oatmeal	1 slice (0.9 oz)	73	1	13	2	1
pan criollo	1 piece (0.9 oz)	69	1	13	tr	tr
pannetone	1 slice (0.9 oz)	86	2	15	5	1
pita	1 sm (1 oz)	77	tr	16	tr	1
pita	1 lg (2 oz)	165	1	33	1	1
pita whole wheat	1 sm (1 oz)	74	1	15	tr	2
pita whole wheat	1 lg (2.2 oz)	170	2	35	1	5
pumpernickel	1 slice (0.9 oz)	65	1	12	tr	2
raisin	1 slice (1.1 oz)	88	1	17	2	1
rye	1 slice (1.1 oz)	83	1	15	tr	2
seven grain	1 slice (1.1 oz)	80	1	15	3	2
wheat berry	1 slice (0.9 oz)	65	1	12	1	1
wheat bran	1 slice (1.3 oz)	89	1	17	3	1
wheat germ	1 slice (1 oz)	73	1	14	1	1
white cubed	1 cup	93	1	18	2	1
whole wheat	1 slice (1 oz)	69	1	13	6	2
Alvarado Street Bakery						
Sprouted Soy Crunch	1 slice (1.2 oz)	90	1	15	1	2
Sprouted Whole Wheat	1 slice	90	1	19	3	3
Arnold						
100% Natural Soft Honey Wheat	2 slices (2 oz)	150	2	28	4	3

FOOD	PORTION	CAL	FAT	CARB	SUGAR	FIBER
Grains & More Double Omega	1 slice	110	2	19	4	3
Jewish Rye	1 slice	90	2	17	1	1
Sandwich Thins Multi-Grain	1 (1.5 oz)	100	1	22	2	5
Sandwich Thins Whole Grain White	1 (1.5 oz)	100	1	22	2	5
Whole Grains 100% Whole Wheat Double Fiber	1 slice	100	2	21	3	5
Whole Grains 12 Grain	1 slice	110	2	21	3	3
Whole Grains 15 Grain	1 slice	110	2	21	4	3
Aunt Gussie's						
Gluten Free Focaccia Bread Kalamata Olive	1 piece (2.7 oz)	180	2	37	4	4
Gluten Free Focaccia Bread Rosemary	1 piece (2.7 oz)	180	2	38	4	4
Comfort Care						
Cabin Hearth Whole Wheat	1 oz	170	3	31	7	4
Ecce Panis						
Classic Ciabatta	⅛ loaf (2 oz)	180	2	36	tr	tr
Freihofer's						
100% Whole Wheat	1 slice	90	2	17	3	2
French Meadow Bakery						
100% Rye Salt Free	1 slice (1.6 oz)	90	0	23	0	3
100% Spelt	2 slices (2.4 oz)	170	1	33	1	4
European Sourdough Rye	1 slice (1.7 oz)	90	0	22	0	3
Gluten Free Multigrain	1 slice (1.8 oz)	150	5	23	0	3
Hemp	2 slices (2.4 oz)	200	5	24	2	5

FOOD	PORTION	CAL	FAT	CARB	SUGAR	FIBER
Kamut	2 slices (3 oz)	170	1	31	1	1
Men's Bread	2 slices (2.4 oz)	200	8	17	1	3
Our Daily Bread	2 slices (2.4 oz)	160	3	24	1	5
Sprouted Cinnamon Raisin	1 slice (1.5 oz)	100	1	19	4	3
Summer	1 slice (1.2 oz)	90	0	17	1	1
Gillian's Foods						
Gluten Free Cinnamon Raisin	1 slice (2 oz)	130	1	25	3	2
Mrs Baird's						
Acti-Fiber Wheat	2 slices (2.2 oz)	160	3	30	4	4
Whole Grain Wheat Sugar Free	1 slice (1.1 oz)	70	2	13	0	3
Natural Ovens						
100% Sweet Whole	1 slice	90	2	16	4	4
Carb Conscious Original	1 slice	80	2	9	1	4
Healthy Beginnings Better White	1 slice	110	2	20	3	2
Healthy Beginnings Honey Wheat	1 slice	120	2	21	3	3
Hunger Filler Whole Grain	1 slice	100	2	15	2	4
Organic Plus Whole Grain & Flax	1 slice	120	2	22	3	3
Whole Grain Oat Nut Crunch	1 slice	100	3	15	2	4
Nature's Pride						
100% Whole Wheat	1 slice (1.5 oz)	110	1	20	4	3
100% Whole Wheat Double Fiber	1 slice (1.5 oz)	100	1	20	4	6

FOOD	PORTION	CAL	FAT	CARB	SUGAR	FIBER
Country Buttermilk	1 slice (1.5 oz)	110	2	21	4	tr
Healthy Multi-Grain	1 slice (1.5 oz)	110	9	20	4	3
Honey Wheat	1 slice (1 oz)	70	1	13	3	tr
Nutty Oat	1 slice (1.5 oz)	110	2	19	4	2
Oroweat						
100% Whole Wheat	1 slice (1.3 oz)	100	1	19	4	3
Country Potato	1 slice (1.3 oz)	100	1	20	3	tr
Country Whole Grain White	1 slice (1.3 oz)	90	2	17	4	1
Double Fiber	1 slice (1.3 oz)	70	1	16	2	6
Honey Fiber Whole Grain	1 slice (1.3 oz)	80	1	18	3	4
Russian Rye	1 slice (1 oz)	80	1	13	tr	tr
Seven Grain	1 slice (1.3 oz)	100	1	20	4	2
Whole Grain & Flax	1 slice (1.3 oz)	100	2	17	3	3
Pepperidge Farm						
Breakfast Apple & Grains	1 slice	90	2	18	5	3
Farmhouse Whole Grain White	1 slice (1.5 oz)	110	2	21	4	3
Fruit & Grain Cranberry Orange	1 slice (1.4 oz)	90	2	19	5	3
Honey Flax Whole Grain	1 slice (1.5 oz)	100	2	19	4	3
Jewish Rye Whole Grain Seeded	1 slice	70	1	14	tr	2
Light Style 7 Grain	1 slice	45	0	9	1	1
Vitality Oats & Barley	1 slice (1.5 oz)	120	2	21	4	5
Whole Grain 100% Soft Whole Wheat Double Fiber	1 slice	100	2	21	3	6
Whole Grain Soft Honey Oat	1 slice (1.5 oz)	100	2	19	3	4
Whole Grain Swirl Cinnamon w/ Raisins	1 slice (1 oz)	80	1	13	4	2

FOOD	PORTION	CAL	FAT	CARB	SUGAR	FIBER
Roman Meal						
Muesli	1 slice (1.5 oz)	110	2	19	5	2
Original Whole Grain	2 slices (2 oz)	130	2	25	5	2
S. Rosen's						
Hawaiian	1 slice	110	2	21	4	0
Rye Black Bavarian	1 slice	100	2	19	0	1
Stroehmann						
Dutch Country Twelve Grain	1 slice	100	2	18	3	2
Sun-Maid						
Raisin Cinnamon Swirl	1 slice (1.2 oz)	100	2	18	8	1
The Baker						
Yoga Bread	1 slice	70	1	13	2	2
Thomas'						
Breakfast Original	1 slice	90	1	17	tr	1
Sahara Pita Pockets Mini Whole Wheat	1 (1 oz)	70	1	13	1	2
Swirl Cinnamon Raisin	1 slice	120	2	21	9	1
Wonder						
Classic White	1 slice (1 oz)	70	1	2	14	0
Classic White Sandwich	1 slice (0.9 oz)	60	1	13	2	0
REFRIGERATED						
Pillsbury						
Italian	1/8 pkg (1.6 oz)	110	2	21	2	tr
TAKE-OUT						
banana	1 slice (2 oz)	196	6	33	–	1
chapati as prep w/ fat	1 (1.6 oz)	95	2	18	1	3
chapati as prep w/o fat	1 (2.5 oz)	141	1	31	–	5
cornbread	1 piece (2.3 oz)	183	6	27	4	2
cornstick	1 (1.4 oz)	118	4	18	3	1
focaccia onion	1 piece (4.6 oz)	282	10	43	2	2

FOOD	PORTION	CAL	FAT	CARB	SUGAR	FIBER
focaccia rosemary	1 piece (3.5 oz)	251	7	40	1	2
focaccia tomato olive	1 piece (4.7 oz)	270	8	42	1	2
garlic bread	1 slice (1 oz)	96	4	13	tr	1
irish soda bread	1 slice (3 oz)	247	4	48	–	2
italian garlic	1 loaf (11 oz)	990	38	137	1	8
naan	1 bread (3.5 oz)	286	9	43	3	2
papadum fried	1 (6 g)	30	2	2	–	tr
paratha plain	1 (1.6 oz)	136	5	19	–	2
poori indian puffed bread	1 piece (1.3 oz)	112	4	16	tr	2
zucchini	1 slice (1.4 oz)	150	7	19	10	1

BREAD COATING
Zatarain's
Crispy Seasoned Fish-Fri	2 tbsp	50	0	11	0	1

BREADCRUMBS
dry seasoned	¼ cup	115	2	21	2	2
fresh	¼ cup	30	tr	6	tr	tr
plain	¼ cup	107	1	19	2	1

Gillian's Foods
Plain Gluten Free	¼ cup (1.2 oz)	60	1	14	1	1

Krasdale
Seasoned	¼ cup	120	2	21	4	2

Progresso
Garlic & Herb	¼ cup (1 oz)	110	2	19	2	1
Plain	¼ cup (1 oz)	110	2	20	2	1

Southern Homestyle
Corn Flake Crumbs	2 tbsp	40	0	9	1	0
Tortilla Crumbs	2 tbsp	40	0	9	1	0

FOOD	PORTION	CAL	FAT	CARB	SUGAR	FIBER
BREADFRUIT						
fresh	1 sm (13.5 oz)	396	1	104	42	19
fried	1 cup	379	21	52	21	9
raw	1 cup	227	1	60	24	11
BREADNUTTREE SEEDS						
dried	1 oz	104	tr	23	–	–
BREADSTICKS						
plain	1 lg	41	1	7	tr	tr
plain	1 sm	21	tr	3	tr	tr
Fattorie & Pandea						
Fornini w/ Sea Salt	5 (1.2 oz)	140	5	21	1	1
Ferrara						
Slim Thin Torinese Style	6 (0.5 oz)	60	1	11	1	0
Pillsbury						
Cornbread Twists	1 (1.4 oz)	140	6	18	4	0
Original Soft	2 (1.8 oz)	140	3	25	3	tr
BREAKFAST BARS (*see* CEREAL BARS, ENERGY BARS)						
BROCCOFLOWER						
fresh raw	½ cup (1.8 oz)	16	tr	3	–	–
BROCCOLI						
FRESH						
chinese broccoli (gai lan) cooked	½ cup	10	tr	2	tr	1
raab cooked	½ cup	28	tr	3	1	2
raw	1 bunch (1.3 lbs)	207	2	40	10	16
raw flower	1 piece	3	tr	1	–	–
raw flowers	1 cup	20	tr	4	–	–
Mann's						
Broccoli Wokly	1 serv (3 oz)	25	0	4	2	2
Broccolini	8 stalks (3 oz)	35	0	6	2	1

FOOD	PORTION	CAL	FAT	CARB	SUGAR	FIBER
Ocean Mist						
Rapini Broccoli Rabe Chopped Raw	1 cup	9	0	1	0	1
FROZEN						
chopped cooked	½ cup	26	tr	5	1	3
spears cooked	1 pkg (10 oz)	70	tr	13	4	8
spears cooked	½ cup	26	tr	5	1	3
Birds Eye						
Steamfresh Florets	1 cup (2.3 oz)	30	0	4	2	2
Cascadian Farm						
Organic Florets	⅔ cup	20	0	4	2	2
Dr. Praeger's						
Broccoli Bites	2 (2 oz)	110	4	17	2	2
Green Giant						
Broccoli & Cheese Sauce	⅔ cup	60	3	7	2	2
Cuts as prep	⅔ cup	25	0	4	2	2
TAKE-OUT						
batter dipped & fried	4 pieces	77	5	6	1	1
w/ cheese sauce	1 cup	242	15	16	5	5
BROWNIE						
brownie	1 (2 oz)	227	9	36	21	1
butterscotch	1 (1.2 oz)	151	8	19	12	tr
Betty Crocker						
Dark Chocolate as prep	1	160	7	24	17	tr
Dark Chocolate as prep	1	170	7	25	17	tr
Fudge Low Fat as prep	1	140	3	28	19	1
Original Supreme as prep	1	160	6	26	18	tr
Triple Chunk as prep	1	180	8	25	18	1
Walnut as prep	1	170	9	22	15	tr
Warm Delights Hot Fudge	1 pkg (3 oz)	370	12	61	41	3

FOOD	PORTION	CAL	FAT	CARB	SUGAR	FIBER
Duncan Hines						
Chocolate Fudge frzn	1/12 pkg (1.4 oz)	170	8	23	16	0
Dark Chocolate Chunk Mix as prep	1/16 pkg	170	7	25	18	1
Milk Chocolate Mix as prep	1/20 pkg	180	9	23	16	0
Peanut Butter Cup Mix as prep	1/16 pkg	170	8	23	16	1
Turtle Mix as prep	1/16 pkg	160	7	23	15	1
Walnut Mix as prep	1/16 pkg	180	8	24	16	2
Erin Baker's						
Organic Bites	1 (1 oz)	100	3	18	10	2
Organic Bites Double Chocolate Chip	1 (1 oz)	90	2	19	10	2
French Meadow Bakery						
Gluten Free Fudge Bites	2 (1.3 oz)	170	7	26	14	2
Hershey's						
Brownie	1/2 pkg (1.5 oz)	190	9	28	14	1
Pillsbury						
Traditional Chocolate Fudge	1 (1.4 oz)	150	6	24	16	tr
Turtle Supreme Bars	1 (1.4 oz)	180	9	23	15	tr
BRUSSELS SPROUTS						
FRESH						
cooked	6 pieces	45	1	9	2	3
Ocean Mist						
Brussels Sprouts	4 (2 oz)	40	1	6	2	3
FROZEN						
cooked	1 cup	65	1	13	3	6
Birds Eye						
Steamfresh Baby	10 (2.9 oz)	45	0	8	2	3
Steamfresh Singles Baby	1 pkg (3.2 oz)	50	0	9	3	3

FOOD	PORTION	CAL	FAT	CARB	SUGAR	FIBER
Green Giant						
Baby & Butter Sauce as prep	½ cup	60	1	9	3	3
BUCKWHEAT						
groats roasted cooked	1 cup (6 oz)	155	1	33	2	5
groats roasted uncooked	½ cup	292	3	61	–	9
BUFFALO (see also JERKY)						
burger	3 oz	202	13	0	0	0
chuck braised	4 oz	205	6	0	0	0
top round steak broiled	3 oz	313	9	0	0	0
water buffalo roasted	3 oz	111	2	0	0	0
Natural Frontier Foods						
Burgers	1 (5 oz)	170	9	0	0	0
Ground	4 oz	170	9	0	0	0
Steaks	1 (4 oz)	160	3	0	0	0
BULGUR						
cooked	½ cup	76	tr	17	tr	4
uncooked	½ cup	239	1	53	tr	13
Near East						
Whole Grain Wheat Pilaf as prep	1 cup	200	4	40	2	8
TAKE-OUT						
tabbouleh	1 cup	198	15	16	2	4
BURBOT (FISH)						
fresh baked	3 oz	98	1	0	0	0
BURDOCK ROOT						
cooked w/o salt	1 root (5.8 oz)	146	tr	35	6	3
cooked w/o salt	1 cup	110	tr	26	4	2
BUTTER						
clarified butter	1 tbsp (0.4 oz)	112	13	0	0	0

FOOD	PORTION	CAL	FAT	CARB	SUGAR	FIBER
clarified butter	¼ cup (1.8 oz)	449	51	0	0	0
honey butter	1 tbsp (0.6 oz)	85	6	9	9	0
honey butter	¼ cup (2.5 oz)	338	23	36	35	tr
light butter whipped salted	1 tbsp (0.3 oz)	48	5	0	0	0
stick salted	1 tbsp (0.5 oz)	102	12	tr	tr	0
stick salted	1 stick (4 oz)	810	92	tr	tr	0
stick salted	¼ cup (2 oz)	407	46	tr	tr	0
stick unsalted	1 (4 oz)	810	92	tr	tr	0
stick unsalted	1 tbsp (0.5 oz)	102	12	tr	tr	0
stick unsalted	¼ cup (2 oz)	407	46	tr	tr	0
whipped salted	¼ cup (1.3 oz)	271	31	tr	tr	0
whipped salted	1 tbsp (0.3 oz)	67	8	tr	tr	0
Cabot						
Salted	1 tbsp	100	11	0	0	0
Country Crock						
Spreadable Butter w/ Canola Oil	1 tbsp (0.4 oz)	80	9	0	0	0
Earth Balance						
Butter Blend Unsalted	1 tbsp	100	11	0	0	0
Land O Lakes						
Light Salted	1 tbsp (0.5 oz)	50	6	0	0	0
Light Whipped Salted	1 tbsp (0.4 oz)	45	5	0	0	0
Salted	1 tbsp (0.5 oz)	100	11	0	0	0
Spreadable w/ Canola Oil	1 tbsp (0.5 oz)	100	11	0	0	0
Whipped Salted	1 tbsp (0.2 oz)	50	6	0	0	0
Molly McButter						
Natural Butter	1 tsp (2 g)	5	0	1	–	0

FOOD	PORTION	CAL	FAT	CARB	SUGAR	FIBER
Straus						
Organic European Style Lightly Salted	1 tbsp (0.5 oz)	110	12	0	0	0
Organic European Style Sweet Butter	1 tbsp (0.5 oz)	110	12	0	0	0
BUTTER SUBSTITUTES						
stick	1 stick	811	91	1	–	–
BUTTERBUR						
canned fuki chopped	1 cup	3	tr	tr	–	–
fresh fuki	1 cup	13	tr	3	–	–
BUTTERNUTS						
dried	1 oz	174	16	3	–	–
BUTTERSCOTCH (*see also* CANDY)						
Hershey's						
Chips	1 tbsp (0.5 oz)	80	4	9	9	–
CABBAGE (*see also* COLESLAW)						
chinese bok choy shredded cooked w/o salt	1 cup	20	tr	3	1	2
chinese pe-tsai shredded cooked w/o salt	1 cup	17	tr	3	–	2
green raw shredded	1 cup	19	tr	4	2	2
green shredded cooked w/o salt	1 cup	34	tr	8	4	3
japanese pickled	½ cup	22	tr	4	1	2
red raw shredded	1 cup	22	tr	5	3	2
red shredded cooked w/o salt	1 cup	44	tr	10	5	4
savoy shredded cooked w/o salt	1 cup	35	tr	8	–	4

FOOD	PORTION	CAL	FAT	CARB	SUGAR	FIBER
Glory						
Country Cabbage	½ cup	25	0	6	3	1
TAKE-OUT						
creamed	1 cup	158	10	13	7	2
kimchee	1 cup	32	tr	6	2	2
stuffed cabbage w/ rice & beef	1 (3.6 oz)	117	5	9	4	1
sweet & sour red cabbage	4 oz	61	3	8	–	3

CACAO
Kopali

FOOD	PORTION	CAL	FAT	CARB	SUGAR	FIBER
Organic Dark Chocolate Covered Cacao Nibs	½ pkg (1 oz)	140	10	15	12	2

CACTUS

FOOD	PORTION	CAL	FAT	CARB	SUGAR	FIBER
fresh cooked w/ fat	1 pad (1 oz)	11	1	1	tr	1
fresh cooked w/o fat	1 cup (5.2 oz)	22	tr	5	2	3
pricklypear	1 (3.6 oz)	42	1	10	–	4
pricklypear resh	1 cup (5.2 oz)	61	1	14	–	5

CAKE (see also CAKE MIX)

FOOD	PORTION	CAL	FAT	CARB	SUGAR	FIBER
battenburg cake	1 slice (2 oz)	204	10	28	–	1
cream puff shell	1 (2.3 oz)	239	17	15	–	–
crumpet	1 (2.3 oz)	131	1	31	–	2
dutch honey cake	1 slice (0.8 oz)	70	0	17	8	0
eccles cake	1 slice (2 oz)	285	16	36	–	1
madeira cake	1 slice (1 oz)	98	4	15	–	1
sponge	1 piece (1.3 oz)	110	1	23	14	tr
sponge cake dessert shell	1 (0.8 oz)	70	2	12	7	0
treacle tart	1 slice (2.5 oz)	258	10	42	–	1

FOOD	PORTION	CAL	FAT	CARB	SUGAR	FIBER
Amy's						
Organic Chocolate	1 slice	170	6	27	16	1
Toaster Pops Apple	1 (2.1 oz)	150	4	27	10	1
Aunt Trudy's						
Organic Baklava Soy Nut	1 (1.8 oz)	190	6	29	17	2
Bellino						
Pandoro	1 (2.8 oz)	330	16	39	16	1
Betty Crocker						
Warm Delights Cinnamon Swirl	1 (3.3 oz)	390	10	72	49	1
Earth Cafe						
Cheesecake Vegan Blueberry Thrill	1 slice (2 oz)	193	15	12	7	1
Cheesecake Vegan Coconut Carob	1 slice (2 oz)	206	16	13	8	1
Cheesecake Vegan Rockin' Raspberry	1 slice (2 oz)	194	15	12	7	2
El Monterey						
Cheesecake Bites Caramel	1 (2 oz)	180	10	23	9	0
Cheesecake Bites Raspberry	1 (2 oz)	200	11	21	6	0
Fillo Factory						
Organic Apple Strudel	1 (4.4 oz)	290	10	47	15	2
Organic Apple Turnovers	1 (3 oz)	180	6	30	9	1
French Meadow Bakery						
Gluten Free Cupcake Chocolate	1 (2 oz)	220	8	35	27	1
Gluten Free Cupcake Yellow	1 (2 oz)	230	9	35	28	0
Vegan Carrot	¼ cake (2.6 oz)	13	0	38	21	1

FOOD	PORTION	CAL	FAT	CARB	SUGAR	FIBER
Gourmet Pastries						
Baklava Walnut	1 piece (1.8 oz)	240	11	30	18	0
Guiltless Gourmet						
Dessert Bowl Bananas Foster Cake	1 pkg (2 oz)	200	2	42	26	tr
Dessert Bowl Black Velvet Cake	1 pkg (2 oz)	200	3	42	30	3
Hostess						
100 Calorie Pack Mini Carrot Cake	1 pkg (1.2 oz)	100	3	20	11	4
100 Calorie Pack Mini Chocolate Cupcakes	1 pkg (1.3 oz)	100	3	22	10	5
100 Calorie Pack Mini Coffee Cake Cinnamon Streusel	1 pkg (1.2 oz)	100	3	21	7	5
100 Calorie Pack Mini Golden Cupcakes	1 pkg (1.2 oz)	100	3	20	11	3
Cup Cakes Chocolate	1 (1.8 oz)	170	6	30	21	1
Ho Ho's	1	120	6	18	14	0
Twinkies	1 (1.5 oz)	150	5	27	19	0
Lance						
Honey Bun	1 (3 oz)	320	13	47	13	4
Mrs. Freshley's						
Golden Cupcakes Creme Filled	1 pkg (1.3 oz)	100	3	24	4	5
Mrs. Smith's						
Singles Heavenly 100 New York Cheesecake	1 (0.9 oz)	100	6	9	6	0
Pillsbury						
Caramel Rolls	1 (1.7 oz)	170	7	24	10	tr
Cinnamon Rolls w/ Icing	1 (3.5 oz)	310	9	54	23	1

FOOD	PORTION	CAL	FAT	CARB	SUGAR	FIBER
Cinnamon Rolls w/ Icing Reduced Fat	1 (1.5 oz)	140	4	24	10	tr
Toaster Strudel	1 (2 oz)	200	9	28	9	1
Toaster Strudel Blueberry	1 (2 oz)	190	9	26	9	tr
Toaster Strudel Cream Cheese	1 (2 oz)	200	11	23	8	tr
Toaster Strudel Raspberry	1 (2 oz)	190	9	26	9	tr
Toaster Strudel Wildberry	1 (2 oz)	190	9	25	9	tr
Turnovers Cherry	1 (2 oz)	180	8	24	12	0
TAKE-OUT						
angelfood	1 slice (2 oz)	143	tr	33	17	tr
apple crisp	1 serv (8.6 oz)	384	8	76	49	4
apple turnover	1 (6.6 oz)	661	34	83	30	3
baklava	1 piece (2.7 oz)	334	23	29	10	2
basbousa namoura	1 piece (1 oz)	60	3	10	10	2
bean cake	1 cake (1.1 oz)	130	7	16	7	1
black forest chocolate cherry	1 piece (2.5 oz)	187	9	27	23	1
boston cream pie	1 slice (3.2 oz)	232	8	39	33	1
cannoli w/ cannoli cream	1	369	21	42	28	–
carrot w/ icing	1 slice (4.7 oz)	543	28	70	52	2
cheesecake	1 slice (4.5 oz)	410	25	37	28	tr
cheesecake chocolate	1 slice (4.5 oz)	489	32	49	29	2

FOOD	PORTION	CAL	FAT	CARB	SUGAR	FIBER
chinese moon cake	1 (4.8 oz)	458	6	92	49	4
coconut mochiko filipino cake	1 piece (2.7 oz)	252	12	35	11	2
coffee cake iced	1 piece (1.6 oz)	175	8	24	15	1
cream puff custard filled chocolate frosted	1 (3.9 oz)	293	18	27	7	1
eclair	1 (3.5 oz)	262	16	24	7	1
french apple tart	1 (3.5 oz)	302	15	37	15	2
fruitcake	1 slice (1.5 oz)	139	4	26	13	2
funnel cake	1 (3.2 oz)	276	14	29	4	1
gingerbread	1 piece (2.4 oz)	213	7	35	22	1
jelly roll	1 slice (1.8 oz)	146	2	28	20	tr
jelly roll lemon filled	1 slice (3 oz)	210	2	48	29	tr
napoleon	1 mini (1 oz)	123	9	9	1	tr
napoleon	1 (3 oz)	348	25	25	4	1
panettone	1/12 cake (2.9 oz)	300	12	43	21	2
petit fours	2 (0.9 oz)	120	7	15	12	0
pineapple upside down	1 piece (4.2 oz)	387	15	61	41	1
pound	1 slice (1 oz)	120	5	15	–	–
pound fat free	1 slice (2 oz)	160	1	35	19	1
sacher torte	1 slice (2.2 oz)	240	11	30	11	4
sacher torte chocolate + apricot jam	1 serv	430	12	23	–	–
strawberry shortcake	1 serv (4.1 oz)	211	5	40	35	1
strudel apple	1 piece (2.2 oz)	175	7	26	16	1
strudel cheese	1 piece (2.2 oz)	195	8	24	14	tr

FOOD	PORTION	CAL	FAT	CARB	SUGAR	FIBER
strudel cherry	1 piece (2.2 oz)	179	6	29	18	1
sweet potato w/ glaze	1 piece (2.7 oz)	275	12	39	26	1
tiramisu	1 cake (4.4 lbs)	5732	421	439	234	3
tiramisu	1 piece (5.1 oz)	409	30	31	17	tr
torte chocolate ganache	1 slice (3.5 oz)	400	26	40	24	6
trifle w/ cream	6 oz	291	16	34	–	1
white w/ coconut icing	1 slice (3.9 oz)	399	12	71	64	1
zucchini bread	1 slice (1.4 oz)	150	7	19	10	1
CAKE ICING						
chocolate	¼ cup	269	7	53	51	1
vanilla	¼ cup	322	8	64	62	0
Betty Crocker						
HomeStyle Mix Fluffy White as prep	6 tbsp	100	0	24	23	–
Rich & Creamy Butter Cream	2 tbsp (1.3 oz)	140	5	15	19	–
Rich & Creamy Chocolate	2 tbsp (1.2 oz)	130	5	21	17	tr
Rich & Creamy Creamy White	2 tbsp (1.2 oz)	140	5	23	20	–
Rich & Creamy Lemon	2 tbsp (1.2 oz)	140	5	23	19	–
Rich & Creamy Vanilla	2 tbsp (1.2 oz)	140	5	23	19	–
Whipped Fluffy White	2 tbsp (0.8 oz)	100	5	15	14	–
Duncan Hines						
Chocolate Butter Cream	2 tbsp (1.2 oz)	140	6	22	20	0
Chocolate Fudge	2 tbsp (1.2 oz)	130	6	21	19	0
Classic Vanilla prep	2 tbsp	140	6	23	22	0

FOOD	PORTION	CAL	FAT	CARB	SUGAR	FIBER
Cream Cheese	2 tbsp (1.2 oz)	140	6	23	22	0
Milk Chocolate	2 tbsp (1.2 oz)	140	6	22	20	0
Manischewitz						
Dairy Free Chocolate	2 tbsp (1.2 oz)	138	5	22	19	0
Naturally Nora						
Frosting Mix Chocolate as prep	1/12 pkg	150	7	24	21	0
Frosting Mix Vanilla as prep	1/12 pkg	170	8	25	23	0

CAKE MIX
Betty Crocker

FOOD	PORTION	CAL	FAT	CARB	SUGAR	FIBER
Gingerbread as prep	1	220	6	39	19	–
Pineapple Upside Down as prep	1/6 cake	390	13	66	43	–
Pound Cake as prep	1/8 cake	260	8	45	26	–
SuperMoist Carrot as prep	1/12 cake	260	12	35	19	–
SuperMoist Chocolate as prep	1/12 cake	250	11	35	18	1
SuperMoist Devil's Food as prep	1/12 cake	260	12	35	18	1
SuperMoist Lemon as prep	1/12 cake	240	9	35	19	–
SuperMoist Milk Chocolate as prep	1/12 cake	240	9	35	19	tr
SuperMoist Spice as prep	1/12 cake	270	13	34	19	1
SuperMoist Vanilla as prep	1/12 cake	230	9	35	18	–
SuperMoist White as prep	1/12 cake	220	8	35	18	–
SuperMoist Yellow	1/12 cake	230	9	35	19	–

FOOD	PORTION	CAL	FAT	CARB	SUGAR	FIBER
Bisquick						
Heart Smart	⅓ cup	140	3	27	3	1
Duncan Hines						
Angel Food as prep	1/12 cake	140	0	31	23	0
Cupcake Mix Classic Yellow as prep	1	130	6	17	10	0
Decadent Carrot as prep	1/12 cake	260	11	37	22	1
Golden Butter Recipe as prep	1/12 cake	270	14	35	23	0
Lemon Supreme as prep	1/12 cake	270	12	36	20	–
Red Velvet as prep	1/12 cake	270	13	35	20	1
Yellow Classic as prep	1/12 cake	270	12	36	20	–
Naturally Nora						
Cheerful Chocolate as prep	1/12 pkg	300	14	39	21	1
Sunny Yellow as prep	1/12 pkg	280	12	39	23	tr
Surprising Stars as prep	1/12 pkg	300	12	42	22	tr

CALABAZA

FOOD	PORTION	CAL	FAT	CARB	SUGAR	FIBER
fresh	½ cup	32	tr	8	–	–

CALZONE (see SANDWICHES)

CANADIAN BACON

FOOD	PORTION	CAL	FAT	CARB	SUGAR	FIBER
grilled	2 slices (1.6 oz)	87	4	1	0	0
Applegate Farms						
Natural	2 slices (2 oz)	90	4	1	1	0

CANDY

FOOD	PORTION	CAL	FAT	CARB	SUGAR	FIBER
butterscotch	1 piece (6 g)	24	tr	6	–	–
candied cherries	1 (4 g)	12	tr	3	–	–
candied citron	1 oz	89	tr	23	–	–
candied lemon peel	1 oz	90	tr	23	–	–
candied orange peel	1 oz	90	tr	23	–	–
candied pineapple slice	1 slice (2 oz)	179	tr	45	–	–

FOOD	PORTION	CAL	FAT	CARB	SUGAR	FIBER
candy corn	1 oz	105	0	27	–	–
caramels	1 piece (8 g)	31	1	6	–	–
caramels chocolate	1 piece (6 g)	22	tr	6	–	–
carob bar	1 (3.1 oz)	453	28	42	–	–
dark chocolate	1 oz	150	10	16	–	–
fondant	1 piece (0.6 oz)	57	0	15	–	–
fondant chocolate coated	1 piece (0.4 oz)	40	1	9	–	–
fondant mint	1 oz	105	0	27	–	–
fruit pastilles	1 tube (1.4 oz)	101	0	25	–	–
fudge brown sugar w/ nuts	1 piece (0.5 oz)	56	1	11	–	–
fudge chocolate marshmallow	1 piece (0.7 oz)	84	3	14	–	–
fudge chocolate marshmallow w/ nuts	1 piece (0.8 oz)	96	4	15	–	–
fudge chocolate w/ nuts	1 piece (0.7 oz)	81	3	14	–	–
fudge peanut butter	1 piece (0.6 oz)	59	1	13	–	–
fudge vanilla w/ nuts	1 piece (0.5 oz)	62	2	11	–	–
gumdrops	10 lg (3.8 oz)	420	0	108	–	–
gumdrops	10 sm (0.4 oz)	135	0	35	–	–
hard candy	1 oz	106	0	28	–	–
jelly beans	10 lg (1 oz)	104	tr	26	–	–
jelly beans	10 sm (0.4 oz)	40	tr	10	–	–
lollipop	1 (6 g)	22	0	6	–	–
marzipan	1 oz	128	7	15	–	2
milk chocolate	1 bar (1.55 oz)	226	14	26	–	–
milk chocolate crisp	1 bar (1.45 oz)	203	11	28	–	–
milk chocolate w/ almonds	1 bar (1.45 oz)	215	14	22	20	–
nougat nut cream	0.5 oz	49	4	8	–	–

FOOD	PORTION	CAL	FAT	CARB	SUGAR	FIBER
organic dark chocolate w/ raisins & pecans	1.4 oz	220	14	22	16	3
peanut bar	1 (1.4 oz)	209	14	19	–	–
peanut brittle	1 oz	128	5	20	–	–
peanuts chocolate covered	10 (1.4 oz)	208	13	20	–	–
peanuts chocolate covered	1 cup (5.2 oz)	773	50	74	–	–
praline	1 piece (1.4 oz)	177	10	24	–	–
pretzels chocolate covered	1 (0.4 oz)	50	2	8	–	–
pretzels chocolate covered	1 oz	130	5	20	–	–
sesame crunch	20 pieces (1.2 oz)	181	12	18	–	–
sweet chocolate	1 oz	143	10	17	–	–
sweet chocolate	1 bar (1.45 oz)	201	14	25	–	–
taffy	1 piece (0.5 oz)	56	1	14	–	–
toffee	1 piece (0.4 oz)	65	4	8	–	–
truffles	1 piece (0.4 oz)	59	4	5	–	–
3 Musketeers						
Bar	1 (2.1 oz)	260	8	46	40	1
Fun Size	3 bars (1.6 oz)	190	6	34	30	1
Minis	7 (1.4 oz)	170	5	32	27	1
Mint	1 bar (1.2 oz)	150	5	26	22	1
5th Avenue						
Bar	1 (2 oz)	260	12	37	28	2

FOOD	PORTION	CAL	FAT	CARB	SUGAR	FIBER
Almond Joy						
Bar	1 (1.6 oz)	220	13	26	20	2
Annabelle's						
Skinny Hunk Chewy Nougat	1 bar (1 oz)	100	1	24	25	0
Baskin-Robbins						
Soft Candy Mint Chocolate Chip	2 (0.3 oz)	40	1	7	5	0
Sugar Free Hard Candy Cookies 'N Cream	4 (0.6 oz)	40	1	15	0	–
Betty Crocker						
Fruit Gushers Rockin' Blue Raspberry	1 pkg (0.9 oz)	90	1	20	13	–
Brach's						
Mellowcreme Pumpkins	6 pieces (1.5 oz)	150	0	38	33	–
Breath Savers						
Peppermint	1 (1.8 g)	5	0	2	0	–
Bubble Chocolate						
Dark Chocolate	1 bar (1.41 oz)	200	15	22	15	3
Milk Chocolate	1 bar (1.41 oz)	220	15	21	20	tr
Cadbury						
Caramello	1 (1.6 oz)	220	10	29	25	tr
Dairy Milk	7 blocks (1.4 oz)	200	11	23	22	tr
Milk Chocolate Roast Almond	7 blocks (1.4 oz)	210	13	21	19	1
Royal Dark	7 blocks (1.4 oz)	170	12	23	20	3
Choward's						
Mints All Flavors	3 (5 g)	20	0	5	5	0

FOOD	PORTION	CAL	FAT	CARB	SUGAR	FIBER
Chuao Chocolatier						
Choco Pod Banana	1 (0.4 oz)	50	3	6	5	–
Choco Pod Passion	1 (0.4 oz)	50	4	5	5	–
Dove						
Dark Chocolate Cranberry Almond	⅓ pkg (1.2 oz)	170	10	20	16	2
Milk Chocolate Roasted Almond	⅓ bar (1.2 oz)	180	12	18	16	1
Emily's						
Espresso Beans Dark Chocolate Covered	26 (1.4 oz)	220	19	24	21	3
Enjoy Life						
Boom Choco Boom Dark Chocolate Dairy Nut Soy Free	1 bar (1.4 oz)	200	15	22	17	3
Ferrero						
Rocher	3 pieces (1.3 oz)	220	16	16	15	1
Rondnoir	3 pieces (1.4 oz)	220	14	21	16	2
Ghirardelli						
Luxe Milk Chocolate	4 sq (1.5 oz)	220	13	26	24	tr
Good & Plenty						
Licorice	33 (1.4 oz)	140	0	35	25	–
Hammond's						
Root Beer Drops	3 (0.6 oz)	60	0	14	12	0
Heath						
Bar	1 (1.4 oz)	210	13	24	23	tr
Hershey's						
Bar Milk Chocolate w/ Almonds	1 (1.4 oz)	210	14	21	19	2
Bar Special Dark	1 (1.4 oz)	180	12	25	21	3
Bliss Dark Chocolate Bar	1 (1.3 oz)	160	12	21	17	3

FOOD	PORTION	CAL	FAT	CARB	SUGAR	FIBER
Bliss Milk Chocolate	6 (1.5 oz)	210	14	24	22	1
Bliss Milk Chocolate Meltaway	6 (1.5 oz)	220	15	24	33	1
Bliss Milk Chocolate Raspberry Meltaway	6 (1.5 oz)	220	14	24	23	tr
Kisses Cherry Cordial	9 (1.5 oz)	180	7	30	26	–
Kisses Hugs	9 (1.4 oz)	210	12	23	21	–
Kisses Milk Chocolate	9 (1.4 oz)	230	13	24	21	1
Kisses Special Dark	9 (1.4 oz)	180	12	25	21	3
Milk Chocolate Bar	1 (1.5 oz)	210	13	26	24	1
Milk Chocolate w/ Almonds Bar	1 (1.5 oz)	210	13	25	22	2
Nuggets Milk Chocolate	4 (1.4 oz)	200	12	25	23	1
Nuggets Milk Chocolate w/ Almonds	4 (1.3 oz)	200	13	20	17	2
Pieces All Flavors	51 (1.4 oz)	190	9	25	21	1
Ice Breakers						
Coolmint	1 (0.8 g)	0	0	tr	–	–
Jolly Rancher						
Gummies	9 (1.4 oz)	120	0	28	22	–
Original Assortment	3 (0.5 oz)	50	0	13	7	–
KitKat						
Bar	1 (1.5 oz)	210	11	28	22	tr
Kopali						
Organic Dark Chocolate Covered Espresso Beans	½ pkg (1 oz)	120	7	17	15	2
Lance						
Chewz Strawberry	1 pkg (1.1 oz)	120	1	28	26	–
Peanut Bar	1 (2.3 oz)	340	19	29	19	3
Lindt						
Lindor Truffles 60% Extra Dark	3 pieces (1.3 oz)	210	19	15	11	tr

FOOD	PORTION	CAL	FAT	CARB	SUGAR	FIBER
Lindor Truffles Swiss Dark Chocolate	3 (1.4 oz)	240	18	17	16	2
Petits Desserts Assorted	4 (1.3 oz)	210	15	20	17	tr
Love Candy						
Dark Chocolate	1 bar (1.5 oz)	190	11	21	15	1
Milk Chocolate	1 bar (1.5 oz)	200	11	22	15	tr
Yogurt Supreme	1 bar (1.5 oz)	190	11	23	7	tr
Mama's Goodies						
Butter Nut Crunch Almond	1 piece (1.33 oz)	220	15	20	18	1
Butter Nut Crunch Sesame Seed	1 piece (1.33 oz)	220	14	20	18	1
Nut Butter Crunch Macadamia & Coconut	1 piece (1.33 oz)	220	17	20	18	1
Mamba						
Fruit Flavor	6 (0.9 oz)	170	3	36	19	0
Sour	6 (0.9 oz)	100	2	22	11	0
Mike & Ike						
All Flavors	1 pkg (2 oz)	200	0	50	–	–
Milk Duds						
Chocolate	13 (1.4 oz)	170	6	28	20	–
Milkfuls						
Candy	6 (1.4 oz)	170	3	35	23	0
Milky Way						
Fun Size	2 bars (1.2 oz)	150	6	24	20	0
Mounds						
Bar	1 (1.7 oz)	230	13	29	21	3
Mr.Goodbar						
Bar	1 (1.7 oz)	250	17	26	23	2
Necco						
Banana Splits	4 (1.4 oz)	150	2	36	21	0
Clark Junior Bar	1 (0.5 oz)	60	3	10	8	0

FOOD	PORTION	CAL	FAT	CARB	SUGAR	FIBER
Conversation Hearts Tiny	40 (1.4 oz)	160	0	39	38	0
Double Dipped Peanuts	15 (1.4 oz)	200	11	25	22	1
Junior Assorted Wafers	1 roll (0.5 oz)	50	0	13	12	–
Mary Janes	5 (1.4 oz)	160	4	32	20	0
Mint Juleps	4 (1.4 oz)	150	2	36	21	0
Nonpareils	10 (1.4 oz)	190	9	29	23	0
Squirrel Nut Caramel	5 (1.6 oz)	170	3	37	25	0
PayDay						
Peanut Caramel	1 (1.8 oz)	240	13	27	21	2
Pot Of Gold						
Nut Assortment	4 (1.4 oz)	210	13	23	20	2
Pecan Caramel Clusters	4 (1.4 oz)	200	12	23	21	1
Truffle Assortment	3 (1.5 oz)	200	9	27	23	1
Pure Fun						
Organic Vegan Barrels Of Fun Root Beer Float	2 (0.5 oz)	60	0	13	3	0
Organic Vegan Candy Canes	1 (0.5 oz)	62	0	14	3	1
Organic Vegan Chocolate Meltdowns All Flavors	3 (0.6 oz)	70	0	16	4	0
Organic Vegan Citrus Slices All Flavors	3 (0.6 oz)	60	0	15	3	0
Organic Vegan Cotton Candy All Flavors	¼ pkg (0.5 oz)	60	0	15	15	0
Organic Vegan Jaw Boulders All Flavors	2 (0.5 oz)	58	0	13	3	0
Organic Vegan Pure Pops All Flavors	3 (0.6 oz)	60	0	15	3	0
Reese's						
Crispy Crunchy Bar	1 (1.7 oz)	250	14	29	22	2
FastBreak	1 (2 oz)	260	12	35	30	2

FOOD	PORTION	CAL	FAT	CARB	SUGAR	FIBER
NutRageous	1 (1.8 oz)	260	16	28	22	2
Pieces Peanut Butter	1 pkg (1.5 oz)	210	10	26	24	1
ReeseSticks						
Wafer Bar Chocolate & Peanut Butter	1 (1.5 oz)	210	13	23	17	1
Riesen						
Candy	4 (1.3 oz)	170	4	28	15	0
Rolo						
Chewy Caramels In Milk Chocolate	3 pkg (1.7 oz)	220	10	33	29	–
Russell Stover						
Private Reserve Triple Chocolate Mousse	3 pieces (1.3 oz)	220	17	19	15	2
See's						
Assorted Chocolates	2 (1.2 oz)	160	9	20	16	tr
Nuts & Chews	3 (1.6 oz)	240	16	25	18	2
Soft Centers	2 (1.4 oz)	170	9	25	22	tr
Sencha Naturals						
Green Tea Mints All Flavors	3	5	0	1	0	0
Shaman Chocolates						
Organic Extra Dark Chocolate 82% Cacao	½ bar (1 oz)	158	14	7	1	4
Organic Milk Chocolate w/ Macadamia Nuts & Hawaiian Pink Sea Salt	½ bar (1 oz)	91	1	13	13	2
Skittles						
Original Fruit	1 pkg (2.2 oz)	250	3	56	47	0
Sour	1 pkg (1.8 oz)	200	0	44	37	0
Skor						
Toffee & Milk Chocolate	1 (1.4 oz)	200	12	25	24	tr

FOOD	PORTION	CAL	FAT	CARB	SUGAR	FIBER
Smile Chocolatiers						
Choclatea Ginger Tea Milk Chocolate 37% Cacao	½ bar (1.5 oz)	230	15	23	21	1
Choclatea Herbal Chai Tea Dark Chocolate 64% Cacao	½ bar (1.5 oz)	220	17	22	15	5
Choclatea Pistachio Green Tea White Chocolate	½ bar (1.5 oz)	240	16	22	22	1
Choclatea Pomegranate White Tea Very Dark Chocolate 72% Cacao	½ bar (1.5 oz)	220	16	16	14	2
Choclatea White Tea Very Dark Chocolate 72% Cacao	½ bar (1.5 oz)	220	17	22	15	5
Sour Patch						
Kids Soft & Chewy	1 pkg (1 oz)	100	0	25	17	–
Starbucks						
Truffles Caffe Mocha	3 (1.3 oz)	200	14	19	17	1
Symphony						
Almonds & Toffee	1 (1.5 oz)	220	14	23	22	tr
Take 5						
Original	1 pkg (1.5 oz)	200	11	25	18	1
Thorntons						
Chocolates Summer Collection	1	65	4	7	–	–
Toblerone						
Bittersweet w/ Honey & Almond Nugget	⅓ bar (1.2 oz)	170	9	20	16	2
Milk Chocolate w/ Honey & Almond Nougat	⅓ bar (1.2 oz)	170	9	21	18	1

FOOD	PORTION	CAL	FAT	CARB	SUGAR	FIBER
White w/ Honey & Almond Nougat	1/3 bar (1.2 oz)	180	10	20	20	1
Toffifay						
Candy	5 (1.4 oz)	200	11	25	18	1
Twizzlers						
Licorice	4 (1.6 oz)	150	1	35	18	–
Strawberry	4 (1.6 oz)	160	1	36	19	–
Werther's						
Caramel Milk Chocolate	6 (1.3 oz)	230	16	18	17	0
Original	3 (0.5 oz)	60	1	13	11	0
Original Sugar Free	5 (0.5 oz)	40	1	14	0	0
Whoppers						
Malted Milk Balls	18 (1.4 oz)	190	7	31	26	–
Wolfgang						
Blueberries Dipped In Dark Chocolate	2 (0.7 oz)	80	4	13	12	tr
Cranberries Dipped In Dark Chocolate	2 (1 oz)	130	6	18	16	1
Raspberries Dipped In Dark Chocolate	2 (1.1 oz)	130	6	21	19	1
York						
Peppermint Patty	1 (1.4 oz)	140	3	31	25	tr
Young & Smylie						
Licorice Black	11 (1.5 oz)	140	2	32	19	–
Licorice Strawberry	11 (1.5 oz)	150	2	33	20	–
Zagnut						
Peanut Butter & Coconut	3 (1.5 oz)	200	8	31	22	1
Zero						
Bar	1 (1.8 oz)	230	8	37	31	–
CANTALOUPE						
dried	3.5 pieces (1.4 oz)	140	0	34	32	1
fresh cubed	1 cup	57	tr	13	–	1
fresh half	1/2	94	1	22	–	2

FOOD	PORTION	CAL	FAT	CARB	SUGAR	FIBER
Chiquita						
Fresh Cup Up	1 cup (6.2 oz)	60	0	16	14	2
CAPERS						
capers	1 tbsp	2	tr	tr	tr	tr
CARAWAY						
seed	1 tbsp	22	1	3	tr	3
CARDAMOM						
ground	1 tsp	6	tr	1	–	1
CARDOON						
fresh cooked w/o salt	1 serv (3.5 oz)	22	tr	5	–	2
fresh shredded	1 cup (6.2 oz)	30	tr	7	–	3
Ocean Mist						
Cardone Fresh Shredded	1 cup (6.2 oz)	36	tr	9	0	3
CARIBOU						
roasted	3 oz	142	4	0	0	0
CARISSA						
fresh	1	12	tr	3	–	–
CAROB						
carob mix	3 tsp	45	0	11	–	–
carob mix as prep w/ whole milk	9 oz	195	8	23	–	–
flour	1 cup	185	1	92	–	–
flour	1 tbsp	14	tr	7	–	–
Tree Of Life						
Chips Malt Sweetened	50 (0.5 oz)	70	4	9	1	1
CARP						
fresh cooked	3 oz	138	6	0	0	0
fresh cooked	1 fillet (6 oz)	276	12	0	0	0
fresh raw	3 oz	108	5	0	0	0
roe raw	1 oz	37	tr	tr	–	–
roe salted in olive oil	2 tbsp (1 oz)	40	–	6	–	0

FOOD	PORTION	CAL	FAT	CARB	SUGAR	FIBER
CARROT JUICE						
canned	6 oz	73	tr	17	–	–
CARROTS						
CANNED						
slices	½ cup	17	tr	4	–	1
slices low sodium	½ cup	17	tr	4	–	1
Allens						
Tiny Sliced	½ cup	35	0	8	3	3
S&W						
Julienne	½ cup (4.3 oz)	35	0	8	5	3
FRESH						
baby raw	1 (0.5 oz)	6	tr	1	–	–
raw	1 (2.5 oz)	31	tr	7	–	2
raw shredded	½ cup	24	tr	6	–	2
slices cooked	½ cup	35	tr	8	–	–
Chiquita						
Carrot Bites w/ Ranch Dressing	1 pkg (2.5 oz)	50	3	7	5	2
FROZEN						
slices cooked	½ cup	26	tr	6	–	–
Birds Eye						
Steam & Serve Carrots & Cranberries	1 cup	130	5	20	15	3
Green Giant						
Honey Glazed	1 cup	90	3	15	11	3
Joy Of Cooking						
Bite Size	½ cup (3.3 oz)	70	3	12	3	2
CASABA						
cubed	1 cup (6 oz)	46	tr	11	10	2
melon fresh	¼ (14 oz)	115	tr	27	23	4

FOOD	PORTION	CAL	FAT	CARB	SUGAR	FIBER
CASHEW JUICE						
O.N.E.						
Cashew Fruit	1 bottle (11 oz)	140	0	34	33	1
CASHEWS						
cashew butter w/o salt	1 tbsp	94	8	4	–	–
dry roasted w/ salt	1 oz	163	13	9	–	–
dry roasted w/ salt	18 nuts (1 oz)	160	13	9	–	1
oil roasted w/ salt	1 oz	163	14	8	–	–
oil roasted w/o salt	1 oz	163	14	8	–	–
Back To Nature						
Jumbo Sea Salt Roasted	1 oz	160	13	9	2	1
Lance						
Cashews	1 pkg (1.5 oz)	270	22	11	4	3
Tree Of Life						
Cashew Butter Creamy	2 tbsp	180	15	9	2	1
Yumnuts						
Chili Lime	¼ cup (1 oz)	170	13	7	2	3
Chocolate	¼ cup (1 oz)	160	11	12	6	2
Honey	¼ cup (1 oz)	170	12	10	6	1
Toasted Coconut	½ cup (1 oz)	170	13	9	4	2
CASSAVA						
diced cooked w/o fat	1 cup (4.6 oz)	213	tr	51	2	2
root raw	1 (14.3 oz)	653	1	155	7	7
TAKE-OUT						
fritter crab meat stuffed	1 (4.4 oz)	341	16	38	7	2
CATFISH						
channel breaded & fried	3 oz	194	11	7	–	–
wolffish atlantic baked	3 oz	105	3	0	0	0
CAULIFLOWER						
flowerets fresh	1 (0.5 oz)	3	tr	1	tr	tr

FOOD	PORTION	CAL	FAT	CARB	SUGAR	FIBER
flowerets fresh cooked w/o salt	3 (2 oz)	12	tr	2	1	1
fresh	1 cup	25	tr	5	2	3
fresh cooked w/o salt	1 cup	29	1	5	3	3
fresh head small	1 (9.2 oz)	66	tr	14	6	7
frzn cooked w/o salt	1 cup	34	tr	7	2	5
green fresh	1 cup	20	tr	4	2	2
green fresh small head	1 (11.4 oz)	101	1	20	10	10
pickled	¼ cup	14	tr	3	2	1
pickled chow chow	¼ cup	74	1	16	15	1
Birds Eye						
Steamfresh Garlic Cauliflower	1 cup (2.4 oz)	40	2	5	2	1
Mann's						
Cauliettes Fresh	1 serv (3 oz)	20	0	4	2	2
TAKE-OUT						
batter dipped fried	1 cup	178	13	12	1	2
batter dipped fried	1 piece (0.9 oz)	55	4	4	tr	1
w/ cheese sauce	1 cup	249	18	12	6	3
CAVIAR						
black or red	2 tbsp	81	6	1	0	0
CELERY						
fresh	1 lg stalk (2.2 oz)	9	tr	2	1	1
pickled	½ cup	10	tr	2	1	1
raw diced	½ cup	8	tr	2	1	1
seed	1 tsp	1	tr	tr	–	tr
strips	1 cup	17	tr	4	2	2
TAKE-OUT						
creamed	½ cup	87	6	7	4	1
stir fried	½ cup	30	2	3	2	1
stuffed w/ cheese	1 (5 inch)	38	3	1	tr	tr

FOOD	PORTION	CAL	FAT	CARB	SUGAR	FIBER
CELERY JUICE						
juice	1 cup	42	tr	9	6	4
CELERY ROOT						
fresh cooked w/o salt	1 cup (5.4 oz)	42	tr	9	–	2
fresh cut up	1 cup (5.5 oz)	66	tr	14	3	3
CELTUCE						
raw	3.5 oz	22	tr	4	–	–
CEREAL						
bran flakes	¾ cup	90	1	22	–	–
corn flakes	1¼ cups	110	tr	24	–	–
farina as prep w/ water	¾ cup	88	tr	19	–	2
granola	½ cup	285	15	32	–	6
oatmeal instant as prep w/ water	1 cup (8.2 oz)	138	2	24	–	4
oatmeal regular & quick as prep w/ water	¾ cup (6.1 oz)	149	2	19	–	3
oatmeal regular & quick not prep	⅓ cup (0.9 oz)	104	2	18	–	3
puffed rice	1 cup	56	tr	13	–	tr
puffed wheat	1 cup	44	tr	10	–	1
shredded mini wheats	1 cup	107	1	24	–	3
shredded wheat rectangular	1 biscuit (0.8 oz)	85	tr	19	–	2
Amy's						
Bowls Organic Cream Of Rice	1 pkg (8.9 oz)	170	1	39	8	2
Bowls Organic Multigrain	1 pkg (8.9 oz)	190	2	40	12	5
Back To Nature						
Granola Apple Blueberry	½ cup (1.8 oz)	200	3	39	13	4

FOOD	PORTION	CAL	FAT	CARB	SUGAR	FIBER
Granola Chocolate Delight	½ cup (1.75 oz)	220	6	37	13	4
Granola Classic	½ cup (1.8 oz)	200	3	39	12	4
Granola Sunflower & Pumpkin Seed	½ cup (1.6 oz)	290	7	31	11	4
Granola To Go Ginger Roasted Almonds w/ Flax Seed	1 serv (1.5 oz)	190	7	29	10	4
Granola To Go Wild Blueberry Walnut w/ Flax Seed	1 serv (1.5 oz)	190	6	30	11	4
Bakery On Main						
Granola Apple Cinnamon Walnut	½ cup (2 oz)	240	12	29	9	4
Granola Fiber Power Cinnamon Raisin	½ cup (2 oz)	230	6	40	9	9
Granola Maple Raisin Almond	½ cup (2 oz)	240	12	30	12	4
Granola Super Fruit & Nut	½ cup (2 oz)	250	13	29	20	4
Barbara's Bakery						
Alpen No Sugar Added	⅔ cup	200	3	40	7	4
Organic Breakfast O's Fruit Juice Sweetened	1 cup	120	2	22	1	3
Organic Brown Rice Crisps Fruit Juice Sweetened	1 cup	120	1	25	2	1
Organic Corn Flakes Fruit Juice Sweetened	1 cup	110	1	25	3	1
Organic Wild Puffs	1 cup	100	1	23	12	tr
Organic Wild Puffs Fruity Punch	1 cup	110	1	26	9	1

FOOD	PORTION	CAL	FAT	CARB	SUGAR	FIBER
Organic Ultima High Fiber	½ cup	90	1	24	5	8
Organic Ultima Pomegranate	½ cup	100	1	24	5	5
Puffins Cinnamon	⅔ cup	100	1	26	6	6
Puffins Originals	¾ cup (0.9 oz)	90	1	23	5	5
Shredded Oats Bite Size	1¼ cups (2 oz)	220	3	46	12	5
Shredded Wheat	2 biscuits (2 oz)	140	1	31	0	5
Cascadian Farm						
Organic Clifford Crunch	1 cup	100	1	25	6	5
Organic Granola Oats & Honey	⅔ cup	230	6	42	14	3
Chappaqua Crunch						
Original Granola	⅓ cup	115	2	20	4	3
Simply Granola w/ Raisins	⅓ cup	120	2	22	6	3
Simply Granola w/ Raspberries	⅓ cup	110	2	21	4	3
Chia Goodness						
Apple Almond Cinnamon	2 tbsp (1 oz)	130	6	16	4	4
Cranberry Ginger	2 tbsp (1 oz)	130	7	16	3	4
Original	2 tbsp (1 oz)	140	8	14	0	5
Country Choice Organic						
Multigrain Hot Cereal not prep	½ cup	130	1	29	0	5
Oats Old Fashioned not prep	½ cup	150	3	27	1	4
Oats Quick not prep	½ cup	150	3	27	1	4
Dorset Cereals						
Berries & Cherries	½ cup	150	1	40	23	3

FOOD	PORTION	CAL	FAT	CARB	SUGAR	FIBER
Simply Delicious Muesli	½ cup	200	5	37	7	4
Super Cranberry Cherry & Almond	½ cup	200	5	39	17	4
Erin Baker's						
Granola Fruit & Nut	½ cup (1.6 oz)	190	8	27	10	4
Granola Oatmeal Raisin	½ cup (1.6 oz)	180	6	30	11	4
Granola Ultra Protein Power Crunch	½ cup (1.6 oz)	200	6	25	6	4
Farina						
Original as prep	1 cup	120	0	22	0	tr
General Mills						
Cheerios Crunch Oat Cluster	¾ cups	100	1	22	8	2
Fiber One Raisin Bran Clusters	1 cup (2 oz)	170	1	45	13	11
Total Whole Grain	¾ cup (1 oz)	100	1	23	5	3
Trix	1 cup (1.1 oz)	120	2	28	12	1
Health Valley						
Empower	1 cup	200	3	42	11	6
Granola Low Fat Tropical Fruit	⅔ cup	180	1	43	10	6
Heart Wise	1 cup	200	3	37	11	5
Organic Cherry Lemon Blast Ems	¾ cup	120	1	25	7	2
Organic Golden Flax	¾ cup	190	3	38	9	6
Organic Multigrain Apple Cinnamon Square Ems	1¼ cup	210	3	44	12	8
Organic Oat Bran O's	¾ cup	100	0	23	14	3
Rice Crunch-Ems	1 cup	110	0	26	2	2
Honest Foods						
Granola Planks Maple Almond Crunch	½ bar (2 oz)	250	10	37	19	5

FOOD	PORTION	CAL	FAT	CARB	SUGAR	FIBER
Kashi						
Honey Sunshine	¾ cup (1.1 oz)	100	2	25	6	6
McCann's						
Irish Oatmeal Instant Apples & Cinnamon not prep	1 pkg (1.2 oz)	130	2	27	12	3
Irish Oatmeal Instant Maple & Brown Sugar not prep	1 pkg (1.5 oz)	160	2	32	13	3
Irish Oatmeal Instant Regular not prep	1 pkg (1 oz)	100	2	18	1	3
Irish Oatmeal Quick Cooking not prep	½ cup (1.4 oz)	150	2	26	0	4
Irish Oatmeal Steel Cut not prep	¼ cup (1.4 oz)	150	2	26	0	4
Natural Ovens						
Great Granola	½ cup	250	9	38	8	3
Newman's Own						
Sweet Enough Honey Flax Flakes	¾ cup	100	1	24	8	4
Sweet Enough Honey Nut O's	¾ cup	110	2	22	7	2
Sweet Enough Wheat Puffs	¾ cup	100	1	22	8	1
Post						
Great Grains Raisins Dates & Pecans	¾ cup (2 oz)	210	5	40	14	4
Raisin Bran	1 cup (2 oz)	190	1	46	19	8
Ralston						
Corn Flakes	1 cup (1 oz)	100	0	24	2	tr
Raisin Bran	1 cup (2 oz)	190	1	46	19	7

FOOD	PORTION	CAL	FAT	CARB	SUGAR	FIBER
Roman Meal						
Cream Of Rye not prep	1/3 cup (1.4 oz)	130	0	27	2	6
Elements Cranberry Passion	1 cup (1.6 oz)	160	3	33	9	5
Hot Cereal not prep	1/3 cup (1.3 oz)	120	2	26	1	6
Silhouette Solution						
Oatmeal Cinnamon Apple	1 pkg. (1.39 oz)	150	2	17	4	4
South Beach						
Crunch Strawberry Harvest	1 cup	170	2	37	9	8
Crunch Vanilla Almond	1 cup	180	4	35	8	8
Granola Clusters Cherry Almond	1 pkg (1 oz)	130	4	18	6	6
Granola Clusters Mixed Berry	1 pkg (1 oz)	130	4	18	6	6
Udi's						
Granola BanaBerry	1/4 cup (1.1 oz)	120	4	19	5	3
Granola Hawaiian	1/4 cup (1.1 oz)	120	5	19	5	3
Granola Muesli	1/4 cup (1.1 oz)	120	4	18	1	4
Granola Nuggets	1/4 cup (1.1 oz)	150	6	22	6	3
Granola Original	1/4 cup (1.1 oz)	130	5	18	5	2
Uncle Sam						
Original	3/4 cup (1.9 oz)	190	5	38	tr	10
Weetabix						
Organic	2 biscuits (1.2 oz)	120	1	28	2	4
Organic Crispy Flakes	3/4 cup	110	1	24	4	4
Wheatena						
Toasted Wheat	1/3 cup	160	1	33	0	5

FOOD	PORTION	CAL	FAT	CARB	SUGAR	FIBER
YogActive						
Probiotic High Fibre Wheat Strawberry Raspberry	²/₃ cup	160	3	29	8	6
Probiotic Kiwi	²/₃ cup	120	2	23	7	1
Probiotic Strawberry	²/₃ cup	130	2	25	7	1
Probiotic Strawberry Dark Chocolate	²/₃ cup	130	3	26	9	2
CEREAL BARS (see also ENERGY BARS)						
Aristo						
Acai Blueberry Lime	1 (1.3 oz)	130	4	22	6	3
Pomegranate & Cranberry	1 (1.3 oz)	140	5	21	6	3
Bakery On Main						
Granola Gluten Free Extreme Trail Mix	1 (1.3 oz)	140	5	23	7	1
Granola Gluten Free Peanut Butter Chocolate Chip	1 (1.2 oz)	140	5	24	7	1
Barbara's Bakery						
Fruit & Yogurt Cherry Apple	1	150	3	29	15	1
Nature's Choice Blueberry	1 (1.3 oz)	150	2	29	15	2
Organic Crunchy Granola Cinnamon Crisp	2 (1.5 oz)	190	8	27	10	3
Cascadian Farm						
Organic Chewy Granola Fruit & Nut	1 (1.2 oz)	140	4	24	11	1
Country Choice Organic						
Oatmeal Squares Apple Cinnamon	1 (2 oz)	210	3	41	16	1
Oatmeal Squares Maple	1 (2 oz)	210	3	41	14	4

FOOD	PORTION	CAL	FAT	CARB	SUGAR	FIBER
Granola Gourmet						
Brownie	1 (1.25 oz)	150	6	20	10	3
Chocolate Espresso	1 (1.25 oz)	150	6	20	10	3
Spiced Orange Cranberry	1 (1.25 oz)	140	5	20	10	3
Health Valley						
Cafe Creations Cinnamon Danish	1 (1.4 oz)	130	3	27	17	2
Date Almond Low Fat	1 (1.5 oz)	150	3	32	15	tr
Granola Chocolate Chip Low Fat	1 (1.5 oz)	160	3	32	13	1
Granola Moist & Chewy Dutch Apple	1 (1 oz)	100	2	20	10	tr
Granola Trail Mix Cranberries Nuts & Yogurt Chips	1 (1.2 oz)	140	4	23	12	1
Organic Fig Cobbler	1 (1.4 oz)	130	3	26	14	2
Organic Raspberry Tarts	1 (1.4 oz)	150	3	30	16	tr
Organic Strawberry Cobbler	1 (1.3 oz)	130	3	26	14	1
Peanut Butter & Grape	1 (1.3 oz)	130	3	26	16	1
Hershey's						
Sweet & Salty Granola Bar Reese's w/ Chocolate	1 (1.2 oz)	160	9	18	8	1
Sweet & Salty Granola Bar w/ Pretzels	1 (1.2 oz)	140	5	22	8	1
Honest Foods						
Cran Lemon Zest	1 (2.2 oz)	240	9	35	17	4
Farmer's Trail Mix	1 (2.2 oz)	240	9	35	17	4

FOOD	PORTION	CAL	FAT	CARB	SUGAR	FIBER
Jungle Grub						
Berry Bamboozle w/ Vanilla Icing Gluten Free	1 (0.9 oz)	100	4	14	8	1
Chocolate Chip Cookie Dough w/ Chocolate Coating Gluten Free	1 (0.9 oz)	100	4	13	8	4
Peanut Butter Groove w/ Vanilla Icing Gluten Free	1 (0.9 oz)	100	4	13	8	1
Kashi						
TLC Chewy Granola Dark Mocha Almond	1 (1.2 oz)	130	4	21	6	4
TLC Soft Baked Apple Spice	1 (1.2 oz)	110	3	21	9	3
TLC Soft Baked Blackberry Graham	1 (1.2 oz)	110	1	21	9	3
TLC Soft Baked Ripe Strawberry	1 (1.2 oz)	110	3	21	9	3
Kellogg's						
FiberPlus Antioxidants Chocolate Chip	1 (1.2 oz)	120	4	26	7	9
FiberPlus Antioxidants Dark Chocolate Almond	1 (1.2 oz)	130	5	24	7	9
KeriBar						
Vegan Apple Peanut Butter	1 (1.4 oz)	140	6	21	10	5
Vegan Cherry Almond	1 (1.4 oz)	140	6	21	10	5
Vegan Strawberry Chocolate Chip	1 (1.4 oz)	130	5	23	12	5
Kudos						
Granola Chocolate Chip	1 (1 oz)	120	4	20	11	1

FOOD	PORTION	CAL	FAT	CARB	SUGAR	FIBER
Lean Body						
Hi-Protein Granola Peanuts 'N Chocolate	1 (2.8 oz)	340	11	39	13	4
Natural Ovens						
Great Granola Mixed Fruit	1 (1.4 oz)	150	3	27	15	2
Quaker						
Chewy Granola w/Protein Peanut Butter & Chocolate	1 (1 oz)	110	3	18	7	1
Reese's						
SnackBarz Peanut Butter	1 (0.9 oz)	120	5	16	11	tr
Revolution Foods						
Jammy Sammy Apple Cinnamon & Oatmeal	1 (1 oz)	100	2	21	10	1
Organic Jammy Sammy PB & Grape	1 (1 oz)	110	3	19	10	1
Organic Jammy Sammy PB & Strawberry	1 (1 oz)	110	3	19	10	1
Roman Meal						
Whole Grain & Fruit	1 (2 oz)	190	2	43	21	6
Silhouette Solution						
Blueberry Pomegranate	1 (1.3 oz)	130	3	14	7	3
Peanut Passion	1 (1.3 oz)	130	4	14	5	3
South Beach						
Fiber Fit Granola Mocha	1 (1.2 oz)	120	4	25	7	9
Fiber Fit Granola S'Mores	1 (1.2 oz)	120	4	25	7	9
Yotta						
Apple Cinnamon	1 (1.2 oz)	120	1	25	11	2
Cherry	1 (1.2 oz)	120	1	26	11	1
Orange	1 (1.2 oz)	120	1	26	11	2

FOOD	PORTION	CAL	FAT	CARB	SUGAR	FIBER
CHAMPAGNE						
champagne	1 serv (3.5 oz)	84	0	3	1	0
mimosa	1 serv	117	tr	12	–	tr
punch	1 serv (4 oz)	73	tr	8	6	0
sekt german champagne	1 serv (3.5 oz)	84	0	5	–	–
CHAYOTE						
fresh cooked	1 cup	38	1	8	–	–
raw	1 (7 oz)	49	1	11	–	–
raw cut up	1 cup	32	tr	7	–	–
CHEESE (see also CHEESE DISHES, CHEESE SUBSTITUTES, COTTAGE CHEESE, CREAM CHEESE, NEUFCHATEL)						
american	1 oz	93	7	2	–	–
american cheese spread	1 oz	82	6	2	–	–
beaufort	1 oz	115	9	tr	tr	0
bel paese	1 oz	112	9	0	0	0
blue	1 oz	100	8	1	–	–
blue crumbled	1 cup (4.7 oz)	477	39	3	–	–
bocconcini smoked	1 oz	90	6	1	0	0
brick	1 oz	105	8	1	–	–
brie	1 oz	95	8	tr	–	–
cacio di roma sheep's milk cheese	1 oz	130	10	0	0	0
caerphilly	1.4 oz	150	13	0	–	0
camembert	1 oz	85	7	tr	–	–
cantal	1 oz	105	9	tr	tr	0
caraway	1 oz	107	8	1	–	–
chabichou	1 oz	95	8	tr	tr	0
chaource	1 oz	83	7	tr	tr	0
cheddar	1 oz	114	9	tr	–	–
cheddar low sodium	1 oz	113	9	1	–	–
cheddar lowfat	1 oz	49	2	1	–	–
cheddar reduced fat	1.4 oz	104	6	0	–	0

FOOD	PORTION	CAL	FAT	CARB	SUGAR	FIBER
cheddar shredded	1 cup	455	37	1	–	–
cheshire	1 oz	110	9	1	–	–
cheshire reduced fat	1.4 oz	108	6	tr	–	0
colby	1 oz	112	9	1	–	–
colby low sodium	1 oz	113	9	1	–	–
colby lowfat	1 oz	49	2	1	–	–
comte	1 oz	114	9	tr	tr	0
coulommiers	1 oz	88	7	tr	tr	0
crottin	1 oz	105	9	tr	tr	0
derby	1.4 oz	161	14	0	–	0
edam reduced fat	1.4 oz	92	4	tr	–	0
emmentaler	1 oz	115	9	tr	–	–
feta	1 oz	75	6	1	–	–
fontina	1 oz	110	9	tr	–	–
frais	1.6 oz	51	3	3	–	0
gjetost	1 oz	132	8	12	–	–
gloucester double	1.4 oz	162	14	0	–	0
goat fresh	1 oz	23	2	tr	tr	0
goat hard	1 oz	128	10	1	–	–
gorgonzola	1 oz	107	9	tr	–	–
gouda	1 oz	101	8	1	–	–
grana padano parmesan shaved	1 tbsp	20	2	0	0	0
gruyere	1 oz	117	9	tr	–	–
lancashire	1.4 oz	149	12	0	–	0
leicester	1.4 oz	160	14	0	–	0
limburger	1 oz	93	8	tr	–	–
lymeswold	1.4 oz	170	16	tr	–	0
maroilles	1 oz	97	8	tr	tr	0
monterey	1 oz	106	9	tr	–	–
morbier	1 oz	99	8	tr	tr	0
mozzarella	1 oz	80	6	1	–	–
mozzarella fresh	1 oz	80	6	tr	0	0

FOOD	PORTION	CAL	FAT	CARB	SUGAR	FIBER
mozzarella part skim	1 oz	72	5	1	–	–
muenster	1 oz	104	9	tr	–	–
parmesan grated	1 tbsp	23	2	tr	–	–
parmesan hard	1 oz	111	7	1	–	–
picodon	1 oz	99	8	tr	tr	0
pimento	1 oz	106	9	tr	–	–
pont l'eveque	1 oz	86	7	tr	tr	0
port du salut	1 oz	100	8	tr	–	–
provolone	1 oz	100	8	1	–	–
pyrenees	1 oz	101	8	tr	tr	0
quark 20% fat	1 oz	33	1	1	–	–
quark 40% fat	1 oz	48	3	1	–	–
quark made w/ skim milk	1 oz	22	tr	1	–	–
queso anejo	1 oz	106	9	1	–	–
queso asadero	1 oz	101	8	1	–	–
queso chihuahua	1 oz	106	8	2	–	–
queso fresco	1 oz	41	2	1	–	0
queso manchego	1 oz	107	8	tr	–	0
queso panela	1 oz	74	5	1	–	0
raclette	1 oz	102	8	tr	tr	0
reblochon	1 oz	88	7	tr	tr	0
ricotta part skim	½ cup (4.4 oz)	171	10	6	–	–
ricotta whole milk	½ cup (4.4 oz)	216	16	4	–	–
romadur 40% fat	1 oz	83	6	tr	–	–
romano	1 oz	110	8	1	–	–
roquefort	1 oz	105	9	1	–	–
rouy	1 oz	95	8	tr	tr	0
saint marcellin	1 oz	94	8	tr	tr	0
saint nectaire	1 oz	97	8	tr	tr	0
saint paulin	1 oz	85	6	tr	tr	0
sainte maure	1 oz	99	8	tr	tr	0
selles sur cher	1 oz	93	8	tr	tr	0

FOOD	PORTION	CAL	FAT	CARB	SUGAR	FIBER
stilton blue	1.4 oz	164	14	0	–	0
stilton white	1.4 oz	145	13	0	–	0
swiss	1 oz	107	8	1	–	–
swiss processed	1 oz	95	7	1	–	–
tilsit	1 oz	96	7	1	–	–
tome	1 oz	92	7	tr	tr	0
triple creme	1 oz	113	11	tr	tr	0
vacherin	1 oz	92	8	tr	tr	0
wensleydale	1.4 oz	151	13	0	–	0
whey cheese	1 oz	126	8	9	0	0
yogurt cheese	1 oz	80	7	0	0	0
Alpine Lace						
Reduced Fat Provolone	1 slice (0.8 oz)	70	5	1	0	0
Reduced Fat Swiss	1 slice (0.8 oz)	70	5	1	1	0
Reduced Fat White American	1 slice (0.8 oz)	70	5	1	1	0
Reduced Sodium Muenster	1 slice (0.8 oz)	90	7	0	0	0
Applegate Farms						
Organic Cheddar Milk	1 slice (0.7 oz)	85	6	0	0	0
Organic Muenster Kase	1 slice (0.8 oz)	85	7	0	0	0
Yogurt Cheese w/ Probiotics	1 slice (0.7 oz)	80	6	tr	0	–
Athenos						
Traditional	¼ cup	90	7	2	0	tr
Traditional Reduced Fat	¼ cup	70	5	1	0	tr
Cabot						
Cheddar	1 oz	110	9	tr	0	0
Cheddar Horseradish	1 oz	110	9	1	0	0
Cheddar Tomato Basil	1 oz	110	9	tr	0	0
Cheddar Light 50% Reduced Fat	1 oz	70	5	tr	0	0

FOOD	PORTION	CAL	FAT	CARB	SUGAR	FIBER
Cheddar Light 50% Reduced Fat Omega-3	1 oz	70	5	tr	0	0
Cheddar Light 75% Reduced Fat	1 oz	60	3	tr	0	0
Cheddar Shake	2 tsp	25	2	1	1	0
Monterey Jack	1 oz	110	9	tr	0	0
Pepper Jack 50% Reduced Fat	1 oz	70	5	tr	0	0
Swiss Slices	1 (1 oz)	110	8	1	0	0
DiGiorno						
Shredded Three Cheese Parmesan Romano & Asiago	¼ cup (1 oz)	110	8	1	0	0
Dragone						
Mozzarella Whole Milk	1 oz	90	7	tr	0	0
Parmesan Wedge	1 oz	100	7	tr	tr	0
Ricotta Part Skim	¼ cup (2.2 oz)	90	6	4	3	0
Finlandia						
Swiss Thin Sliced	1 slice (0.5 oz)	55	4	0	0	0
Fresh Made						
Farmers Cheese Nonfat	2 tbsp	15	0	1	0	0
Friendship						
Farmer	2 tbsp (1 oz)	50	3	0	0	0
Farmer No Salt Added	2 tbsp (1 oz)	50	3	0	0	0
Frigo						
Mozzarella Part Skim	1 oz	80	6	tr	0	0
Parmesan Shredded	¼ cup (1 oz)	100	7	1	1	tr
Ricotta Whole Milk	¼ cup (2.2 oz)	110	8	2	2	0
Romano Shredded	¼ cup (1 oz)	100	7	1	tr	tr
Haolam						
Cheddar Sliced	1 slice (1 oz)	114	9	1	0	0
Kraft						
Crumbles Three Cheese	¼ cup (1 oz)	110	9	tr	0	0

FOOD	PORTION	CAL	FAT	CARB	SUGAR	FIBER
Land O Lakes						
American	1 slice (0.7 oz)	70	5	2	1	0
Chedarella	1 oz	110	9	0	0	0
Cheddar	1 oz	110	9	0	0	0
Snack 'N Cheese To Go Cheddar Mild	1 serv (0.7 oz)	80	7	0	0	0
Snack 'N Cheese To Go Cheddar Mild Reduced Fat	1 serv (0.5 oz)	60	5	0	0	0
Snack 'N Cheese To Go Co-Jack	1 serv (0.7 oz)	80	7	0	0	0
Snack 'N Cheese To Go Co-Jack Reduced Fat	1 serv (0.7 oz)	60	5	0	0	0
Swiss	1 oz	110	8	1	1	0
Molly McButter						
Natural Cheese	1 tsp (2 g)	5	0	1	–	0
Rosenborg						
Danish Camembert	1 oz	80	7	0	0	0
Rouge Et Noir						
Breakfast	1 oz	90	7	0	0	0
Brie Garlic	1 oz	90	7	0	0	0
Brie Pesto	1 oz	90	7	0	0	0
Brie Tomato Basil	1 oz	90	7	0	0	0
Brie Triple Creme	1 oz	110	10	0	0	0
Camembert	1 oz	90	7	0	0	0
Le Petit Bleu	1 oz	110	10	0	0	0
Le Petit Chevre	1 oz	90	6	0	0	0
Marin French Blue	1 oz	110	10	0	0	0
Marin French Gold	1 oz	110	10	0	0	0
Schlosskranz	1 oz	85	7	0	0	0
Saladena						
Goat Crumbles	¼ cup	80	7	tr	0	0

FOOD	PORTION	CAL	FAT	CARB	SUGAR	FIBER
Sap Sago						
Fat Free Cheese Grated	1 tsp	10	0	0	0	0
Stella						
3 Cheese Italian Shredded	¼ cup	100	7	1	tr	tr
Asiago Wedge	1 oz	110	9	tr	tr	0
Gorgonzola Wedge	1 oz	100	9	tr	0	0
Kasseri Wedge	1 oz	110	9	tr	tr	0
The Greek Gods						
Kefir Cheese	2 tbsp (1 oz)	80	5	2	1	0
Treasure Cave						
Blue Cheese Crumbled	¼ cup (1 oz)	100	8	tr	–	–
Feta Crumbled	¼ cup (1 oz)	60	5	tr	–	–
Gorgonzola Crumbled	¼ cup (1 oz)	100	8	tr	–	–
Weight Watchers						
String Light	1 stick (0.8 oz)	50	3	tr	0	0
Wholesome Valley						
Organic American	1 slice (0.7 oz)	50	4	tr	0	0
CHEESE DISHES						
Banquet						
Mozzarella Nuggets	7	270	16	21	tr	tr
Fillo Factory						
Tyropita Cheese Fillo Appetizers	3 (3 oz)	230	14	19	2	0
TAKE-OUT						
fondue	½ cup (3.8 oz)	247	15	4	–	–
fried mozzarella sticks	3 (4.6 oz)	503	32	20	2	1
souffle	1 serv (7 oz)	504	38	18	5	1
welsh rarebit	1 slice	228	16	14	–	1
CHEESE SUBSTITUTES						
mozzarella	1 oz	70	3	7	–	–
soya cheese	1.4 oz	128	11	tr	–	0

FOOD	PORTION	CAL	FAT	CARB	SUGAR	FIBER
Playfood						
Cheesey Cheese	1 oz	60	5	4	0	1
Rice						
American Flavor	1 slice (0.7 oz)	50	3	tr	0	0
American Flavor Vegan	1 slice (0.7 oz)	45	3	0	0	0
Shreds Mozzarella Flavor	⅓ cup (1 oz)	70	4	3	0	0
Super Stix						
Mozzarella Flavor	1 (1 oz)	70	5	0	0	0
Vegan Gourmet						
Cheese Alternative Cheddar	1 oz	50	4	2	0	2
Cheese Alternative Monterey Jack	1 oz	70	7	2	0	2
Cheese Alternative Mozzarella	1 oz	70	8	1	0	1
Cheese Alternative Nacho	1 oz	45	4	2	0	2
Veggie						
American Flavor	1 slice (0.6 oz)	40	3	tr	0	0
Grated Parmesan Flavor	2 tsp	15	1	0	0	0
Pepper Jack Flavor	1 oz	60	4	2	0	0
Shreds Cheddar Flavor	1 oz	70	4	0	0	0
Veggy						
Mozzarella Flavor	1 slice (0.7 oz)	40	3	tr	0	0
CHERIMOYA						
fresh	1	515	2	131	–	–
CHERRIES						
CANNED						
maraschino	¼ cup (1.4 oz)	66	tr	17	16	1
maraschino	1 (4 g)	7	tr	2	2	tr
sour in heavy syrup	½ cup	116	tr	30	28	1

FOOD	PORTION	CAL	FAT	CARB	SUGAR	FIBER
sour in light syrup	½ cup	94	tr	24	–	1
sour water packed	½ cup	44	tr	11	9	1
sweet juice pack	½ cup	68	tr	17	15	2
sweet pitted in heavy syrup	½ cup	105	tr	27	25	2
sweet water pack	½ cup	57	tr	15	13	2
Chukar Cherries						
Cherry Jubilee Dessert Sauce	1 tbsp	40	0	10	8	tr
Del Monte						
Sweet Dark Pitted In Heavy Syrup	½ cup (4.2 oz)	100	0	24	24	tr
S&W						
Sliced	½ cup (4.7 oz)	140	0	34	26	1
The Gracious Gourmet						
Spiced Sour Cherry Spread	1 tbsp (0.5 oz)	15	0	4	3	0
DRIED						
bing unsulfured	¼ cup	130	0	31	21	2
montmorency tart pitted	⅓ cup	160	1	36	24	2
tart	½ cup	200	1	49	41	2
yogurt covered	¼ cup	170	6	29	22	5
Chukar Cherries						
Bing	3 tbsp	130	1	33	29	3
Bing Chocolate Covered	3 tbsp (1.4 oz)	180	9	24	19	2
Cabernet Dark Chocolate Covered	2 tbsp (1.5 oz)	180	9	26	17	3
Columbia River Tart	⅓ cup	120	1	36	24	2
Rainier	3 tbsp	130	1	33	29	3
Totally Tart	⅓ cup	140	1	33	16	3
Emily's						
Dark Chocolate Covered	11 (1.4 oz)	180	9	27	23	2

FOOD	PORTION	CAL	FAT	CARB	SUGAR	FIBER
Raisinets						
Dark & Milk Chocolate	¼ cup (1.6 oz)	200	8	32	28	2
Stoneridge Orchards						
Bing	⅓ cup (1.4 oz)	130	0	32	31	1
Organic Montmorency Whole	⅓ cup (1.4 oz)	135	1	33	27	2
FRESH						
sour	1 cup	52	tr	13	9	2
sour pitted	1 cup	78	tr	19	13	3
sweet	20	86	1	22	17	3
Chiquita						
Cherries	1 cup (4.8 oz)	87	0	22	18	3
FROZEN						
sour unsweetened	½ cup	36	tr	9	7	1
sweet sweetened	½ cup	115	tr	29	26	3
CHERRY JUICE						
tart cherry concentrate	1 cup	140	0	34	27	0
Froose						
Cheerful Cherry	1 box (4.2 oz)	80	0	19	7	3
Santa Cruz						
Organic 100% Juice Red Tart	8 oz	120	0	30	30	0
Smart Juice						
Organic 100% Juice Tart Cherry	8 oz	130	0	32	24	1
Tart Is Smart						
Tart Cherry Concentrate	1 oz	80	0	19	15	0
CHERVIL						
seed	1 tsp	1	tr	tr	–	–
CHESTNUTS						
chinese steamed	3 (1 oz)	43	tr	10	–	–

FOOD	PORTION	CAL	FAT	CARB	SUGAR	FIBER
creme de marrons	1 oz	73	tr	18	10	1
japanese roasted	1 oz	57	tr	13	–	–
ready-to-eat vacuum packed	5 (1 oz)	40	0	8	0	0
roasted	3 (1 oz)	70	1	15	3	1
Gefen						
Whole Roasted & Peeled	¼ cup (1.4 oz)	52	0	11	11	1

CHEWING GUM

FOOD	PORTION	CAL	FAT	CARB	SUGAR	FIBER
bubble gum	1 block	20	tr	5	5	tr
stick	1 piece	7	tr	2	2	tr
sugarless	1 piece	5	tr	2	0	0
Bubble Yum						
Original	1 piece (8 g)	25	0	6	5	–
Sugarless	1 piece (5 g)	10	0	3	–	–
Choward's						
Scented Gum	3 pieces	10	0	3	3	0
Orbit						
Sugarfree Citrusmint	1 piece	<5	0	1	0	–
Trident						
Extra Care	1 piece	<5	0	1	0	–
Splash Strawberry Lime	1 piece	<5	0	2	0	–

CHIA SEEDS

FOOD	PORTION	CAL	FAT	CARB	SUGAR	FIBER
dried	1 oz	134	7	14	–	–

CHICKEN (see also CHICKEN DISHES, CHICKEN SUBSTITUTES, DINNER, HOT DOG)
CANNED

FOOD	PORTION	CAL	FAT	CARB	SUGAR	FIBER
chicken spread	1 serv (2 oz)	88	10	2	tr	tr
meat drained	1 can (5 oz)	230	10	1	0	0
w/ broth	½ can (2.5 oz)	117	6	0	0	0
Hormel						
Chunk White & Dark	2 oz	70	3	0	0	0
Premium Chunk Breast	2 oz	60	2	0	0	0

FOOD	PORTION	CAL	FAT	CARB	SUGAR	FIBER
FRESH						
back w/ skin roasted bones removed	1 (3.7 oz)	318	22	0	0	0
back w/o skin roasted bones removed	1 (2.8 oz)	191	11	0	0	0
breast roasted diced	1 cup (5 oz)	231	5	0	0	0
breast w/ skin battered fried bones removed	½ breast (4.9 oz)	364	18	13	0	tr
breast w/ skin floured fried bones removed	1 (3.4 oz)	218	9	2	–	tr
breast w/ skin roasted bones removed	½ breast (3.4 oz)	193	8	0	0	0
breast w/ skin stewed bones removed	½ breast (3.9 oz)	202	8	0	0	0
breast w/o skin fried bones removed	½ breast (3 oz)	161	4	tr	0	0
breast w/o skin roasted bones removed	½ breast (3 oz)	142	3	0	0	0
breast w/o skin stewed bones removed	1 (3.3 oz)	143	3	0	0	0
broiler/fryer w/ skin roasted bones removed	½ (10.5 oz)	715	41	0	0	0
capon meat & skin roasted bones removed	½ (1.4 lbs)	1459	74	0	0	0
cornish hen w/ skin roasted	1 (9 oz)	668	47	0	0	0
cornish hen w/ skin roasted	½ (4.5 oz)	335	23	0	0	0
cornish hen w/o skin roasted	½ (4 oz)	147	4	0	0	0
cornish hen w/o skin roasted	1 (7.7 oz)	295	9	0	0	0

FOOD	PORTION	CAL	FAT	CARB	SUGAR	FIBER
dark meat w/o skin roasted diced	1 cup (5 oz)	287	14	0	0	0
drumstick w/ skin battered floured & fried bones removed	1 (1.7 oz)	120	7	1	–	0
drumstick w/ skin battered fried bones removed	1 (2.5 oz)	193	11	6	–	tr
drumstick w/ skin roasted bones removed	1 (1.8 oz)	112	6	0	0	0
drumstick w/ skin stewed bones removed	1 (2 oz)	116	6	0	0	0
drumstick w/o skin fried bones removed	1 (1.5 oz)	82	3	0	0	0
drumstick w/o skin roasted bones removed	1 (1.5 oz)	76	2	0	0	0
drumstick w/o skin stewed bones removed	1 (1.6 oz)	78	3	0	0	0
feet cooked	1 (1.2 oz)	73	5	tr	0	0
ground crumbled fried	3 oz	161	9	0	0	0
ground patty cooked	1 sm (1.7 oz)	114	6	0	0	0
ground patty cooked	1 med (2.1 oz)	142	8	0	0	0
ground patty cooked	1 lg (2.8 oz)	190	11	0	0	0
meat & skin stewed bones removed	¼ chicken (4.6 oz)	372	25	0	0	0
neck w/ skin battered fried	1 (1.8 oz)	172	12	5	–	–
neck w/ skin fried	1 (1.3 oz)	120	9	2	–	–
neck w/ skin simmered	1 (1.3 oz)	94	7	0	0	0
roaster meat & skin roasted bones removed	¼ chicken (8.4 oz)	535	32	0	0	0

FOOD	PORTION	CAL	FAT	CARB	SUGAR	FIBER
skin battered fried from ½ chicken	6.7 oz	749	55	44	–	–
skin floured fried from ½ chicken	2 oz	281	24	5	–	–
skin roasted from ½ chicken	2 oz	254	23	0	0	0
skin stewed from ½ chicken	2.5 oz	261	24	0	0	0
tail cooked	1 (1 oz)	84	5	3	0	tr
thigh w/ skin battered & fried bones removed	1 (3 oz)	238	14	8	–	tr
thigh w/ skin floured fried bones removed	1 (2.2 oz)	162	9	2	–	tr
thigh w/ skin roasted bones removed	1 (2.2 oz)	153	10	0	0	0
thigh w/ skin stewed bones removed	1 (2.4 oz)	158	10	0	0	0
thigh w/o skin fried bones removed	1 (1.8 oz)	113	5	1	–	0
thigh w/o skin roasted bones removed	1 (1.8 oz)	109	6	0	0	0
thigh w/o skin stewed bones removed	1 (1.9 oz)	107	5	0	0	0
wing w/ skin battered fried bones removed	1 (1.7 oz)	159	11	5	–	tr
wing w/ skin floured fried bones removed	1 (1.1 oz)	103	7	1	–	0
wing w/ skin roasted bones removed	1 (1.4 oz)	100	7	0	0	0
wing w/o skin fried bones removed	1 (0.7 oz)	42	2	0	0	0
wing w/o skin roasted bones removed	1 (0.7 oz)	43	2	0	0	0

FOOD	PORTION	CAL	FAT	CARB	SUGAR	FIBER
wing w/o skin stewed bones removed	1 (0.8 oz)	43	2	0	0	0
Perdue						
Boneless Skinless Breasts cooked	3 oz	110	1	0	0	0
Breast Boneless Herb & Pepper	1 piece (4.8 oz)	140	2	0	0	0
Breast Boneless Roasted Garlic w/ White Wine	1 piece (4.8 oz)	110	2	1	0	–
Breast Boneless Skinless cooked	3 oz	100	1	0	0	0
Breast Perfect Portions Boneless Skinless	1 (4.8 oz)	130	2	0	0	–
Ground cooked	3 oz	170	11	0	0	0
Ground Breast cooked	3 oz	80	1	0	0	0
Oven Ready Cornish Hen Seasoned	4 oz	160	10	1	0	–
Oven Ready Roaster Bone-In Breast	4 oz	140	7	1	0	0
Oven Ready Roaster Seasoned	4 oz	210	15	1	1	–
Oven Stuffer Drumstick	1 (3.6 oz)	190	11	0	0	0
Patties cooked	1 (3 oz)	170	11	0	0	0
Thigh Filets Boneless Skinless	4 oz	150	8	0	0	0
Thighs Tender & Tasty Boneless Skinless cooked	3 oz	150	9	0	0	0
Whole Dark Meat cooked	3 oz	210	15	0	0	0
Whole White Meat cooked	3 oz	170	9	0	0	0

FOOD	PORTION	CAL	FAT	CARB	SUGAR	FIBER
Whole Chicken Tender & Tasty cooked	3 oz	150	8	0	0	0
Wingettes cooked	3 oz	170	10	0	0	0
Wings cooked	3 oz	170	10	0	0	0
FROZEN						
breast roll roasted	2 oz	75	4	1	tr	0
fajita strips	1 (0.3 oz)	13	1	tr	0	0
patty cooked	1 (3.5 oz)	287	20	13	0	tr
Banquet						
Wings Hot & Spicy	¼ pkg (3 oz)	260	17	8	0	5
Health Is Wealth						
Nuggets	4 (3 oz)	130	4	11	0	0
Perdue						
Breast Chunks Breaded BBQ Glazed	3 oz	190	8	17	9	–
Breast Chunks Breaded General Tso's Glazed	3 oz	190	8	16	10	–
Breast Chunks Breaded Honey BBQ Glazed	3 oz	180	8	17	1	–
Breast Chunks Breaded Honey Dijon Glazed	3 oz	200	11	16	3	–
READY-TO-EAT						
Applegate Farms						
Organic Roasted	2 oz	60	2	1	1	0
Butterball						
Breast Oven Roasted Thin Sliced	4 slices (2 oz)	50	1	1	0	0
Breast Strips Oven Roasted	½ pkg (3 oz)	90	2	1	–	–
Carl Buddig						
Chicken Sliced	2 oz	85	5	1	–	–

FOOD	PORTION	CAL	FAT	CARB	SUGAR	FIBER
Hormel						
Natural Choice Carved Breast Grilled	½ pkg (2 oz)	60	1	0	0	0
Oscar Mayer						
Breast Oven Roasted Thin Sliced	⅓ pkg (2 oz)	60	2	1	1	0
Breast Strips Breaded	½ pkg (3 oz)	170	6	14	–	–
Breast Strips Grilled	½ pkg (3 oz)	110	3	1	–	–
Perdue						
Breast Bites Popcorn Breaded	12 (3 oz)	190	12	14	1	–
Breast Strips Breaded Original	2 (2.6 oz)	160	10	12	1	–
Cutlets Breaded Original	1 (3 oz)	200	13	13	0	–
Nuggets Original	5 (2.9 oz)	200	13	13	0	–
Nuggets w/ Whole Grain Breading	4 (2.8 oz)	160	8	13	1	–
Short Cuts Carved Chicken Breast Original Roasted	½ cup (2.5 oz)	90	2	1	–	–
Short Cuts Chicken Breast Grilled	½ cup (2.5 oz)	90	2	1	0	–
Sara Lee						
Breast Oven Roasted	4 slices (2 oz)	45	1	0	0	0
TAKE-OUT						
chicken tenders	4 (2.2 oz)	180	10	11	1	tr

CHICKEN DISHES
FROZEN

FOOD	PORTION	CAL	FAT	CARB	SUGAR	FIBER
Banquet						
Boneless Popcorn Chicken	11 pieces	180	9	18	tr	tr
Wings Honey BBQ	¼ pkg (3 oz)	270	17	12	tr	5

FOOD	PORTION	CAL	FAT	CARB	SUGAR	FIBER
MIX						
Chicken Helper						
Asian Chicken Fried Rice as prep	1 cup	250	8	22	1	1
Classic Creamy Chicken & Noodles as prep	1 cup	280	8	24	1	tr
Jambalaya as prep	1 cup	280	8	15	tr	1
TAKE-OUT						
arroz con pollo	1 serv (16 oz)	579	14	62	3	2
barbecued pulled chicken	1 serv (9 oz)	312	2	37	27	2
boneless breast w/ apple stuffing	1 serv (5 oz)	260	9	10	2	1
breast & wing breaded & fried	2 pieces (5.7 oz)	494	30	20	–	–
buffalo wing + sauce	2 (1.7 oz)	147	10	tr	tr	0
cacciatore breast + sauce	1 serv (5.9 oz)	323	18	9	3	1
cacciatore drumstick + sauce	1 serv (3.2 oz)	172	9	5	2	1
cacciatore thigh + sauce	1 serv (3.8 oz)	204	11	6	2	1
cacciatore wing + sauce	1 serv (2.1 oz)	113	6	3	1	tr
chicharrones de pollo	3 (2.6 oz)	289	18	14	tr	1
chicken & dumplings	1 cup (8.6 oz)	368	19	22	1	1
chicken & noodles in cream sauce	1 cup (8 oz)	323	11	32	5	1
chicken a la king	1 cup (8.5 oz)	465	34	16	4	1
chicken cordon bleu + sauce	1 roll (8 oz)	504	29	11	1	1
chicken meatloaf	1 lg slice (5 oz)	243	9	11	3	1

FOOD	PORTION	CAL	FAT	CARB	SUGAR	FIBER
chicken pie w/ top crust	1 slice (5.6 oz)	472	31	32	–	1
chicken satay + peanut sauce	2 skewers	239	12	6	4	1
chicken breast parmigiana	1 serv (5.8 oz)	278	14	13	3	1
chicken creole w/o rice	1 cup (8.6 oz)	187	4	8	5	2
chicken kiev breast meat	1 serv (9 oz)	653	34	11	1	1
creamed chicken	1 cup (8.5 oz)	388	23	14	8	tr
croquette	1 (2.2 oz)	159	9	8	2	tr
curry	1 cup (8.3 oz)	288	16	9	5	2
curry breast half + sauce	1 (7 oz)	244	14	8	4	2
curry drumstick + sauce	1 (3.7 oz)	129	7	4	2	1
curry thigh + sauce	1 (4.4 oz)	154	9	5	3	1
curry wing + sauce	1 (2.4 oz)	84	5	3	1	1
drumstick & thigh breaded & fried	2 pieces (5.2 oz)	431	27	16	–	–
fricassee	1 cup (8.6 oz)	322	18	8	tr	tr
groundnut stew hkatenkwan	1 serv (15.7 oz)	576	40	18	3	4
jamaican jerk wings	4 wings (9.9 oz)	709	51	3	tr	tr
jambalaya w/ sausage & rice	1 cup (8.6 oz)	393	21	23	2	1
sancocho de pollo dominican chicken stew	1 serv	702	30	34	4	1
stew	1 cup (8.8 oz)	176	5	19	4	3
tandoori chicken breast	1 serv	260	13	5	–	–
tandoori chicken leg & thigh	1 serv	300	17	6	–	–
tetrazzini	1 cup (8.6 oz)	369	18	29	2	2

FOOD	PORTION	CAL	FAT	CARB	SUGAR	FIBER
CHICKEN SUBSTITUTES						
Chicken Free Chicken						
Country Smoked	2 oz	80	2	5	1	0
Health Is Wealth						
Chicken-Free Nuggets	3 pieces (2.9 oz)	120	2	14	0	2
Veat						
Chick'n Free Nuggets	1 serv (2.5 oz)	140	5	5	2	2
Vegetarian Breast	1 (1.8 oz)	90	3	5	1	tr
CHICKPEAS						
CANNED						
chickpeas	1 cup	285	3	54	–	–
Allens						
Garbanzo Beans	½ cup	120	3	19	0	8
Progresso						
ChickPeas	½ cup	100	2	17	2	4
DRIED						
cooked	1 cup	269	4	45	–	–
CHICORY						
endive fresh chopped	½ cup	4	tr	1	–	–
greens raw chopped	½ cup	21	tr	4	–	–
root raw	1 (2.1 oz)	44	tr	11	–	–
roots raw cut up	½ cup (1.6 oz)	33	tr	8	–	–
witloof head raw	1 (1.9 oz)	9	tr	2	–	–
witloof raw	½ cup (1.6 oz)	8	tr	2	–	–
CHILI						
powder	1 tbsp	24	1	4	1	3
Ahh!Gourmet						
Wriggly Sambal Chili Sauce Paste	4 tbsp	170	9	15	11	4
Allergaroo						
Gluten Free Chili Mac	1 pkg (8 oz)	240	4	50	8	3

FOOD	PORTION	CAL	FAT	CARB	SUGAR	FIBER
Amy's						
Organic Black Bean Medium	1 cup	200	2	31	3	15
Whole Meals Chili & Cornbread	1 pkg	340	6	59	14	10
Comfort Care						
Vegetarian White	1 cup (8 oz)	150	2	26	4	5
Dennison's						
Con Carne	1 cup	350	15	31	2	11
Fat Free w/ Beans	1 cup	210	2	29	2	8
Turkey	1 cup	210	3	29	3	7
Vegetarian	1 cup	190	2	34	6	9
Dynasty						
Thai Chili Garlic Paste	1 tsp (5 g)	0	0	0	0	0
Health Valley						
Chunky Spicy Vegetarian No Salt Added	1 cup	150	1	31	5	10
Vegetarian Spicy	1 cup	150	1	31	5	10
Heinz						
Chili Sauce	1 tbsp (0.6 oz)	20	0	5	3	0
Hormel						
Chili Mac	1 pkg (9.9 oz)	270	7	34	10	6
Chili No Beans	1 pkg (7.3 oz)	190	8	16	3	2
Chili No Beans Less Sodium	1 serv (8.3 oz)	220	9	18	3	3
Chili w/ Beans	1 serv (8.7 oz)	260	7	33	5	7
Chili w/ Beans Less Sodium	1 serv (8.7 oz)	260	7	33	5	7
Turkey Chili w/ Beans	1 serv (8.7 oz)	210	3	28	6	6
Vegetarian Chili w/ Beans	1 serv (8.7 oz)	190	1	35	6	10

FOOD	PORTION	CAL	FAT	CARB	SUGAR	FIBER
Master Chili						
Chipotle Chicken No Bean	1 serv (8.3 oz)	230	10	18	7	3
Roasted Tomato w/ Bean	1 serv (8.7 oz)	210	6	25	7	7
Mimi's Gourmet						
Organic Vegan Gluten Free 3 Bean w/ Rice	1 pkg (11.5 oz)	270	6	46	9	10
Organic Vegan Gluten Free Black Bean & Corn	1 pkg (10.5 oz)	250	6	40	9	11
Organic Vegan Gluten Free White Bean	1 pkg (10.5 oz)	230	6	35	11	9
Thai Kitchen						
Roasted Red Chili Paste	1 tbsp (0.5 oz)	50	3	6	4	0
TAKE-OUT						
chiles rellenos cheese filled	1 (5 oz)	365	30	8	5	1
chili con carne w/ beans	1 cup	264	11	22	6	7
chili con carne w/ beans & chicken	1 cup (8.9 oz)	218	7	19	6	6
chili con carne w/ beans & rice	1 cup	298	9	45	2	7
vegetarian con carne	1 cup	272	7	35	7	11

CHILI PEPPER (see PEPPERS)

CHINESE FOOD (see ASIAN FOOD)

CHINESE PRESERVING MELON

cooked	½ cup	11	tr	3	–	–

CHIPS (see also SNACKS)

apple chips	10 (0.8 oz)	101	5	16	14	2

FOOD	PORTION	CAL	FAT	CARB	SUGAR	FIBER
banana	1 oz	147	10	17	10	2
carrot	28 (1 oz)	95	tr	22	11	7
corn	1 oz	147	8	18	tr	2
plantain	1 oz	158	10	16	–	1
potato salted	1 oz	155	11	14	tr	1
potato sticks	1 pkg (1 oz)	148	10	15	tr	1
potato sticks	½ cup (0.6 oz)	94	6	10	tr	1
potato unsalted	1 oz	152	10	15	tr	1
potato unsalted reduced fat	1 oz	138	6	19	tr	2
soy	1 oz	107	2	15	1	1
sweet potato	1 oz	141	7	18	2	1
taro	10 (0.8 oz)	115	6	16	1	2
tortilla lowfat baked	1 oz	118	2	23	tr	2
tortilla lowfat unsalted	1 oz	118	2	23	tr	2
tortilla white corn	1 oz	139	7	19	tr	2
tortilla yellow corn	1 oz	139	6	19	tr	1
Athenos						
Pita Chips Original	11 (1 oz)	120	4	19	tr	0
Beanitos						
Pinto Bean & Flax	10 (1 oz)	150	8	14	0	5
Betty Crocker						
Potato Kettle Cooked Lightly Salted	1 oz	120	5	15	0	1
Boulder Canyon						
Potato 50% Reduced Salt	14 (1 oz)	150	8	17	0	2
Potato Sour Cream & Chive	14 (1 oz)	150	8	15	1	2
Potato Spinach & Artichoke	14 (1 oz)	150	8	17	0	2

FOOD	PORTION	CAL	FAT	CARB	SUGAR	FIBER
Brothers-All-Natural						
Potato Crisps Fresh Onion & Fresh Garlic	1 pkg	45	0	10	0	1
Potato Crisps Original w/ Sea Salt	1 pkg	45	0	10	0	1
Burger King						
Potato Flame Broiled	16 (1 oz)	150	8	19	1	1
Potato Ketchup & Fries	16 (1 oz)	150	8	19	1	1
Butterfield						
Potato Sticks Shoestring	1 pkg (1.7 oz)	250	15	26	0	3
Deep River Snacks						
Potato Baked Fries Sweet Maui Onion	1 oz	135	5	19	2	1
Potato Kettle Cooked Asian Sweet & Spicy	1 oz	150	8	15	3	1
Potato Kettle Cooked Original Salted	1 oz	150	8	16	0	1
Potato Kettle Cooked Rosemary & Olive Oil	1 oz	150	8	16	1	1
Potato Kettle Cooked Salt & Vinegar	1 oz	150	8	15	0	1
Potato Zesty Jalapeno	1 oz	150	8	15	0	1
FoodShouldTasteGood						
Tortilla Buffalo	10 (1 oz)	130	6	18	1	3
Tortilla Chocolate Gluten Free	1 pkg (1 oz)	140	7	19	4	3
Tortilla Multigrain Gluten Free	1 pkg (1 oz)	140	7	18	2	3
Tortilla Sweet Potato Gluten Free	10 (1 oz)	130	6	18	2	3
Guiltless Gourmet						
Tortilla Blue Corn	18 (1 oz)	120	3	23	0	2
Tortilla Chili Lime	18 (1 oz)	120	3	19	0	2

FOOD	PORTION	CAL	FAT	CARB	SUGAR	FIBER
Tortilla Chipotle	18 (1 oz)	123	3	22	1	2
Tortilla Yellow Corn	18 (1 oz)	120	3	22	0	2
Tortilla Yellow Corn Unsalted	18 (1 oz)	120	2	22	1	2
Hippie Chips						
Baked Potato Chive-Talkin' Sour Cream	1 pkg (0.7 oz)	90	3	14	1	tr
Baked Potato Height AshBerry Japapeno	1 pkg (0.7 oz)	90	3	15	2	tr
Baked Potato Memphis Blues Barbeque	1 pkg (0.7 oz)	90	3	15	2	tr
Baked Potato Sea Of Love Salt	1 pkg (1 oz)	125	4	21	0	1
Baked Potato Woodstock Ranch	1 pkg (0.7 oz)	90	3	14	1	tr
Little Wings						
Multi Grain Hot Buffalo Wing w/ Bleu Cheese Drizzle	1 pkg (0.5 oz)	60	3	10	2	2
Mexi-Snax						
Tortilla Multi-Grain Blue	15 (1 oz)	140	7	17	0	2
Tortilla Pico De Gallo	15 (1 oz)	140	7	18	0	2
Tortilla Salted	15 (1 oz)	140	7	18	0	2
Tortilla Tamari	15 (1 oz)	130	6	17	0	2
Michael Season's						
Potato Kettle Style Reduced Fat	18	130	6	18	1	1
Potato Reduced Fat	20	140	7	17	0	1
Potato Reduced Fat Unsalted	20	140	7	17	0	1
Potato Crisps Thin Baked Low Fat	14	120	2	23	2	2

FOOD	PORTION	CAL	FAT	CARB	SUGAR	FIBER
Poore Brothers						
Original	14 (1 oz)	140	9	15	tr	1
Salt & Vinegar	15 (1 oz)	150	9	15	1	1
Sweet Maui Onion	14 (1 oz)	140	9	15	2	1
Revolution Foods						
Organic Popalongs Whole Grains Cheesy Cheese	16 (0.7 oz)	90	3	14	1	1
Organic Popalongs Whole Grains Original	16 (0.7 oz)	100	3	15	1	1
Organic Popalongs Whole Grains Simply Cinnamon	16 (0.7 oz)	100	3	16	3	1
Robert's American Gourmet						
Soy Crisps Country Barbecue	1 oz	130	4	15	3	3
Salba Smart						
Organic Blue Corn Omega-3 Enriched	1 oz	104	6	19	0	4
SunChips						
Original	16 (1 oz)	140	6	18	2	2
T.G.I. Friday's						
Potato Cheese Pizza	16 (1 oz)	160	9	17	1	1
Tater Skins						
Cheddar Bacon	16 (1 oz)	150	8	19	1	1
Original	16 (1 oz)	150	8	19	1	1
Thunder						
Potato Buffalo Wing w/ Blue Cheese	22 (1 oz)	150	8	16	tr	tr
Sour Cream & Onion	22 (1 oz)	150	9	15	tr	tr
Utz						
Pita Natural w/ Sea Salt	1 oz	120	5	18	1	tr
Potato	20 (1 oz)	150	9	14	0	1

FOOD	PORTION	CAL	FAT	CARB	SUGAR	FIBER
Potato Baked	1 oz	110	2	23	2	2
Potato BBQ	20 (1 oz)	150	10	14	1	1
Potato Grandma Kettle	1 oz	140	8	14	0	1
Potato Homestyle Kettle	1 oz	140	8	14	0	1
Potato Kettle Classics	20 (1 oz)	150	9	15	0	1
Potato Mystic Kettle	1 oz	150	9	15	0	1
Potato Mystic Kettle Reduced Fat	1 oz	130	6	18	0	1
Potato Natural Lightly Salted Kettle	1 oz	140	8	15	0	1
Potato No Salt Added	20 (1 oz)	150	9	14	0	1
Potato Onion & Garlic	1 oz	150	9	14	tr	1
Potato Ripple	20 (1 oz)	150	10	14	0	1
Sweet Potato Kettle Classics	20 (1 oz)	150	9	16	3	2
Tortilla Baked	10	120	2	23	0	1
Tortilla Organic Yellow Corn	1 oz	140	6	19	0	2
Vegetable Natural Exotic Medley	1 oz	160	10	15	2	2
Zapp's						
Potato Cajun Dill	1 oz	150	8	17	0	1
Potato No Salt	1 oz	150	9	18	0	1
Potato Original	1 oz	150	8	17	0	1
Potato Sizzlin Steak	1 oz	150	8	17	tr	1
Sweet Potato Lightly Salted	1 oz	150	8	17	6	1

CHITTERLINGS

FOOD	PORTION	CAL	FAT	CARB	SUGAR	FIBER
pork cooked	3 oz	258	24	0	0	0

CHIVES

FOOD	PORTION	CAL	FAT	CARB	SUGAR	FIBER
freeze-dried	1 tbsp	1	tr	tr	–	–
fresh chopped	1 tsp	0	tr	tr	–	–
fresh chopped	1 tbsp	1	tr	tr	–	–

FOOD	PORTION	CAL	FAT	CARB	SUGAR	FIBER

CHOCOLATE (see also CANDY, CHOCOLATE SYRUP, COCOA, HOT CHOCOLATE, ICE CREAM TOPPINGS, MILK DRINKS)

BAKING

FOOD	PORTION	CAL	FAT	CARB	SUGAR	FIBER
baking	1 oz	145	15	8	–	–
grated unsweetened	¼ cup	165	17	10	tr	6
liquid unsweetened	1 oz	134	14	10	0	5
mexican baking	1 sq (0.7 oz)	85	3	15	14	1
squares unsweetened	1 sq (1 oz)	145	15	9	tr	5

Hershey's

FOOD	PORTION	CAL	FAT	CARB	SUGAR	FIBER
Unsweetened Block	1 (0.5 oz)	70	7	4	–	2

CHIPS

FOOD	PORTION	CAL	FAT	CARB	SUGAR	FIBER
milk chocolate	1 cup (6 oz)	862	52	100	–	–
semisweet	60 pieces (1 oz)	136	9	18	–	–
semisweet	1 cup (6 oz)	804	50	106	–	–

Hershey's

FOOD	PORTION	CAL	FAT	CARB	SUGAR	FIBER
Milk Chocolate	1 tbsp (0.5 oz)	70	5	9	8	1
Premier White	1 tbsp (0.5 oz)	80	4	9	9	–
Semi-Sweet	1 tbsp (0.5 oz)	70	4	10	8	tr
Special Dark	1 tbsp (0.5 oz)	70	5	9	8	1
Sugar Free	1 tbsp (0.5 oz)	70	5	9	–	1

MIX

FOOD	PORTION	CAL	FAT	CARB	SUGAR	FIBER
drink mix powder	2–3 heaping tsp	75	1	20	–	–
drink mix powder as prep w/ whole milk	9 oz	226	9	31	–	–

Nesquik

FOOD	PORTION	CAL	FAT	CARB	SUGAR	FIBER
Chocolate Powder	2 tbsp (0.6 oz)	60	1	14	13	tr
Chocolate Powder No Sugar Added	2 tbsp (0.4 oz)	35	1	7	3	1

CHOCOLATE MILK (see MILK DRINKS)

FOOD	PORTION	CAL	FAT	CARB	SUGAR	FIBER
CHOCOLATE SYRUP						
chocolate fudge	1 cup (11.9 oz)	1176	46	200	–	–
chocolate fudge	1 tbsp (0.7 oz)	73	3	12	–	–
syrup	2 tbsp	82	tr	22	–	–
syrup	1 cup	653	3	177	–	–
syrup as prep w/ whole milk	1 cup (9.9 oz)	254	8	36	32	1
Hershey's						
Lite	2 tbsp (1.2 oz)	45	0	11	10	tr
Sugar Free	2 tbsp (1.1 oz)	15	0	5	–	tr
Sundae Syrup Double Chocolate	2 tbsp (1.3 oz)	100	0	24	21	1
Syrup	2 tbsp (1.4 oz)	100	0	24	20	1
Nesquik						
Calcium Fortified	2 tbsp (1.3 oz)	100	0	25	23	tr
Santa Cruz						
Organic	2 tbsp	110	0	27	25	tr
U-Bet						
Original	2 tbsp (1.4 oz)	128	0	29	23	–
CHUTNEY						
apple	1.2 oz	68	0	18	–	1
coconut	2 oz	87	9	1	1	3
fresh mint	2 oz	18	0	3	3	1
mango	¼ cup (2 oz)	227	5	43	16	10
tomato	1 oz	90	7	6	6	2
Chukar Cherries						
Curried Cherry	1 tbsp	30	0	8	7	tr
The Gracious Gourmet						
Mango Pineapple	2 tbsp (1 oz)	45	1	9	7	0
Wild Thymes Farm						
Apricot Cranberry Walnut	1 tbsp	16	0	4	3	tr
Plum Currant Ginger	1 tsp	20	0	5	4	tr

FOOD	PORTION	CAL	FAT	CARB	SUGAR	FIBER
CILANTRO						
fresh	¼ cup	1	tr	tr	tr	tr
fresh sprigs	5 (5 g)	1	tr	tr	tr	tr
CINNAMON						
cinnamon sugar	1 tsp	16	tr	4	4	tr
ground	1 tsp	6	tr	2	tr	1
sticks	0.5 oz	39	tr	8	0	3
CISCO						
raw	3 oz	84	2	0	0	0
smoked	1 oz	50	3	0	0	0
CLAMS						
CANNED						
liquid only	3 oz	2	tr	tr	–	–
liquid only	1 cup	6	tr	tr	–	–
meat only	3 oz	126	2	4	–	–
meat only	1 cup	236	3	8	–	–
Polar						
Baby	¼ cup	30	0	3	0	0
FRESH						
cooked	20 sm	133	2	5	–	–
cooked	3 oz	126	2	4	–	–
raw	20 sm (6.3 oz)	133	2	5	–	–
raw	9 lg (6.3 oz)	133	2	5	–	–
raw	3 oz	63	1	2	–	–
TAKE-OUT						
breaded & fried	20 sm	379	21	19	–	–
CLEMENTINE JUICE						
Izze						
Sparkling Clementine	1 bottle (12 oz)	120	0	30	27	–

FOOD	PORTION	CAL	FAT	CARB	SUGAR	FIBER
CLEMENTINES						
Cuties						
fresh	2 (6 oz)	80	1	17	13	4
Disney Garden						
Clementines	1	35	0	9	7	1
CLOVES						
ground	1 tsp	7	tr	1	tr	1
COCOA (*see also* HOT CHOCOLATE)						
cocoa butter	1 tbsp	120	14	0	0	0
powder unsweetened	1 tbsp	12	1	3	tr	2
Hershey's						
Cocoa	1 tbsp (5 g)	10	1	3	–	2
COCONUT						
dried sweetened shredded	¼ cup	116	8	11	10	1
dried toasted	1 oz	168	13	13	–	–
dried unsweetened	1 oz	187	18	7	2	5
fresh from 1 coconut	14 oz	1405	133	60	25	36
fresh shredded	¼ cup	71	7	3	1	2
Mounds						
Sweetened Flakes	2 tbsp (0.5 oz)	70	5	6	5	1
COCONUT JUICE						
coconut water fresh	½ cup	23	tr	4	3	1
creamed sweetened canned	½ cup	264	12	39	38	tr
milk canned	½ cup	276	29	7	4	3
O.N.E.						
Natural Coconut Water	1 box (11 oz)	60	0	15	14	0
Thai Kitchen						
Lite Coconut Milk	2 oz	45	4	1	1	0

FOOD	PORTION	CAL	FAT	CARB	SUGAR	FIBER
Zico						
Coconut Water All Flavors	1 pkg (11 oz)	60	0	15	14	0
COD						
atlantic canned	3 oz	89	1	0	0	0
atlantic canned	1 can (11 oz)	327	3	0	0	0
atlantic dried	3 oz	246	2	0	0	0
atlantic fresh cooked	3 oz	89	1	0	0	0
atlantic fresh cooked	1 fillet (6.3 oz)	189	2	0	0	0
atlantic fresh raw	3 oz	70	1	0	0	0
pacific fresh baked	3 oz	95	1	0	0	0
roe canned	1 oz	34	1	tr	–	–
roe tarama	3.5 oz	547	55	6	tr	–
TAKE-OUT						
roe baked w/ butter & lemon juice	1 oz	36	1	tr	–	–
COFFEE (*see also* COFFEE BEVERAGES)						
INSTANT						
decaffeinated as prep	8 oz	2	0	0	0	0
decaffeinated powder	1 rounded tsp	4	0	1	0	0
regular powder	1 rounded tsp	4	tr	1	0	0
REGULAR						
brewed	8 oz	2	tr	0	0	0
roasted beans	1 oz	64	4	18	–	2
COFFEE BEVERAGES						
Click						
Espresso Protein Drink as prep	2 scoops (1.1 oz)	120	2	12	7	tr
N.O. Brew						
Iced Coffee not prep	1 serv (2.6 oz)	10	0	1	0	0

FOOD	PORTION	CAL	FAT	CARB	SUGAR	FIBER
O.N.E.						
Coffee Fruit	1 bottle (11 oz)	107	1	26	25	1
Wolfgang Puck						
Culinary Iced All Flavors	1 bottle (8.5 oz)	120	3	23	21	–
TAKE-OUT						
cafe amaretto w/ alcohol	1 serv	192	9	15	–	0
cafe au lait	1 cup (8 oz)	77	4	6	7	–
cafe brulot	1 cup	48	0	3	3	–
cafe brulot w/ alcohol	1 serv	130	tr	16	–	3
cappuccino	1 cup (8 oz)	77	4	6	7	–
coffee con leche	1 cup (6 oz)	104	4	16	17	0
cuban coffee w/ rum & creme de cacao	1 (9 oz)	112	2	6	–	0
dutch coffee w/ gin	1 (7 oz)	181	10	6	5	0
espresso	1 cup (4 oz)	2	tr	0	0	0
french coffee w/ orange liqueur & kahlua	1 (8 oz)	232	10	24	–	0
irish coffee	1 serv (8 oz)	209	11	5	4	0
italian coffee w/ strega	1 (7 oz)	163	10	12	10	0
latte w/ skim milk	1 serv (13 oz)	88	tr	12	11	0
latte w/ whole milk	1 serv (14 oz)	143	6	15	14	0
mocha	1 serv (17 oz)	403	9	69	54	2
puerto rican coffee w/ rum & kahlua	1 (8 oz)	166	10	9	–	0
turkish	1 cup (4 oz)	50	1	12	12	0
COFFEE WHITENERS						
Silk						
French Vanilla	1 tbsp (0.5 oz)	20	1	3	3	0
Original	1 tbsp (0.5 oz)	15	1	1	1	0

FOOD	PORTION	CAL	FAT	CARB	SUGAR	FIBER
COLESLAW						
Fresh Express						
3 Color Deli	1½ cups	20	0	5	3	2
Kit w/ Sweet & Creamy Dressing	3 cups	120	8	12	10	2
Old Fashioned	2 cups	25	0	5	3	2
Mann's						
Broccoli Cole Slaw w/o Dressing	1 serv (3 oz)	25	0	5	2	3
TAKE-OUT						
coleslaw w/ dressing	¾ cup	147	11	13	–	–
vinegar & oil coleslaw	3.5 oz	150	9	16	–	–
COLLARDS						
fresh cooked	½ cup	17	tr	4	–	–
frzn chopped cooked	½ cup	31	tr	6	–	–
raw chopped	½ cup	6	tr	1	–	–
Allens						
Seasoned Southern Style	½ cup (4.1 oz)	35	0	6	3	2
COOKIES						
MIX						
chocolate chip	1 (0.56 oz)	79	4	10	–	–
oatmeal	1 (0.6 oz)	74	3	10	–	tr
oatmeal raisin	1 (0.6 oz)	74	3	10	–	tr
Betty Crocker						
Caramelita Bars as prep	1	190	8	28	17	1
Chocolate Chip as prep	2	170	8	21	13	tr
Oatmeal as prep	2	160	7	22	11	tr
Peanut Butter as prep	2	150	7	20	12	–
Reese's Dessert Bar Mix No Bake as prep	1	180	10	20	13	1
Sugar as prep	2	160	8	21	12	0

FOOD	PORTION	CAL	FAT	CARB	SUGAR	FIBER
Sunkist Lemon Bars as prep	1	140	4	24	17	–
Turtle Cookie Bars as prep	1	180	8	27	16	tr
Duncan Hines						
Chocolate Chip as prep	2 (1.1 oz)	180	9	23	14	0
READY-TO-EAT						
animal crackers	1 (2.5 g)	11	tr	2	–	–
animal crackers	11 (1 oz)	126	4	21	–	–
animal crackers	1 box (2.4 oz)	299	9	51	–	–
australian anzac biscuit	1	98	3	17	–	1
butter	1 (5 g)	23	1	3	–	tr
chocolate chip	1 box (1.9 oz)	233	12	36	–	–
chocolate chip	1 (0.4 oz)	48	2	7	–	tr
chocolate chip low sugar low sodium	1 (0.24 oz)	31	1	5	–	–
chocolate chip lowfat	1 (0.25 oz)	45	2	7	–	–
chocolate chip soft-type	1 (0.5 oz)	69	4	9	–	tr
chocolate w/ creme filling	1 (0.35 oz)	47	2	7	–	tr
chocolate w/ creme filling chocolate coated	1 (0.60 oz)	82	5	11	–	–
chocolate w/ creme filling sugar free low sodium	1 (0.35 oz)	46	2	7	–	–
chocolate w/ extra creme filling	1 (0.46 oz)	65	3	9	–	–
chocolate wafer	1 (0.2 oz)	26	1	4	–	–
cream cheese	1 (1.1 oz)	141	9	14	6	tr
digestive biscuits plain	2	141	7	21	–	1
fig bars	1 (0.56 oz)	56	1	11	–	1
fortune	1 (0.28 oz)	30	tr	7	–	tr
fudge	1 (0.73 oz)	73	1	17	–	tr

FOOD	PORTION	CAL	FAT	CARB	SUGAR	FIBER
gingersnaps	1 (0.24 oz)	29	1	5	–	–
graham	1 sq (0.24 oz)	30	1	5	–	–
graham chocolate covered	1 (0.49 oz)	68	3	9	–	–
graham honey	1 (0.24 oz)	30	1	5	–	tr
hermits	1 (1 oz)	117	5	18	10	1
jumbles coconut	1 (1 oz)	121	7	13	7	1
ladyfingers	1 (0.38 oz)	40	1	7	–	–
macaroons	1 (0.8 oz)	97	3	17	–	–
madeleines	1 (0.8 oz)	86	5	10	5	tr
marshmallow chocolate coated	1 (0.46 oz)	55	2	9	–	–
marshmallow pie chocolate coated	1 (1.4 oz)	165	7	26	–	–
molasses	1 (0.5 oz)	65	2	11	–	–
neapolitan tri-color cookie	1 (0.6 oz)	79	5	8	5	tr
oatmeal	1 (0.6 oz)	81	3	12	–	1
oatmeal soft-type	1 (0.5 oz)	61	2	10	–	tr
oatmeal raisin	1 (0.6 oz)	81	3	12	–	1
oatmeal raisin low sugar no sodium	1 (0.24 oz)	31	1	5	–	–
oatmeal raisin soft-type	1 (0.5 oz)	61	2	10	–	tr
peanut butter sandwich	1 (0.5 oz)	67	3	9	–	–
peanut butter sandwich sugar free low sodium	1 (0.35 oz)	54	3	5	–	–
peanut butter soft-type	1 (0.5 oz)	69	4	9	–	tr
pinenut cookies	1 (1.1 oz)	134	9	11	8	1
raisin soft-type	1 (0.5 oz)	60	2	10	–	–
reginette queen's biscuit	1 (0.8 oz)	86	3	13	4	tr
shortbread	1 (0.28 oz)	40	2	5	–	–
shortbread pecan	1 (0.49 oz)	79	5	8	–	tr
spritz	1 (0.4 oz)	42	2	6	3	tr

FOOD	PORTION	CAL	FAT	CARB	SUGAR	FIBER
sugar	1 (0.52 oz)	72	3	10	–	–
sugar low sugar sodium free	1 (0.24 oz)	30	1	5	–	–
sugar wafers w/ creme filling	1 (0.12 oz)	18	1	3	–	–
sugar wafers w/ creme filling sugar free sodium free	1 (0.14 oz)	20	1	3	–	–
toll house original	1 (0.8 oz)	105	6	13	9	tr
vanilla sandwich	1 (0.35 oz)	48	2	7	–	tr
vanilla wafers	1 (0.21 oz)	28	1	4	–	–
zeppole	1 (0.8 oz)	78	6	6	4	tr
Almond Joy						
Cookies	2 (1 oz)	140	8	17	12	tr
Anna's Swedish Thins						
Almond Cinnamon	6 (1 oz)	140	7	18	5	1
Cappuccino	6 (1 oz)	140	7	18	6	2
Chocolate Mint	6 (1 oz)	150	8	17	6	2
Orange	6 (1 oz)	140	7	19	6	3
Archway						
Coconut Macaroon	2 (1.3 oz)	160	8	22	16	2
Frosty Lemon	1 (0.9 oz)	110	5	18	10	0
Fruit Filled Raspberry	1 (0.8 oz)	90	3	15	7	0
Aunt Gussie's						
Biscotti Almond	1 (0.8 oz)	110	6	13	5	1
Biscotti Almond Sugar Free	2 (1 oz)	150	10	14	3	1
Biscotti Cinnamon Raisin No Sugar Added	1 (0.8 oz)	110	6	14	2	1
Biscotti Italian w/ Olive Oil	2 (1.2 oz)	160	5	25	13	1
Coconut Crisp	2 (1.1 oz)	170	9	18	9	1
Latte Sugar Free	1 (0.9 oz)	110	6	18	0	0

FOOD	PORTION	CAL	FAT	CARB	SUGAR	FIBER
Lemon Sugar Free	3 (1.2 oz)	160	9	22	0	1
Mexican Wedding Cakes	3 (1.2 oz)	160	10	19	8	1
Snickerdoodle	2 (1.1 oz)	180	12	16	4	1
Vanilla Spritz Sugar Free Gluten Free	2 (0.9 oz)	110	5	17	0	0
Back To Nature						
Granola Cranberry Pecan	1 (1.1 oz)	130	6	20	10	2
Granola Honey Nut	1 (1.1 oz)	140	7	18	8	2
Bahlsen						
Delice	6 (1.1 oz)	150	8	19	6	tr
Hannover Wafflen	6 (1.1 oz)	180	11	19	8	1
Hit Minis Chocolate Filled	5 (1.2 oz)	170	8	23	11	tr
Waffeletten	4 (1 oz)	160	9	18	10	1
Barbara's Bakery						
Fig Bars Traditional	1	60	1	14	8	–
Fig Bars Wheat Free	1	60	0	13	8	1
Organic 100 Calorie Mini Ginger	1 pkg (0.9 oz)	100	2	19	9	–
Snackimals Chocolate Chip	10	120	4	19	8	–
Snackimals Wheat Free Oatmeal	10	120	5	17	6	1
Barry's Bakery						
French Twists Wild Raspberry	2 (0.5 oz)	60	2	9	4	0
Breaktime						
Ginger	4 (1 oz)	130	4	23	10	0
Oatmeal	4 (1 oz)	130	4	22	9	tr
Brown & Haley						
Almond Roca	6 (1 oz)	110	4	19	10	0

FOOD	PORTION	CAL	FAT	CARB	SUGAR	FIBER
Buzz Strong's						
Real Coffee	1 (1.2 oz)	150	7	22	13	1
Comfort Care						
Cabin Hearth Chocolate Chip	1 (2 oz)	250	11	38	23	1
Cabin Hearth Oatmeal Peach	1 (2 oz)	200	7	31	17	3
Cabin Hearth Oatmeal Raisin	1 (2 oz)	200	7	31	17	3
Country Choice Organic						
Fit Kids Snackin' Grahams Chocolate	18 (1 oz)	110	3	20	7	2
Oatmeal Chocolate Chip	1 (0.8 oz)	100	4	15	8	1
Oatmeal Raisin	1 (0.8 oz)	100	3	16	9	1
Dare						
Lemon Creme	1 (0.7 oz)	100	4	14	7	0
Maple Leaf Creme	1 (0.6 oz)	80	4	12	6	0
Divvies						
Chocolate Chip Vegan	1	130	7	17	11	tr
Oatmeal Raisin Vegan	1	120	5	17	8	tr
Emily's						
Fortune Dark Chocolate Covered	2 (1.4 oz)	140	6	23	15	2
Graham Cracker Milk Chocolate Covered	1 (1 oz)	150	9	17	13	tr
Erin Baker's						
Breakfast Banana Toasted Flax	1 (3 oz)	300	5	55	12	6
Breakfast Caramel Apple	1 (3 oz)	290	4	57	21	6
Breakfast Mocha Cappuccino	1 (3 oz)	300	6	54	19	6
Breakfast Morning Glory	1 (3 oz)	310	8	54	17	6

FOOD	PORTION	CAL	FAT	CARB	SUGAR	FIBER
Breakfast Peanut Butter & Jelly	1 (3 oz)	320	9	52	21	5
Breakfast Vegan Chocolate Chip	1 (3 oz)	310	6	57	22	6
Organic Breakfast Mini Oatmeal Raisin	1 (1 oz)	100	2	18	9	2
Organic Breakfast Mini Peanut Butter	1 (1 oz)	110	3	16	7	2
French Meadow Bakery						
Coconutty Macaroons	2 (1.1 oz)	150	8	17	11	1
Gluten Free Chocolate Chip	1 (2.1 oz)	320	16	43	23	1
Rhubarb Bar	1 (2.7 oz)	250	11	34	18	1
Vegan Peanut Butter Bliss	2 (1.2 oz)	150	7	19	3	1
Girl Scout						
Lemon Chalet Cremes	3 (1.3 oz)	170	7	26	13	tr
Gourmet Pastries						
Kourabiethes Butter Almond	1 (1.1 oz)	150	9	15	5	1
Phoenicia Honey & Spice	1 (1.3 oz)	140	5	20	12	0
Health Valley						
Mini Mint Chocolate Chip	4 (1 oz)	120	6	16	7	1
Oatmeal Raisin	1 (0.8 oz)	90	4	14	8	1
Raisin Oatmeal Low Fat	3	110	2	23	13	1
White Chocolate Chunk	1 (1 oz)	140	7	17	10	0
Home Free						
Organic Chocolate Chip	1 (1 oz)	140	6	21	11	1
Organic Oatmeal	1 (1 oz)	120	4	19	9	2
Kedem						
Tea Biscuits Chocolate	2 (0.3 oz)	32	1	6	2	tr
Tea Biscuits Vanilla	2 (0.3 oz)	32	1	6	2	tr

FOOD	PORTION	CAL	FAT	CARB	SUGAR	FIBER
Keebler						
100 Calorie Right Bites Fudge Shoppe Fudge Grahams	1 pkg (0.7 oz)	100	4	15	7	tr
100 Calorie Pack RightBites Sandies Shortbread	1 pkg (0.7 oz)	100	3	17	7	tr
Animal Crackers Frosted	8	150	7	22	13	tr
Chips Deluxe Chocolate Lovers	1	90	5	10	5	0
Chips Deluxe Coconut	2	150	9	18	9	1
Chips Deluxe Fudge Stripes	1	100	6	13	8	tr
Chips Deluxe Original	1 pkg (2 oz)	300	16	37	18	1
Danish Wedding	4	130	6	18	10	tr
Dipping Delights Cheesecake	1	90	4	13	8	0
E.L. Fudge Original	1	90	4	13	6	tr
Fudge Shoppe Fudge Stripes	3	150	7	21	10	tr
Fudge Shoppe Grasshoppers	4	140	7	19	11	tr
Fudge Shoppe Mint Creme Filled	2	160	9	20	14	tr
Graham Honey	8 (1 oz)	110	2	22	7	tr
Graham Original	8 (1 oz)	130	4	22	7	tr
Oatmeal Country Style	2	130	6	18	8	1
Sandies Drops Butter Pecan	4	140	7	18	10	tr
Sandies Pecan Shortbread Reduced Fat	1	80	4	11	4	0
Scooby-Doo Graham Sticks	9	130	4	21	8	tr

FOOD	PORTION	CAL	FAT	CARB	SUGAR	FIBER
Soft Batch Chocolate Chip	1	80	4	11	6	tr
Vanilla Wafers	8	140	6	21	9	tr
Vienna Fingers	2 (1.1 oz)	150	6	23	10	tr
Vienna Fingers Reduced Fat	2	140	5	24	12	tr
Khaya						
Krunchi Orange & Chocolate	5 (1.53 oz)	240	12	29	14	2
Shortbread Grapeseed	13 (1.15 oz)	193	10	27	6	tr
Shortbread Orange Rooibos	13 (1.15)	259	14	36	8	tr
La Choy						
Fortune	4 (1 oz)	110	0	25	9	0
Lance						
Oatmeal Creme	1 (2.5 oz)	300	12	45	26	2
Van-O-Lunch	1 pkg (1.6 oz)	230	10	34	14	0
Late July						
Organic Sandwich Dark Chocolate	3 (1.2 oz)	150	6	21	9	2
Organic Sandwich Vanilla Bean w/ Green Tea	2 (0.8 oz)	110	5	16	8	1
Lean Body						
Cookie Bar Hi-Protein S'Mores	1 (3.2 oz)	360	13	30	13	2
Loacker						
Quadratini Dark Chocolate	9 (1.1 oz)	160	8	20	9	2
Lorna Doone						
Shortbread	4 (1 oz)	140	7	20	6	0
LU						
Le Petit Beurre	4 (1.2 oz)	140	4	24	8	tr

FOOD	PORTION	CAL	FAT	CARB	SUGAR	FIBER
Petit Ecolier Dark Chocolate	2 (0.9 oz)	130	6	17	9	1
Petit Ecolier Milk Chocolate	2 (0.9 oz)	130	6	17	10	tr
Shortbread	2 (1 oz)	140	8	16	5	tr
Luna						
Berry Pomegranate	1 (1.4 oz)	140	3	27	11	4
Peanut Butter Chocolate	1 (1.4 oz)	150	6	23	10	3
M&M's						
Milk Chocolate	1 pkg (1.15 oz)	150	5	22	11	1
Mauna Loa						
Macadamia Nut Chocolate Chip	4 (1 oz)	150	9	17	5	<1
Montana Monster Munchies						
Original	½ (1.4 oz)	177	9	21	14	2
Raisin	½ (1.4 oz)	172	9	22	14	2
MoonPie						
Mini All Flavors	1 pkg (1.2 oz)	130	4	23	11	2
Mrs. Fields						
Cookie Dough Snacks Brownie Chocolate Chip	7 (1 oz)	120	3	18	10	0
Cookie Dough Snacks Chocolate Chip	7 (1 oz)	120	4	19	12	tr
Natural Ovens						
Oatmeal Raisin	1 (1.3 oz)	120	4	20	10	2
Nonni's						
Biscotti Cioccolati	1 (0.8 oz)	110	5	17	9	1
Biscotti Limone	1 (0.8 oz)	110	5	17	9	0
Biscotti Original	1 (0.7 oz)	90	3	14	7	0
Oreo						
Cakesters Mini Golden 100 Calorie Pack	1 pkg (0.8 oz)	100	5	15	10	0

FOOD	PORTION	CAL	FAT	CARB	SUGAR	FIBER
Orion						
Choco Pie	1 (1 oz)	120	5	19	10	tr
Pepperidge Farm						
Bordeaux	4 (1 oz)	130	5	19	12	tr
Pirouette						
Sandwich Vanilla Creamed	3 (1.1 oz)	133	4	22	7	0
Polar						
Fortune	2	56	0	12	6	0
Q.bel						
Wafer Rolls Dark Chocolate	1 pkg (0.9 oz)	120	6	18	13	1
Wafer Rolls Milk Chocolate	1 pkg (0.9 oz)	130	6	18	13	tr
Ruger						
Wafers Vanilla	3 (1 oz)	160	9	20	15	0
Snikiddy						
Cherry Oaties	1 pkg (0.8 oz)	110	4	17	6	1
South Beach						
Fiber Fit Double Chocolate Chunk	1 pkg (0.8 oz)	100	5	17	5	5
Fiber Fit Oatmeal Chocolate Chunk	1 pkg (0.8 oz)	100	5	17	5	5
Wafer Sticke Dark Chocolate Hazelnut Creme	1 pkg	100	6	10	tr	3
Wafer Sticke Dark Chocolate Peanut Butter	1 pkg	100	6	10	1	3
Starbucks						
Almond Roca Buttercrunch Toffee	6 (1 oz)	110	4	19	10	0
Biscotti Chocolate Hazelnut	1 (0.9 oz)	100	5	14	7	1

FOOD	PORTION	CAL	FAT	CARB	SUGAR	FIBER
White Chocolate & Raspberry	2 (0.9 oz)	120	6	15	8	tr
Stella D'Oro						
100 Calorie Pack Breakfast Treats Original	1 pkg (0.8 oz)	100	2	19	6	1
Voortman						
Chinese Almond	1 (0.9 oz)	130	7	16	7	0
Coconut Delight	1 (0.6 oz)	90	6	10	5	tr
Dutch Creme	1 (0.8 oz)	110	4	16	8	0
Fudge Swirl	1 (0.6 oz)	80	4	10	4	0
Gingerboy	1 (0.7 oz)	100	4	15	7	0
Maple Leaf	1 (0.6 oz)	90	4	13	7	0
Molasses	1 (1 oz)	110	3	20	10	tr
Oatmeal Apple	1 (0.7 oz)	90	4	13	6	1
Peanut Delight	1 (0.9 oz)	130	7	15	6	tr
Shortbread	1 (0.6 oz)	90	5	11	4	tr
Sugar Free Chocolate Chip	1 (0.7 oz)	80	5	13	0	0
Sugar Free Lemon Wafers	3 (1 oz)	130	8	17	0	0
Sugar Free Vanilla Creme	2 (0.7 oz)	100	6	13	0	0
Sugar Free Wafers Peanut Butter	4 (1 oz)	150	8	17	0	0
Sugar Free Wafers Vanilla	3 (1 oz)	130	8	17	0	0
Turnover Blueberry	1 (0.9 oz)	110	4	18	9	tr
Turnover Cherry	1 (0.9 oz)	110	4	18	9	tr
Turnover Strawberry	1 (0.9 oz)	110	4	18	9	tr
Wafer Chocolate Covered	1 (0.7 oz)	100	5	13	9	0
Wafer Vanilla	3 (1 oz)	140	7	20	12	0
Wafers Mini Chocolate	5 (1 oz)	130	6	19	11	0

FOOD	PORTION	CAL	FAT	CARB	SUGAR	FIBER
Walkers						
Shortbread	1	100	6	11	3	0
Shortbread Chocolate Chip	2 (1 oz)	140	8	17	7	tr
Whippet						
Original	2 (1.2 oz)	150	5	24	16	1
World Of Grains						
Apple Cinnamon	1 pkg	130	4	21	9	3
Cranberry	1 pkg	130	4	21	9	3
Multigrain	1 pkg	130	5	21	6	3
REFRIGERATED						
chocolate chip	1 (0.42 oz)	59	3	8	–	–
chocolate chip dough	1 oz	126	6	17	–	–
oatmeal	1 (0.4 oz)	56	3	8	–	–
oatmeal raisin	1 (0.4 oz)	56	3	8	–	–
peanut butter	1 (0.4 oz)	60	3	7	–	–
peanut butter dough	1 oz	130	7	15	–	–
sugar	1 (0.42 oz)	58	3	8	–	–
sugar dough	1 oz	124	6	17	–	–
Pillsbury						
Chocolate Chip	2 (1.3 oz)	170	9	22	14	tr
Gingerbread	2 (1.1 oz)	170	7	18	9	0
Oatmeal Chocolate Chip	2 (1.3 oz)	170	8	23	14	1
Peanut Butter	2 (1 oz)	130	6	16	9	0
S'Mores	2 (1.3 oz)	160	7	23	25	tr
Sugar	2 (1.3 oz)	170	9	22	12	0
TAKE-OUT						
biscotti w/ nuts chocolate dipped	1 (1.3 oz)	117	6	16	11	1
black & white	1 lg (3 oz)	302	9	52	31	1
finikia	1 (1.2 oz)	171	5	16	5	1
koulourakia butter cookie twist	1 (0.9 oz)	113	6	14	5	tr
linzer tart	1 (2.4 oz)	280	14	34	12	0

FOOD	PORTION	CAL	FAT	CARB	SUGAR	FIBER
CORIANDER						
cilantro fresh	1 tsp (2 g)	tr	tr	tr	–	tr
leaf dried	1 tsp	2	tr	tr	tr	tr
leaf fresh	¼ cup	1	tr	tr	–	–
seed	1 tsp	5	tr	1	–	1
CORN						
CANNED						
cream style	½ cup	93	1	23	–	–
w/ red & green peppers	½ cup	86	1	21	–	–
white	½ cup	66	1	15	–	–
yellow	½ cup	66	1	15	–	1
Green Giant						
Mexicorn	⅓ cup	70	1	14	4	1
Super Sweet Yellow & White	⅓ cup	60	1	12	3	1
Orchids						
Whole Young Spears	½ cup (4.6 oz)	25	0	4	1	2
FRESH						
white cooked	½ cup	89	1	21	–	–
white raw	½ cup	66	1	15	–	–
yellow cooked	½ cup	89	1	21	–	–
yellow cooked	1 ear (2.7 oz)	83	1	19	–	–
yellow raw	½ cup	66	1	15	–	–
yellow raw	1 ear (3 oz)	77	1	17	–	–
FROZEN						
cooked	½ cup	67	tr	17	–	–
on the cob cooked	1 ear (2.2 oz)	59	tr	14	–	–
Birds Eye						
Steamfresh Singles Super Sweet	1 pkg (3.2 oz)	80	1	14	6	2
Steamfresh Southwestern	⅔ cup (2.9 oz)	90	2	16	5	1

FOOD	PORTION	CAL	FAT	CARB	SUGAR	FIBER
Green Giant						
Cream Style	½ cup	110	1	24	7	2
Nibblers On-The-Cob	1 (2.1 oz)	70	1	14	2	1
Health Is Wealth						
Creamed	½ pkg (4.5 oz)	110	2	23	7	1
TAKE-OUT						
fritters	1 (1 oz)	62	2	9	–	1
on the cob w/ butter cooked	1 ear	155	3	32	–	–
scalloped	1 cup	257	11	34	11	3

CORN CHIPS (*see* CHIPS)

CORNISH HEN (*see* CHICKEN)

CORNMEAL

FOOD	PORTION	CAL	FAT	CARB	SUGAR	FIBER
cornmeal mush as prep w/ water	1 cup	223	1	47	tr	5
cornmeal yellow	½ cup (2.2 oz)	236	1	52	tr	1
whole grain blue	½ cup (1.9 oz)	201	3	41	0	5
yellow self-rising	½ cup (3 oz)	296	2	62	–	5
Martha White						
White Self Rising	3 tbsp (1.1 oz)	100	1	22	0	2
White Enriched	3 tbsp (1.2 oz)	120	1	24	0	2
Yellow	3 tbsp (1.1 oz)	110	1	22	0	2
TAKE-OUT						
corn pone	1 piece (2.1 oz)	128	3	23	tr	2
fritter puerto rican style	1 (1.4 oz)	109	7	8	tr	1
harina de maiz con coco	½ cup	383	27	36	21	4
harina de maize con leche	1 cup	295	7	51	32	7
hush puppies	1 (0.8 oz)	74	3	10	tr	1

FOOD	PORTION	CAL	FAT	CARB	SUGAR	FIBER
johnnycake	1 piece (1.7 oz)	134	4	21	4	2

CORNSTARCH

cornstarch	1 tbsp (0.3 oz)	34	0	8	0	tr
cornstarch	¼ cup (1.1 oz)	122	tr	29	0	tr
Argo						
Cornstarch	1 tbsp (0.3 oz)	30	0	7	–	–

COTTAGE CHEESE

creamed large curd	½ cup (4 oz)	110	5	4	3	0
creamed small curd	½ cup (3.7 oz)	103	5	4	3	0
dry curd	½ cup (2.5 oz)	52	tr	5	1	0
lowfat 1%	½ cup (4 oz)	81	1	3	3	0
lowfat 1% lactose reduced	½ cup (4 oz)	84	1	4	3	1
Axelrod						
Lowfat 1%	½ cup (4 oz)	90	2	6	4	0
Cabot						
Cottage Cheese	½ cup	100	5	4	4	0
No Fat	½ cup	70	0	5	4	0
Friendship						
1% Lowfat	½ cup	90	1	3	3	0
1% Lowfat No Salt Added	½ cup	90	1	4	3	1
1% Lowfat Whipped	½ cup	90	1	3	3	0
2% Digestive Health	½ cup	90	3	5	2	3
2% Pot Style	½ cup	90	3	3	2	0
4% California Style	½ cup	110	5	3	2	1
Nonfat	½ cup	80	0	4	4	0
Land O Lakes						
1% Lowfat	½ cup (4 oz)	90	2	5	3	0
2% Lowfat	½ cup (3.7 oz)	100	3	5	3	0

FOOD	PORTION	CAL	FAT	CARB	SUGAR	FIBER
Cottage Cheese	½ cup (3.7 oz)	110	5	5	4	0
Fat Free	½ cup (4 oz)	80	0	6	4	0
Nancy's						
Organic Lowfat	½ cup	80	1	3	3	0

COTTONSEED

FOOD	PORTION	CAL	FAT	CARB	SUGAR	FIBER
kernels roasted	1 tbsp	51	4	2	–	–

COUSCOUS

FOOD	PORTION	CAL	FAT	CARB	SUGAR	FIBER
cooked	1 cup (5.5 oz)	176	tr	36	–	2
dry	1 cup (6.1 oz)	650	1	134	–	9
Near East						
Mediterranean Curry as prep	1 cup	220	4	40	2	3
Original Plain as prep	1 cup	190	2	37	1	3
Parmesan as prep	1 cup	220	4	39	3	2
Toasted Pine Nut as prep	1 cup	230	5	39	2	2
Wild Mushroom & Herb as prep	1 cup	230	4	40	1	3

CRAB
CANNED

FOOD	PORTION	CAL	FAT	CARB	SUGAR	FIBER
blue	½ cup	67	1	0	0	0
blue drained	1 can (6.5 oz)	124	2	0	0	0
Polar						
Claw Meat	¼ cup (2 oz)	37	0	1	1	0
Jumbo Lump Meat	¼ cup (2 oz)	39	1	0	0	0
FRESH						
alaska king meat only steamed	3 oz	82	1	0	0	0
blue cooked flaked	1 cup (4 oz)	120	2	0	0	0
dungeness steamed	3 oz	94	1	1	–	0
queen steamed	3 oz	98	1	0	0	0

FOOD	PORTION	CAL	FAT	CARB	SUGAR	FIBER
FROZEN						
Mama Belle's						
Crab Cakes Maryland Style	1 (2 oz)	100	5	4	1	0
TAKE-OUT						
alaska king leg steamed	1 leg (4.7 oz)	130	2	0	0	0
baked	1 (3.8 oz)	160	2	4	–	–
cakes	2 (4.2 oz)	186	9	1	–	0
crab imperial	1 crab (6.8 oz)	289	15	6	3	0
crab salad	1 serv (5.5 oz)	285	21	3	1	1
crab thermidor	1 serv (6.4 oz)	456	37	8	tr	tr
deviled	1 serv (4.5 oz)	254	13	17	6	1
dungeness steamed	1 crab (4.5 oz)	140	2	1	–	0
empanada de jueyes	1 (4.4 oz)	341	16	38	7	2
fried crab puffs	4 (3.2 oz)	323	18	30	tr	1
kenagi korean crab cooked	1 serv (3 oz)	71	tr	0	0	0
salmorejo de jueyes (in tomato sauce)	1 serv (4.5 oz)	215	14	3	1	tr
soft-shell breaded & fried	1 med (2.3 oz)	216	13	11	1	1
taco de jueyes	1 (4.2 oz)	266	14	18	1	2
CRACKER CRUMBS						
cracker meal	1 cup	440	2	93	tr	3
graham cracker crumbs	1 cup	355	8	65	26	2
Honey Maid						
Graham Cracker Crumbs	2½ tbsp (0.6 oz)	70	2	13	4	0

FOOD	PORTION	CAL	FAT	CARB	SUGAR	FIBER
Keebler						
Graham	¼ cup	93	2	17	4	1
CRACKERS						
melba toast round	1	12	tr	2	tr	tr
oyster cracker	¼ cup	48	1	8	tr	tr
saltines	1	13	tr	2	tr	tr
water biscuits	3	92	3	16	–	1
zwieback	1 oz	107	1	21	–	1
34 Degrees						
Crispbread Sesame	19 (1.1 oz)	140	3	26	1	1
Athenos						
Pita Chips Whole Wheat	11 (1 oz)	120	4	18	tr	2
Aunt Gussie's						
Cracker Flats Spelt Cinnamon Raisin	1 (1 oz)	100	2	19	5	1
Cracker Flats Spelt Everything	1 (0.8 oz)	60	2	12	0	2
Back To Nature						
Poppy Thyme	17 (1 oz)	130	4	21	2	1
Sesame Tarragon	17 (1 oz)	130	5	21	2	1
Barbara's Bakery						
Rite Rounds Lite Original	5 (0.5 oz)	60	2	11	tr	–
Wheatines Original	4	60	1	11	1	tr
Bremner Wafers						
Cracked Wheat	7 (0.5 oz)	70	2	11	0	0
Original	7 (0.5 oz)	70	2	11	0	0
Soup & Chili Crackers	50 (0.5 oz)	60	2	11	0	0
Breton						
Garden Vegetable	4 (0.7 oz)	100	4	13	1	1
Minis Cheddar Cheese	20 (0.7 oz)	100	5	13	1	1
Dare						
Crackers	3 (0.5 oz)	70	4	9	tr	0
Original	4 (0.7 oz)	90	4	13	1	1
Reduced Fat & Salt	5 (0.7 oz)	80	2	16	2	1

FOOD	PORTION	CAL	FAT	CARB	SUGAR	FIBER
GrainsFirst						
Autumn Harvest	7 (1.1 oz)	140	7	16	2	3
Grissol						
Crispy Baguettes Garden Herb	8 (1 oz)	110	2	19	2	1
Health Valley						
Organic Bruschetta Vegetable	4	70	3	10	1	0
Organic Cracked Pepper	4	70	3	10	1	0
Organic Cracker Stix Garlic Herb	8	70	3	9	1	tr
Organic Whole Wheat	4	70	3	9	1	1
Kashi						
Heart To Heart Whole Grain	7 (1 oz)	120	4	22	0	4
TLC Toasted Asiago	15 (1.1 oz)	130	4	21	2	2
Keebler						
Club Multi-Grain	4	70	3	10	2	tr
Club Original	4	70	3	9	1	tr
Club Reduced Fat	5	70	3	12	2	tr
Club Snack Sticks	12	130	6	19	2	tr
Puffed Original	24	140	6	20	3	1
Sandwich Cheese & Peanut Butter	1 pkg (1.4 oz)	200	10	23	4	1
Sandwich Toast & Peanut Butter	1 pkg (1.4 oz)	200	10	23	4	1
Sandwich Wheat & Cheddar	1 pkg (1.3 oz)	190	10	23	5	tr
Toasteds Harvest Wheat	16	130	6	20	3	1
Toasteds Sesame	5	80	4	10	1	tr
Toasteds Wheat	5	80	4	10	1	tr
Town House Bistro	2	80	3	11	1	tr

FOOD	PORTION	CAL	FAT	CARB	SUGAR	FIBER
Town House FlipSides Original	5	70	4	10	1	tr
Town House Original	5	80	5	10	1	tr
Town House Reduced Fat	6	60	2	11	1	tr
Town House Reduced Sodium	5	80	5	10	1	tr
Town House Toppers	3	70	3	9	1	0
Wheatables 33% Less Fat	19	140	4	22	5	1
Wheatables Original	17	140	6	20	4	1
Zesta Saltine Fat Free	5	60	0	13	0	tr
Zesta Saltine Original	5	60	2	11	0	tr
Kellogg's						
All Bran Garlic Herb	18 (1 oz)	120	6	19	3	5
Lance						
Captain Wafers	4	70	3	9	1	0
Nekot	1 pkg (1.7 oz)	240	11	30	13	1
Nipchee	1 pkg (1.4 oz)	190	11	22	3	1
Peanut Butter On Wheat	1 pkg (1.4 oz)	200	9	21	4	1
Toastchee	1 pkg (1.5 oz)	220	11	23	3	2
Toastchee Reduced Fat	1 pkg (1.4 oz)	180	7	23	2	2
Larzaroni						
Bruschette w/ Olives	9 (1.1 oz)	140	5	21	tr	1
Late July						
Organic Classic Rich	4 (0.5 oz)	70	2	11	2	0
Organic Classic Saltine	4 (0.5 oz)	60	3	10	0	0
Mary's Gone Crackers						
Wheat Free Gluten Free Black Pepper	13 (1 oz)	140	5	21	0	3
Wheat Free Gluten Free Onion	13 (1 oz)	140	5	21	0	3

FOOD	PORTION	CAL	FAT	CARB	SUGAR	FIBER
Wheat Free Gluten Free Original Seed	13 (1 oz)	140	5	21	0	3
Nonni's						
Panetini Roasted Garlic	5 (1 oz)	120	4	19	1	tr
Panetini Sun Dried Tomato Basil	5 (1 oz)	120	4	17	1	tr
Orkney						
Oatcakes Thin	4 (1.8 oz)	227	12	25	tr	3
Ritz						
Crackerfuls Classic Cheddar	1 (1 oz)	130	7	17	3	3
Hint Of Salt	0.5 oz	80	4	10	1	0
Original	0.5 oz	80	5	10	1	0
Reduced Fat	5 (0.5 oz)	70	2	11	1	0
Whole Wheat	0.5 oz	70	3	11	2	1
Triscuit						
Cracked Pepper & Olive Oil	6 (1 oz)	120	4	20	0	3
True North						
Peanut Crunches	¼ cup (1 oz)	150	8	13	5	4
Pistachio Crisps	12 (1 oz)	140	7	15	4	2
Utz						
Cheese Peanut Butter	6	200	10	21	3	2
Vegetable Thins						
Original	21 (1.1 oz)	150	7	19	2	1
Vinta						
Original	3 (0.7 oz)	100	5	12	2	1
Wasa						
Hearty	1 (0.5 oz)	45	0	11	0	2
Light Rye	2 (0.6 oz)	60	0	14	0	3
Multi Grain	1 (0.5 oz)	45	0	10	0	2
Sourdough	1 (0.4 oz)	35	0	9	0	2
Whole Grain	1 (0.4 oz)	40	0	10	0	2
Whole Wheat	1 (0.5 oz)	50	1	10	tr	1

FOOD	PORTION	CAL	FAT	CARB	SUGAR	FIBER
Water Crackers						
Original	6 (0.5 oz)	60	2	11	0	0
CRANBERRIES						
cranberry orange relish	¼ cup	118	tr	31	28	2
dried	½ cup	85	tr	23	18	2
fresh chopped	1 cup	13	tr	3	1	1
fresh whole	1 cup	11	tr	3	1	1
sauce	1 slice (2 oz)	86	tr	22	22	1
sauce	¼ cup	109	tr	27	26	1
Chukar Cherries						
North Cove Dried	¼ cup	100	0	24	22	2
Emily's						
Milk Chocolate Covered	¼ cup (1.4 oz)	180	10	24	23	2
Fruitaceuticals						
OmegaCrans Dried	¼ cup	91	1	22	20	1
Ocean Spray						
Whole Berry Sauce	¼ cup (2.5 oz)	110	0	25	22	1
S&W						
Sauce Jellied	¼ cup (2.5 oz)	100	0	26	17	1
Sauce Whole Berry	¼ cup (2.5 oz)	100	0	26	17	1
Stoneridge Orchards						
Dried	⅓ cup (¼ oz)	140	0	33	26	2
Sun-Maid						
Dried Cape Cod	⅓ cup (1.4 oz)	130	0	33	27	2
Tree Of Life						
Organic Jellied	¼ cup (2.5 oz)	100	0	26	17	1
Wild Thymes Farm						
Cranberry Fig Sauce	1 tsp	19	0	5	4	tr
Original Cranberry Sauce	1 tbsp	21	0	5	5	tr
CRANBERRY BEANS						
canned	½ cup	108	tr	20	–	8
dried cooked w/o salt	½ cup	120	tr	22	–	9

FOOD	PORTION	CAL	FAT	CARB	SUGAR	FIBER
Goya						
Roman Beans Dried not prep	¼ cup (1.4 oz)	80	0	24	2	13

CRANBERRY JUICE

FOOD	PORTION	CAL	FAT	CARB	SUGAR	FIBER
cranberry juice cocktail low calorie w/ vitamin C	8 oz	46	tr	11	11	0
cranberry juice cocktail w/ vitamin C	8 oz	137	tr	34	30	0
unsweetened	8 oz	116	tr	31	31	tr
Nantucket Nectars						
Cranberry Cocktail	8 oz	130	0	33	32	0
Northland						
100% Juice No Sugar Added	8 oz	130	0	33	29	–
Ocean Spray						
Cran.Grape	8 oz	120	0	31	31	–
Cran.Pomegranate	8 oz	120	0	30	30	–
Cranberry Juice Cocktail	8 oz	120	0	30	30	–
Santa Cruz						
Organic Nectar	8 oz	110	0	27	26	0

CRAYFISH

FOOD	PORTION	CAL	FAT	CARB	SUGAR	FIBER
cooked	3 oz	97	1	0	0	0
raw	8	24	tr	0	0	0
raw	3 oz	76	1	0	0	0

CREAM (see also WHIPPED TOPPING)

FOOD	PORTION	CAL	FAT	CARB	SUGAR	FIBER
clotted cream	2 tbsp (1 oz)	164	18	1	–	0
creme fraiche	2 tbsp (1 oz)	100	11	1	–	0
half & half	1 cup (8.5 oz)	315	28	10	–	–
half & half	1 tbsp (0.5 oz)	20	2	1	–	–
heavy whipping	1 tbsp (0.5 oz)	52	6	tr	–	–
heavy whipping whipped	1 cup (4.1 oz)	411	44	7	–	–

FOOD	PORTION	CAL	FAT	CARB	SUGAR	FIBER
light coffee	1 cup (8.4 oz)	496	46	9	–	–
light coffee	1 tbsp (0.5 oz)	29	3	1	–	–
light whipping	1 tbsp (0.5 oz)	44	5	tr	–	–
light whipping whipped	1 cup (4.2 oz)	345	37	7	–	–
Cabot						
Whipped	2 tbsp	15	2	1	1	0
Land O Lakes						
Aerosol Whipped Light Cream	2 tbsp (0.2 oz)	20	2	1	1	0
Half & Half	2 tbsp (1.1 oz)	35	4	1	1	0
Half & Half Fat Free	2 tbsp (1.1 oz)	20	0	3	2	0
Heavy Whipping	1 tbsp (0.5 oz)	50	5	0	0	0
Straus						
Organic Whipping Cream	1 tbsp (0.5 oz)	52	6	0	0	0

CREAM CHEESE

FOOD	PORTION	CAL	FAT	CARB	SUGAR	FIBER
cream cheese	1 pkg (3 oz)	297	30	2	–	–
cream cheese	1 oz	99	10	1	–	–
Earth Balance						
Brick	2 tbsp	80	6	2	2	0
Tub	2 tbsp	80	6	2	2	0
Nancy's						
Organic	2 tbsp	95	9	2	2	0
Philadelphia						
1/3 Less Fat	1 oz	70	6	tr	tr	0
Original	1 oz	100	9	1	tr	0

CREAM CHEESE SUBSTITUTES

FOOD	PORTION	CAL	FAT	CARB	SUGAR	FIBER
Vegan Gourmet						
Alternative Cream Cheese	2 tbsp (1 oz)	90	8	3	0	2

CREAM OF TARTAR

FOOD	PORTION	CAL	FAT	CARB	SUGAR	FIBER
cream of tartar	1 tsp	8	0	2	0	0

FOOD	PORTION	CAL	FAT	CARB	SUGAR	FIBER
CREPES						
basic crepe unfilled	1 (7 in)	112	6	11	2	tr
Ekizian						
Chickpea Crepe	1 (7 in) (1.5 oz)	212	13	16	3	3
CROAKER						
atlantic breaded & fried	3 oz	188	11	6	–	–
atlantic raw	3 oz	89	3	0	0	0
CROCODILE						
cooked	3 oz	78	1	0	0	0
CROISSANT						
apple	1 (2 oz)	145	5	21	–	1
butter	1 lg (2.4 oz)	272	14	31	8	2
butter mini	1 (1 oz)	114	6	13	3	1
cheese	1 (1.5 oz)	174	9	20	5	1
chocolate	1 (2 oz)	237	14	25	6	2
TAKE-OUT						
w/ egg & cheese	1 (4.5 oz)	368	25	24	–	–
w/ egg & sausage	1 (5 oz)	497	34	31	8	2
w/ egg cheese & bacon	1 (4.1 oz)	385	24	25	8	1
w/ egg cheese & ham	1 (5.1 oz)	402	24	25	8	1
w/ egg cheese & sausage	1 (5.6 oz)	539	39	26	8	1
w/ ham & cheese	1 (4 oz)	338	20	25	4	1
CROUTONS						
plain	1 cup (1 oz)	122	2	22	–	2
seasoned	1 cup (1.4 oz)	186	7	25	–	2
Fresh Gourmet						
Cheese & Garlic	12 (0.5 oz)	70	3	9	0	0
Classic Caesar	6 (7 g)	35	2	4	0	0
Country Ranch	6 (7 g)	35	2	4	0	–

FOOD	PORTION	CAL	FAT	CARB	SUGAR	FIBER
CUCUMBER						
fresh peeled	1 med (7 oz)	24	tr	4	3	1
fresh sliced	1 cup	14	tr	3	2	1
fresh w/ peel sliced	½ cup	34	tr	2	1	tr
TAKE-OUT						
cucumber & onion salad w/ vinegar	1 cup	52	tr	12	8	1
cucumber raita	1 serv (3.3 oz)	40	3	3	3	1
cucumber salad w/ oil & vinegar	1 cup	183	15	11	8	1
cucumber salad w/ sour cream dressing	1 cup	68	6	3	2	1
kimchee	½ cup (1.8 oz)	36	2	4	3	tr
tzatziki	½ cup (3.4 oz)	72	6	4	3	1
CUMIN						
seed	1 tbsp (6 g)	22	1	3	tr	1
seed	1 tsp (2 g)	8	tr	1	tr	tr
CURRANT JUICE						
black currant nectar	7 oz	110	0	26	–	–
red currant nectar	7 oz	108	tr	26	–	–
CURRANTS						
black fresh	½ cup	36	tr	9	–	–
zante dried	½ cup	204	tr	53	–	–
Sun-Maid						
Zante	¼ cup (1.4 oz)	120	0	30	28	2
CURRY						
curry powder	1 tsp	7	tr	1	tr	1
paste	1 tube (6 oz)	465	36	30	13	12
Ethnic Gourmet						
Gujarati Vegetable Curry	1 pkg (10 oz)	380	11	63	17	4
Malay Chicken Curry	1 pkg (10 oz)	410	11	59	15	2

FOOD	PORTION	CAL	FAT	CARB	SUGAR	FIBER
Simmer Sauce Bombay Curry	4 oz	70	3	10	6	2
Fortun's						
Finishing Sauce Mulligatawny Curry	¼ cup (2 oz)	60	2	10	7	1
French Meadow Bakery						
Fragrant Chicken Curry	1 pkg (12 oz)	280	5	36	2	3
Thai Kitchen						
Green Curry Paste	1 tbsp (0.5 oz)	15	0	3	1	0
TAKE-OUT						
beef curry	1 cup	432	31	14	6	3
beef kurma	1 serv (10 oz)	611	47	6	3	6
chicken curry ½ breast	1 serv	160	9	6	3	1
chicken curry boneless	1 serv (6.2 oz)	219	12	8	4	2
chicken curry leg & thigh	1 serv	180	10	7	3	1
chickpea curry	1 serv (8.3 oz)	305	15	23	1	15
eggplant curry	1 serv (8 oz)	241	19	12	–	5
lamb curry	1 cup	257	14	4	1	1
mixed vegetable curry	1 serv (7.7 oz)	398	33	22	–	–
pea & potato curry	1 serv (7 oz)	284	22	19	–	6
pork vandaloo curry	1 serv	620	47	3	–	–
potato curry	1 serv (5.5 oz)	791	60	35	5	14
sambhar dhal curry	1 serv (10 oz)	177	7	21	–	8

CUSK

FOOD	PORTION	CAL	FAT	CARB	SUGAR	FIBER
fillet baked	3 oz	106	1	0	0	0

CUSTARD
MIX

FOOD	PORTION	CAL	FAT	CARB	SUGAR	FIBER
egg custard as prep w/ 2% milk	1 serv (3.5 oz)	112	3	18	5	0
egg custard as prep w/ whole milk	1 serv (3.5 oz)	122	4	18	5	0

FOOD	PORTION	CAL	FAT	CARB	SUGAR	FIBER
flan as prep w/ 2% milk	1 serv (3.5 oz)	103	2	19	–	0
flan as prep w/ whole milk	1 serv (3.5 oz)	113	3	19	–	0
READY-TO-EAT						
Signature						
Flan Coffee	1 pkg (4.5 oz)	340	12	48	47	0
Flan Vanilla	1 pkg (4.5 oz)	350	13	49	49	0
TAKE-OUT						
baked	½ cup (5 oz)	147	6	16	16	0
flan	½ cup (5.4 oz)	222	6	35	35	0
flan de calabaza	1 serv (3.5 oz)	225	10	30	22	tr
flan de coco	½ cup (4.3 oz)	345	13	49	49	tr
flan de pini	½ cup (4.6 oz)	202	6	31	29	tr
puerto rican corn custard	½ cup (4.9 oz)	553	34	65	51	5
puerto rican style	½ cup (4.3 oz)	204	6	31	29	0
tocino del cielo heaven's delight	1 cup	856	21	156	154	0
zabaione	½ cup (2 oz)	135	5	13	–	0
CUTTLEFISH						
steamed	3 oz	134	1	1	–	–
DANDELION GREENS						
fresh cooked	½ cup	17	tr	3	–	–
raw chopped	½ cup	13	tr	3	–	–
DANISH PASTRY						
TAKE-OUT						
cheese	1 (2.5 oz)	266	16	26	5	1

FOOD	PORTION	CAL	FAT	CARB	SUGAR	FIBER
cinnamon	1 (5 oz)	572	32	63	28	2
fruit	1 (5 oz)	527	27	68	39	3
lemon	1 (2.5 oz)	263	13	34	–	1
raisin nut	1 (2.3 oz)	280	16	30	17	1
DATES						
deglet noor chopped	¼ cup (1.3 oz)	104	tr	28	23	3
deglet noor dried	1 (7 g)	20	tr	5	5	1
jujube dried	1 oz	75	tr	19	–	2
jujube fresh	1 oz	30	tr	7	–	–
jujube preserved in sugar	1 oz	91	tr	22	–	–
medjool	1 (0.8 oz)	66	tr	18	16	2
SunDate						
Fancy Medjool	3 (1.4 oz)	120	0	31	25	3
Sun-Maid						
Pitted	¼ cup (1.4 oz)	110	0	30	21	4
Tree Of Life						
Deglet Noor Pitted	5 (1.5 oz)	120	0	31	28	3
Organic Medjool	5 (1.5 oz)	120	0	31	28	3

DEER (see JERKY, VENISON)

DELI MEATS/COLD CUTS (see also BEEF, CHICKEN, HAM, MEAT SUBSTITUTES, TURKEY)

FOOD	PORTION	CAL	FAT	CARB	SUGAR	FIBER
barbecue loaf pork & beef	1 slice (0.8 oz)	40	2	1	–	0
beerwurst beef	2 oz	155	13	2	0	1
berliner pork & beef	1 slice (0.8 oz)	53	4	1	1	0
blood sausage	1 slice (0.9 oz)	95	9	tr	tr	0
bologna beef	1 slice (1 oz)	88	8	1	0	0
bologna beef & pork low fat	1 slice (1 oz)	64	5	1	0	0
bologna beef lowfat	1 slice (1 oz)	57	4	1	0	0

FOOD	PORTION	CAL	FAT	CARB	SUGAR	FIBER
bologna beef reduced sodium	1 slice (1 oz)	88	8	1	0	0
bologna beef & pork	1 slice (1 oz)	87	7	2	1	0
braunschweiger pork	1 slice (1 oz)	92	8	1	0	0
corned beef brisket	2 oz	90	5	0	0	0
dutch brand loaf pork & beef	1 slice (1.3 oz)	104	9	1	0	tr
headcheese pork	1 slice (1.6 oz)	71	5	0	0	0
honey loaf pork & beef	1 slice (1 oz)	35	1	1	0	0
lebanon bologna beef	2 slices (1 oz)	105	6	tr	0	0
mortadella beef & pork	1 slice (0.5 oz)	47	4	tr	0	0
olive loaf pork	2 slices (2 oz)	134	9	5	0	0
pastrami beef	1 slice (1 oz)	41	2	tr	tr	tr
peppered loaf pork & beef	1 slice (1 oz)	41	2	1	0	0
pepperoni pork & beef	15 slices (1 oz)	135	12	1	tr	tr
picnic loaf pork & beef	1 slice (1 oz)	65	5	1	–	0
salami cooked beef & pork	1 slice (0.8 oz)	58	5	1	0	0
salami hard pork	3 slices (0.9 oz)	14	8	1	0	0
salami hard pork & beef less sodium	1 slice (1 oz)	113	9	2	2	tr
sandwich spread pork & beef	¼ cup	141	10	7	0	tr
summer sausage thuringer cervelat	2 oz	203	17	2	tr	0
Applegate Farms						
Organic Genoa Salami Sliced	1 oz	100	7	0	0	0
Butterball						
Turkey Bologna	1 slice (1 oz)	60	5	3	–	–
Turkey Ham	1 slice (1 oz)	35	2	1	–	–

FOOD	PORTION	CAL	FAT	CARB	SUGAR	FIBER
Carl Buddig						
Beef	2 oz	90	5	1	–	–
Corned Beef	2 oz	90	5	1	–	–
Healthy Ones						
Pastrami 97% Fat Free	4 slices (2 oz)	60	2	3	0	0
Oscar Mayer						
Salami Beef	3 slices (1.8 oz)	150	13	1	0	0
DILL						
seed	1 tsp	6	tr	1	–	tr
sprigs fresh	5 (0.3 oz)	0	tr	tr	–	–
weed dry	1 tbsp	8	tr	2	–	tr

DINNER (see also ASIAN FOOD, CURRY, PASTA DINNERS, POT PIE, SPANISH FOOD)

FOOD	PORTION	CAL	FAT	CARB	SUGAR	FIBER
A La Carte						
Stuffed Zucchini w/ Barley Risotto Chicken Stuffing in Tomato Sauce	1 serv (5 oz)	140	7	14	3	2
Amy's						
Country Dinner Vegetable Salisbury Steak	1 pkg (10.9 oz)	380	16	50	7	7
Banquet						
Boneless Pork Ribs	1 pkg	370	17	47	10	4
Chicken Fingers	1 pkg	460	15	69	32	11
Corn Dog Meal	1 pkg	470	18	68	25	8
Crock Pot Classics Chicken & Dumplings	2/3 cup	200	8	21	4	6
Crock Pot Classics Hearty Beef & Vegetables	2/3 cup	140	6	15	4	4

FOOD	PORTION	CAL	FAT	CARB	SUGAR	FIBER
Crock Pot Classics Meatballs In Stroganoff Sauce	2/3 cup	300	14	29	3	5
Fish Sticks	1 pkg	360	13	46	14	3
Fried Beef Steak	1 pkg	390	19	41	5	3
Meatloaf	1 pkg	300	15	28	tr	5
Original Fried Chicken	1 pkg	380	20	35	3	5
Salisbury Steak	1 pkg	300	16	25	2	5
Swedish Meatballs	1 pkg	430	23	35	0	5
Turkey	1 pkg	200	8	27	3	5
Betty Crocker						
Complete Meals Chicken & Buttermilk Biscuits	1/5 pkg (5.4 oz)	280	11	37	3	2
Complete Meals Stroganoff	1/5 pkg (5 oz)	200	5	30	3	1
Birds Eye						
Steamfresh Meals For Two Asian Chicken Vegetable Medley	1/2 pkg (11.9 oz)	290	6	36	13	10
Steamfresh Meals For Two Grilled Chicken Marinara	1/2 pkg (11.9 oz)	360	10	45	9	4
Steamfresh Meals For Two Sweet & Spicy Chicken	1/2 pkg (11.9 oz)	370	10	53	8	4
Fillo Factory						
Organic Fillo Pie Eggplant & Red Pepper	1 serv (5 oz)	230	9	35	5	3
French Meadow Bakery						
Garlic Ginger Chicken	1 pkg (12 oz)	310	5	42	9	3
Gluten Free Cafe						
Lemon Basil Chicken	1 pkg (9.2 oz)	340	11	42	1	3

FOOD	PORTION	CAL	FAT	CARB	SUGAR	FIBER
Green Giant						
Skillet Meal Chicken Teriyaki as prep	1½ cups	240	1	46	8	3
Healthy Choice						
Beef Pot Roast w/ Gravy	1 pkg (11 oz)	310	7	45	21	5
Beef Tips Portabello	1 pkg	300	8	33	14	7
Cafe Steamers Beef Merlot	1 pkg (10 oz)	220	6	22	6	5
Cafe Steamers Cajun Style Chicken & Shrimp	1 pkg (10.4 oz)	250	3	36	3	3
Cafe Steamers Chicken Margherita	1 pkg (10 oz)	340	8	43	8	4
Cafe Steamers Creamy Dill Salmon	1 pkg (9.8 oz)	240	6	26	1	5
Cafe Steamers Grilled Basil Chicken	1 (10.6 oz)	290	6	37	3	5
Cafe Steamers Grilled Whiskey Steak	1 pkg (9.4 oz)	250	4	34	14	6
Chicken Parmigiana	1 pkg (11.6 oz)	350	9	48	16	7
Country Herb Chicken	1 pkg (11.35 oz)	240	5	34	15	5
Fresh Mixers Southwestern Chicken	1 pkg (7.9 oz)	310	3	60	3	5
Lemon Pepper Fish	1 pkg (10.7 oz)	310	5	53	14	5
Mandarin Chicken	1 pkg (9.1 oz)	240	3	39	9	5
Salisbury Steak	1 pkg (12.5 oz)	360	9	46	19	7
Slow Roasted Turkey Medallions	1 pkg (8.5 oz)	220	5	28	14	5
Sweet & Sour Chicken	1 pkg (12 oz)	430	9	69	29	5
Traditional Turkey Breast	1 pkg	300	4	42	20	6

FOOD	PORTION	CAL	FAT	CARB	SUGAR	FIBER
Hormel						
Compleats Microwave Meals Beef Steak & Peppers w/ Noodles	1 pkg (9.9 oz)	210	5	22	4	2
Compleats Microwave Meals Chicken Breast & Dressing	1 pkg (9.9 oz)	270	7	29	3	2
Compleats Microwave Meals Chicken Breast & Gravy w/ Mashed Potatoes	1 pkg (9.9 oz)	200	3	24	3	2
Compleats Microwave Meals Homestyle Beef w/ Potatoes & Gravy	1 pkg (9.9 oz)	220	6	30	2	3
Compleats Microwave Meals Meatloaf w/ Potatoes & Gravy	1 pkg (9.9 oz)	310	11	34	3	3
Compleats Microwave Meals Salisbury Steak w/ Slice Potato & Gravy	1 pkg (9.9 oz)	280	11	30	1	2
Compleats Microwave Meals Santa Fe Chicken w/ Rice & Beans	1 pkg (9.9 oz)	280	4	41	6	4
Compleats Microwave Meals Swedish Meatballs	1 pkg (9.9 oz)	350	18	32	4	1
Compleats Microwave Meals Sweet & Sour Chicken w/ Rice	1 pkg (9.9 oz)	290	2	54	23	2
Compleats Microwave Meals Tuna Casserole	1 pkg (9.9 oz)	240	7	26	3	2

FOOD	PORTION	CAL	FAT	CARB	SUGAR	FIBER
Compleats Microwave Meals Turkey & Dressing w/ Gravy	1 pkg (9.9 oz)	290	9	31	4	2
Compleats Microwave Meals Turkey & Hearty Vegetables	1 pkg (9.9 oz)	180	4	24	3	4
Compleats Mircowave Meals Teriyaki Chicken w/ Rice	1 pkg (9.9 oz)	270	2	50	20	2
Joy Of Cooking						
Braised Beef Tips & Egg Noodles	1 cup (7.7 oz)	220	7	24	3	1
Roasted Herb Chicken	1 cup (7.7 oz)	170	3	27	4	3
Lean Cuisine						
Cafe Classics Sweet & Sour Chicken	1 pkg (10 oz)	300	3	51	20	2
Marie Callender's						
Chicken Fried Beef	1 meal	540	28	51	11	6
Chicken Teriyaki	1 meal	430	4	78	27	5
Golden Battered Filet Dinner	1 meal	450	16	53	9	4
Herb Roasted Chicken	1 meal	460	25	26	3	5
Meat Loaf w/ Gravy	1 meal	480	22	39	6	3
Old Fashioned Beef Pot Roast	1 meal	330	10	32	tr	9
Salisbury Steak	1 meal	400	16	38	6	7
Slow Roasted Beef	1 meal	370	13	37	6	7
Sweet & Sour Chicken	1 meal	600	20	88	28	10
Turkey w/ Stuffing	1 meal	400	9	45	9	4
Mon Cuisine						
Vegan Moroccan Couscous	1 pkg (10 oz)	280	4	46	10	10

FOOD	PORTION	CAL	FAT	CARB	SUGAR	FIBER
Vegan Veal Schnitzel In Sauce	1 pkg (10 oz)	300	8	38	2	7
Vegetarian Stuffed Cabbage In Tomato Sauce	1 pkg (10 oz)	220	5	36	8	5
Moosewood						
Organic Vegetarian Moroccan Stew	1 pkg (10 oz)	150	3	29	11	5
Organic Bistro						
Chicken Citron	1 pkg (13.5 oz)	490	17	53	15	6
Ginger Chicken	1 pkg (13.25 oz)	490	17	53	15	6
Jamaican Shrimp Cakes	1 pkg (12 oz)	380	8	55	10	7
Savory Turkey	1 pkg (12 oz)	430	14	43	5	8
Sockeye Salmon Cakes	1 pkg (12.2 oz)	600	36	36	7	8
Spiced Chicken Morocco	1 pkg (12.2 oz)	390	11	46	5	7
Wild Salmon	1 pkg (13.1 oz)	500	23	41	7	8
Organic Classics						
Chicken Marsala w/ Mashed Potatoes	1 pkg (9.5 oz)	330	16	31	3	3
Jamaican Style Jerk Chicken w/ Wehani Rice	1 pkg (9.5 oz)	270	7	37	8	4
Lemon Chicken w/ Wehani Rice	1 pkg (9.5 oz)	320	8	49	1	3
South Beach						
Chicken Santa Fe Style Rice & Beans	1 pkg (8.9 oz)	340	12	35	3	4
Meatloaf w/ Gravy	1 pkg (8.9 oz)	210	9	17	5	4
Roasted Turkey	1 pkg (9.4 oz)	240	9	27	2	4

FOOD	PORTION	CAL	FAT	CARB	SUGAR	FIBER
Sukhis						
Tikka Masala Chicken	1 serv (5 oz)	170	6	46	2	0
Taste Above						
Meatless Zesty BBQ w/ Veggie Beef & Rice	1 pkg (10 oz)	280	6	48	18	7
DIP						
spinach sour cream	¼ cup	155	15	4	1	1
Cabot						
French Onion	2 tbsp	50	5	1	0	0
Ranch	2 tbsp	50	5	1	1	0
Cedarlane						
Organic Five Layer Mexican	2 tbsp	60	3	4	2	1
Emerald Valley						
Organic Black Bean	1 tbsp (1 oz)	45	2	6	0	1
Guiltless Gourmet						
Black Bean Mild	2 tbsp (1.1 oz)	40	0	7	0	2
Health Is Wealth						
Vegetarian Spinach & Artichoke	3 tbsp (1 oz)	30	2	3	2	0
Kraft						
Green Onion	2 tbsp	60	5	3	tr	0
LiteHouse						
Avocado	2 tbsp	140	15	2	1	0
Caramel Low Fat	1 tbsp	110	0	27	16	0
Caramel Original	2 tbsp	110	2	25	15	1
Dilly	2 tbsp	150	16	1	1	0
Fruit Dip Chocolate Yogurt	2 tbsp	110	6	14	9	0
Fruit Dip Vanilla Yogurt	2 tbsp	60	2	10	7	0
Lite Ranch Veggie	2 tbsp	70	7	3	1	0
Organic Ranch	2 tbsp	130	13	2	2	0

FOOD	PORTION	CAL	FAT	CARB	SUGAR	FIBER
Naturally Fresh						
Caramel	2 tbsp	100	4	15	13	0
Chocolate	2 tbsp	70	0	17	14	0
Cream Cheese Strawberry	2 tbsp	90	4	14	10	0
Ranch Lite	2 tbsp	80	8	2	1	0
Ranch Vegetable	2 tbsp	120	12	2	1	0
Utz						
Jalapeno Cheddar	2 tbsp	260	4	2	0	0
Sour Cream & Onion	2 tbsp	60	5	2	1	0
Wild Thymes Farm						
Indian Vindaloo Curry	1 tbsp	12	1	1	tr	tr
Indonesian Peanut Sauce	1 tbsp	32	2	2	1	tr
DOCK						
fresh cooked	3½ oz	20	1	3	–	–
raw chopped	½ cup	15	tr	2	–	–
DOUGHNUTS						
chocolate glazed	1 med (1.5 oz)	175	8	24	13	1
chocolate w/ chocolate icing	1 med (2 oz)	218	12	26	13	1
creme filled	1 (3 oz)	307	21	26	12	1
custard filled	1 (2.3 oz)	235	16	20	9	1
french cruller glazed	1 med (1.4 oz)	169	8	24	14	1
jelly filled	1 (3 oz)	289	16	33	18	1
old fashioned plain	1 med (2 oz)	226	13	25	9	1
oriental okinawan	1 (0.6 oz)	75	4	10	4	tr
plain chocolate frosted	1 med (1.5 oz)	194	11	22	11	1
plain glazed	1 med (1.6 oz)	192	10	23	–	1
whole wheat sugared	1 med (1.6 oz)	162	9	19	10	1

FOOD	PORTION	CAL	FAT	CARB	SUGAR	FIBER
Entenmann's						
PoP'ettes Chocolate Frosted	3 (2.2 oz)	330	24	28	16	1
DRINK MIXERS						
whiskey sour mix not prep	1 pkg (0.6 oz)	64	0	16	–	–
whiskey sour mix	2 oz	55	0	14	–	0
Angostura						
Bloody Mary	4 oz	20	0	4	1	0
Daiquiri	2 oz	72	0	18	18	0
Grenadine	1 tsp	10	0	3	3	0
Margarita	4 oz	80	0	30	28	0
Pina Colada	4 oz	60	0	16	16	0
Strawberry Daiquita	8 oz	120	0	31	31	0
Dave's Gourmet						
Bloody Mary Original	2 oz	25	0	5	3	tr
DRUM						
freshwater fillet baked	5.4 oz	236	10	0	0	0
freshwater baked	3 oz	130	5	0	0	0
DUCK						
boneless roasted	½ duck (7.8 oz)	444	25	0	0	0
boneless w/o skin roasted	3.5 oz	201	11	0	0	0
boneless w/o skin roasted diced	1 cup (4.9 oz)	281	16	0	0	0
chinese pressed	1 cup (4.9 oz)	267	14	26	14	1
chinese pressed	3 oz	162	8	16	9	1
pekin breast boneless w/ skin roasted	1 (4.2 oz)	242	13	0	0	0
pekin breast w/o skin broiled	3 oz	133	2	0	0	0

FOOD	PORTION	CAL	FAT	CARB	SUGAR	FIBER
pekin leg w/ skin w/o bone roasted	1 (3.2 oz)	200	10	0	0	0
pekin leg w/o skin & bone roasted	1 (2.6 oz)	134	5	0	0	0
w/ skin & bone roasted	1 serv (6 oz)	583	49	0	0	0
w/ skin & bone roasted	½ duck (13 oz)	1287	108	0	0	0
wing roasted bone removed	1 (1.1 oz)	101	8	0	0	0
Grimaud Farms						
Muscovy Duck Confit	1 serv (3 oz)	170	10	tr	–	–
Muscovy Duck Whole	1 serv (3.7 oz)	200	14	tr	–	–
TAKE-OUT						
breast battered & fried bone removed	½ (3.2 oz)	199	10	6	tr	tr
leg battered & fried bone removed	1 (2.5 oz)	155	8	5	tr	tr

DUMPLING

FOOD	PORTION	CAL	FAT	CARB	SUGAR	FIBER
Health Is Wealth						
Potstickers Vegan	2 (1.6 oz)	90	3	13	tr	2
Joyce Chen						
Chinese Style Potstickers Chicken & Vegetable	6	170	2	30	2	2
Chinese Style Potstickers Pork & Vegetable	6	170	3	30	2	2
TAKE-OUT						
apple	1 (6.7 oz)	661	34	83	30	3
bread dumpling	1 lg	330	10	28	–	–
cherry	1 (2.7 oz)	238	12	31	13	1
cornmeal	1 (2.8 oz)	134	4	20	1	2
fried pork	1 (3.5 oz)	338	21	25	1	1
fried puerto rican style	1 med (1.1 oz)	117	7	11	1	tr

FOOD	PORTION	CAL	FAT	CARB	SUGAR	FIBER
gyoza potstickers vegetable	8 (4.9 oz)	210	4	34	7	5
peach	1 (2.7 oz)	253	12	33	12	1
piroshki meat filled	1 (3.4 oz)	348	22	25	tr	1
steamed meat	1 (1.3 oz)	41	1	4	tr	tr

DURIAN
fresh	3.5 oz	141	2	29	–	–

EDAMAME (see SOYBEANS)

EEL
fresh cooked	3 oz	200	13	0	0	0
fresh cooked	1 fillet (5.6 oz)	375	24	0	0	0
raw	3 oz	156	10	0	0	0
smoked	3.5 oz	330	28	0	0	0

EGG (see also EGG DISHES, EGG SUBSTITUTES)
CHICKEN
hard or soft cooked	1	77	5	1	1	0
pickled	1	72	5	1	1	0
poached	1	73	5	tr	tr	0
scrambled plain	2	199	15	2	–	0
sunny side up	2	155	12	1	1	0
white cooked	1	17	tr	tr	tr	0
yolk cooked	1	55	4	1	tr	0

Egg Innovations
100% Organic Cage Free Large	1 (1.8 oz)	70	5	1	0	0

Good Earth Organics
Organic Instant Whites	1 pkg (0.5 oz)	50	0	1	1	0

Pete & Gerry's
Organic Large	1 (1.8 oz)	70	5	1	–	–

FOOD	PORTION	CAL	FAT	CARB	SUGAR	FIBER
Tree Of Life						
White Large Natural Omega-3	1 (1.8 oz)	70	5	tr	0	0
OTHER POULTRY						
duck 100 year old	1 (1 oz)	49	3	1	–	–
duck cooked	1 (2.5 oz)	129	10	1	1	0
duck preserved hard core	1 (1.8 oz)	80	6	1	0	0
duck preserved soft core	1 (1.8 oz)	80	6	1	0	0
duck salted	1 (1 oz)	54	4	2	–	–
goose cooked	1 (5 oz)	265	19	2	1	0
quail canned	1 (0.3 oz)	14	1	tr	tr	0
quail cooked	1 (0.5 oz)	24	2	0	0	0
turkey raw	1 (2.8 oz)	135	9	1	–	0
EGG DISHES						
Cedarlane						
Zone Omelette Cheese	1 pkg (10.4 oz)	350	14	31	5	2
Jimmy Dean						
Breakfast Skillets Bacon as prep	1 serv (4.5 oz)	370	24	14	2	2
Breakfast Skillets Ham as prep	1 serv (4.5 oz)	270	15	16	1	2
Breakfast Skillets Smoked Sausage as prep	1 serv (4.5 oz)	380	25	20	1	3
Breakfast Bowls D-Lights Sausage	1 pkg	230	7	19	1	2
Breakfast Bowls Eggs Potato & Ham	1 pkg	390	23	23	1	3
Breakfast Bowls Eggs Potatoes Sausage & Cheddar Cheese	1 pkg	490	34	20	1	3

FOOD	PORTION	CAL	FAT	CARB	SUGAR	FIBER
Omelets Ham & Cheese	1 (4.2 oz)	280	19	4	1	0
Omelets Sausage & Cheese	1 (4.3 oz)	270	22	5	1	0
TAKE-OUT						
deviled	1 half	62	5	tr	tr	0
eggs benedict	2	825	64	26	3	2
omelet cheese	3 eggs	387	29	6	6	0
omelet mushroom	3 eggs	251	17	6	4	1
omelet mushroom & onion	3 eggs	294	20	7	5	1
omelet plain	3 eggs	338	25	4	4	0
omelet spanish	3 eggs	496	38	17	11	3
omelet spinach	3 eggs	279	19	6	4	1
omelet western	3 eggs	355	23	6	4	tr
salad	½ cup	353	34	2	1	0
scotch egg	1 (4.2 oz)	301	21	16	–	2
tortilla de amarillo omelet w/ plantain	3 eggs	536	35	43	21	3

EGG ROLLS

FOOD	PORTION	CAL	FAT	CARB	SUGAR	FIBER
egg roll wrapper fresh	1 (1.1 oz)	93	tr	19	–	1
spring roll deep fried	1 (0.8 oz)	70	4	7	–	1
Blue Horizon Organic						
Spring Rolls Chinese Shrimp	3 (2.1 oz)	130	4	16	1	1
Spring Rolls Indian	3 (2.1 oz)	110	4	15	1	1
Spring Rolls Thai	3 (2.1 oz)	110	4	16	1	1
Spring Rolls Thai Shrimp	3 (2.1 oz)	130	4	15	1	1
Health Is Wealth						
Spinach	1 (3 oz)	170	8	18	1	3
Thai Spring Roll	2 (1.6 oz)	90	3	13	1	1
TAKE-OUT						
chicken	1 (3 oz)	140	4	20	5	4

FOOD	PORTION	CAL	FAT	CARB	SUGAR	FIBER
lobster	1 (4.8 oz)	270	7	43	4	6
lumpia vegetable & shrimp	2 (3 oz)	120	0	26	1	2
meat & shrimp	1 (4.8 oz)	320	12	41	3	4
pork & shrimp	1 (5 oz)	300	10	41	6	7
shrimp	1 (3 oz)	170	5	24	5	5
spicy pork	1 (3 oz)	200	9	23	3	3
vegetable	1 (3 oz)	170	4	28	4	4

EGG SUBSTITUTES
Egg Beaters
Original	¼ cup (2.1 oz)	30	0	1	tr	0

Quick Eggs
Fat Free Cholesterol Free	¼ cup	30	0	1	tr	0

EGGNOG
eggnog	1 cup	342	19	34	–	–
eggnog	1 qt	1368	76	138	–	–
eggnog flavor mix as prep w/ milk	9 oz	260	8	39	–	–

Straus
Organic Cream Top	4 oz	160	10	13	13	0

TAKE-OUT
eggnog	1 cup	306	22	16	–	0

EGGNOG SUBSTITUTES
Silk
Nog	½ cup (4 oz)	90	2	15	12	0

EGGPLANT
cubed cooked w/ oil	1 cup	133	8	17	6	5
pickled	½ cup	33	tr	7	3	2
slices grilled	1 (2 oz)	36	2	5	2	1

FOOD	PORTION	CAL	FAT	CARB	SUGAR	FIBER
Cedarlane						
Eggplant Mediterranean	1 pkg (10 oz)	230	10	22	7	6
The Gracious Gourmet						
Tapenade Roasted Eggplant	2 tbsp (1 oz)	35	4	3	1	tr
TAKE-OUT						
baba ghannouj	¼ cup	55	4	5	–	–
caponata	2 tbsp (1 oz)	30	2	3	2	–
iman bayildi eggplant w/ onion & tomato	1 serv (15.6 oz)	345	28	25	6	2
indian eggplant runi	1 serv	180	14	13	1	1
moussaka	1 serv (9 oz)	372	24	18	6	5
papoutsaki little shoes	1 serv (15.5 oz)	245	16	15	1	1
tempura	1 serv (1.5 oz)	118	10	5	0	1
ELDERBERRIES						
fresh	1 cup	105	1	27	–	–
ELDERBERRY JUICE						
elderberry	7 oz	76	0	16	–	–
ELK						
eye of round roasted	3.5 oz	151	3	1	0	0
ground cooked	3.5 oz	143	3	0	0	0
Natural Frontier Foods						
Filet	1 (4 oz)	140	3	0	0	0
ENERGY BARS (*see also* CEREAL BARS, NUTRITION SUPPLEMENTS)						
Balance						
100 Calories Peanut Butter Crisp	1 (1 oz)	100	5	14	4	5
100 Calories Vanilla Crisp	1 (1 oz)	100	4	15	5	5

FOOD	PORTION	CAL	FAT	CARB	SUGAR	FIBER
Carbwell Chocolate Fudge	1 (1.8 oz)	190	6	23	1	2
Gold Chocolate Peanut Butter	1 (1.8 oz)	210	6	23	14	tr
Gold S'mores Crunch	1 (1.8 oz)	210	6	23	12	0
Organic Apricot Mango Crisp	1 (1.6 oz)	180	7	23	11	5
Organic Cranberry Pomegranate Crisp	1 (1.6 oz)	180	7	23	12	5
Original Almond Brownie	1 (1.8 oz)	200	6	22	17	2
Original Mocha Crisp	1 (1.8 oz)	200	6	21	18	tr
Pure Banana Cashew	1 (1.6 oz)	180	6	23	18	2
Pure Cherry Pecan	1 (1.6 oz)	190	7	22	18	2
Clif						
Apricot	1 (2.4 oz)	230	3	45	21	5
Black Cherry Almond	1 (2.4 oz)	250	5	44	20	5
Builders Chocolate	1 (2.4 oz)	270	8	30	20	4
Builders Lemon	1 (2.4 oz)	270	8	31	23	1
Chocolate Almond Fudge	1 (2.4 oz)	250	5	44	20	5
Chocolate Chip Peanut Crunch	1 (2.4 oz)	260	6	42	21	5
Crunchy Peanut Butter	1 (2.4 oz)	250	6	42	20	5
Mojo Chocolate Peanut	1 (1.6 oz)	210	10	22	11	3
Mojo Honey Roasted Peanuts	1 (1.6 oz)	200	10	20	9	2
Mojo Mountain Mix	1 (1.6 oz)	180	8	21	12	2
Mojo Peanut Butter & Jelly	1 (1.6 oz)	220	11	21	12	2
Nectar Cherry Pomegranate	1 (1.6 oz)	150	5	29	20	7

FOOD	PORTION	CAL	FAT	CARB	SUGAR	FIBER
Nectar Dark Chocolate Walnut	1 (1.6 oz)	160	6	27	18	6
Oatmeal Raisin Walnut	1 (2.4 oz)	240	5	43	20	5
Spiced Pumpkin Pie	1 (2.4 oz)	240	5	45	23	5
Vanilla Almond	1 (2.4 oz)	270	8	30	22	3
ZBar Blueberry	1 (1.3 oz)	120	3	23	11	3
ZBar Honey Graham	1 (1.3 oz)	130	3	26	10	3
ZBar Spooky S'mores	1 (1.3 oz)	130	4	23	11	3
Gnu						
Flavor & Fiber Chocolate Brownie Bar	1 (1.4 oz)	140	3	32	9	12
Green SuperFood						
Whole Food	1 (2.1 oz)	220	8	36	25	4
Whole Food Chocolate	1 (2.1 oz)	230	9	37	27	0
LaraBar						
Jocalat Chocolate	1 (1.7 oz)	190	10	24	18	5
Lean Body						
Gold Caramel Cookie Twist	1 (2.9 oz)	330	7	36	10	2
Luna						
Berry Almond	1 (1.7 oz)	170	4	29	11	3
Chai Tea	1 (1.7 oz)	190	5	26	12	3
Dulce De Leche	1 (1.7 oz)	170	4	28	13	3
Mini Caramel Nut Brownie	1 (0.7 oz)	70	3	11	5	2
Mini S'mores	1 (0.7 oz)	80	2	11	5	1
Sunrise Apple Cinnamon	1 (1.7 oz)	180	5	27	11	5
Sunrise Strawberry Crunch	1 (1.7 oz)	170	5	26	12	5
Toasted Nuts 'N Cranberry	1 (1.7 oz)	170	5	26	11	3
Mrs. May's						
Trio Tropical	1 (1.2 oz)	170	12	14	6	2

FOOD	PORTION	CAL	FAT	CARB	SUGAR	FIBER
Sencha Naturals						
Green Tea Bar Lively Lemongrass	1 (2 oz)	220	8	29	12	3
Green Tea Bar Original	1 (2 oz)	220	9	29	12	3
South Beach						
Energy Mix	1 pkg (1 oz)	160	13	8	3	2
Think5						
Red Berry	1 (2.5 oz)	240	4	48	7	3

ENERGY DRINKS

FOOD	PORTION	CAL	FAT	CARB	SUGAR	FIBER
180						
Blue w/ Acai	1 can (8.2 oz)	120	0	31	–	–
Blue w/ Acai Low Calorie	1 can (8.2 oz)	15	0	4	–	–
Orange Citrus Blast	1 can (8.2 oz)	120	0	33	–	–
Orange Citrus Blast Sugar Free	1 can (8.2 oz)	5	0	1	–	–
Red w/ Gogi	1 can (8.2 oz)	130	0	31	–	–
Bai						
Antioxidant Infusion Jamaica Blueberry	8 oz	70	0	18	18	–
Antioxidant Infusion Mango Kauai	8 oz	70	0	18	18	–
Antioxidant Infustion Kenya Peach	8 oz	70	0	17	17	–
Boost						
Beauty	1 bottle (12 oz)	220	0	52	40	tr
Youth	1 bottle (12 oz)	200	0	48	36	tr
Boozer						
Hangover Remedy	1 can (8.4 oz)	110	0	28	28	–
Clif						
Quench Fruit Punch	8 oz	45	0	11	10	0
Quench Orange	8 oz	45	0	11	10	0

FOOD	PORTION	CAL	FAT	CARB	SUGAR	FIBER
Dr. Tim's						
ISO-5	1 bottle (11.2 oz)	60	0	15	15	–
Jungle Juice	1 bottle (4 oz)	20	0	8	4	0
Fuze						
Refresh Banana Coconut	8 oz	90	0	25	23	–
Refresh Peach Mango	8 oz	90	0	23	22	–
Refresh Strawberry Banana	8 oz	100	0	25	24	–
Slenderize Cranberry Raspberry	8 oz	5	0	2	1	–
Slenderize Low Carb Tropical Punch	8 oz	5	0	tr	0	–
Slenderize Tangerine Grapefruit	8 oz	10	0	2	1	–
Vitalize Blackberry Grape	8 oz	100	0	26	25	–
Vitalize Orange Mango	8 oz	100	0	25	25	–
Ginger Boost						
Ginger Orange	8 oz	110	0	24	21	1
Go Girl						
Bliss	1 can (11.5 oz)	35	0	8	8	–
Glo	1 can (12 oz)	35	0	9	8	0
Sugar Free	1 can (12 oz)	<5	0	tr	0	–
Hiro						
Thermo	1 can (8.33 oz)	10	0	2	tr	–
Vitality	1 can (8.33 oz)	10	0	2	1	–
IChill						
Relaxation Shot Blissful Berry	1 bottle (2 oz)	0	0	0	0	0
Kidstrong						
All Flavors	8 oz	30	0	7	3	1

FOOD	PORTION	CAL	FAT	CARB	SUGAR	FIBER
King 888						
Original	8 oz	110	0	28	28	–
Sugar Free	8 oz	0	0	0	0	0
Me						
Curious Blueberry Lime	1 can	70	0	17	16	–
Vivacious Tangerine Pineapple	1 can	70	0	17	17	–
Neuro						
Bliss	1 bottle (14.5 oz)	35	0	9	9	–
Gasm	1 bottle (14.5 oz)	35	0	9	9	–
Sleep	1 bottle (14.5 oz)	35	0	9	9	–
Sonic	1 bottle (14.5 oz)	35	0	9	9	–
Sport	1 bottle (14.5 oz)	35	0	9	9	–
Trim	1 bottle (14.5 oz)	35	0	9	9	1
NOS						
High Performance	1 bottle (11 oz)	150	0	38	37	–
Ocean Spray						
Cranergy Cranberry Lift	1 bottle (12 oz)	50	0	12	12	–
Cranergy Raspberry Cranberry Lift	1 bottle (12 oz)	50	0	13	13	–
OOBA						
All Flavors	8 oz	90	0	22	20	–
Quench Aid						
Berry	1 pkg	10	0	2	2	–
Dragonfruit	1 pkg	10	0	2	2	–

FOOD	PORTION	CAL	FAT	CARB	SUGAR	FIBER
T-Fusion						
Energy Tea	8 oz	0	0	1	0	0
Therafizz						
Vitamin C	1 pkg	5	0	tr	–	–
UnderWay						
Appetite Suppressing All Flavors	8 oz	10	0	2	–	1
Venga						
Brainstorm	8 oz	130	0	31	29	–
Calorie Burn	8 oz	10	0	2	–	–
Energize	8 oz	100	0	24	24	–
Health&Zen	8 oz	80	0	20	20	–
VIB						
Chill-N	1 can (8 oz)	40	0	10	10	0
XOOD						
Endurance Drink All Flavors as prep	1 serv	135	0	30	10	–
Zenergize						
Chill	1 tablet	2	0	1	0	0
Energy+	1 tablet	2	0	1	0	0
Hydrate	1 tablet	2	0	1	0	0
ENGLISH MUFFIN						
READY-TO-EAT						
apple cinnamon	1	138	2	28	–	–
crumpets	1 (1.5 oz)	80	0	16	1	tr
granola	1	155	1	31	–	–
mixed grain	1	155	1	31	–	–
plain	1	134	1	26	–	–
plain toasted	1	133	1	26	–	–
raisin cinnamon	1	138	2	28	–	–
sourdough	1	134	1	26	–	–
wheat	1	127	1	26	–	–
whole wheat	1	134	1	27	–	4

FOOD	PORTION	CAL	FAT	CARB	SUGAR	FIBER
Aunt Gussie's						
Gluten Free Cinnamon Raisin	1 (3 oz)	200	3	41	8	4
Gluten Free Original	1 (3 oz)	200	3	41	6	4
Fiber One						
100% Whole Wheat	1 (2 oz)	100	0	22	3	6
Milton's						
Healthy Multi-Grain	1 (2 oz)	150	1	33	7	3
Roman Meal						
English Muffin	1 (2.3 oz)	140	1	29	4	3
Sun-Maid						
Raisin	1 (2.5 oz)	170	1	36	13	2
Thomas'						
Griller Multi Grain	1 (3.2 oz)	210	2	41	5	3
Griller Onion	1 (3.2 oz)	200	1	40	2	2
TAKE-OUT						
w/ butter	1 (2.2 oz)	189	6	30	–	–
w/ cheese & sausage	1 (4 oz)	393	24	29	–	–
w/ egg cheese & canadian bacon	1 (4.8 oz)	289	13	28	–	2
w/ egg cheese & sausage	1 (5.8 oz)	487	31	31	–	–
EPAZOTE						
fresh	1 tbsp (1 g)	tr	0	tr	–	tr
fresh sprig	1 (2 g)	1	tr	tr	–	tr
EPPAW						
raw	½ cup	75	1	16	–	–
FALAFEL						
Near East						
Falafel Patties Vegetarian as prep	2.5	220	13	18	3	5
TAKE-OUT						
falafel	1 (1.2 oz)	57	3	5	–	–

FOOD	PORTION	CAL	FAT	CARB	SUGAR	FIBER
FAT (*see also* BUTTER, BUTTER SUBSTITUTES, MARGARINE, OIL)						
bacon grease	1 tbsp	116	13	0	0	0
beef shortening	1 tbsp	115	13	0	0	0
beef suet	1 oz	242	27	0	0	0
chicken	1 tbsp (0.4 oz)	115	13	0	0	0
duck	1 tbsp (0.4 oz)	113	13	0	0	0
goose	1 oz	257	29	0	0	0
goose	1 tbsp	115	13	0	0	0
lamb new zealand	1 oz	182	19	0	0	0
lard	1 tbsp (0.5 oz)	115	13	0	0	0
lard	1 cup (7.2 oz)	1849	205	0	0	0
meat pan drippings	½ tbsp	124	14	0	0	0
pork raw	1 oz	230	25	0	0	0
salt pork	1 cube (1 oz)	215	23	0	0	0
shortening	1 tbsp	113	13	0	0	0
shortening	1 cup	1812	205	0	0	0
turkey	1 tbsp	116	13	0	0	0
ucuhuba butter	1 tbsp	120	14	0	0	0
whale blubber	1 oz	248	28	0	0	0
Crisco						
Butter Flavor	1 tbsp	110	12	0	0	0
Shortening	1 tbsp	110	12	0	0	0
Earth Balance						
Natural Shortening	1 tbsp	130	14	0	0	0
FAVA BEANS						
canned	½ cup	91	tr	16	–	–
fava fresh cooked	½ cup	94	tr	17	2	5
Progresso						
Fava Beans	½ cup (4.6 oz)	100	1	17	–	5

FOOD	PORTION	CAL	FAT	CARB	SUGAR	FIBER
FEIJOA						
fresh	1 (1.75 oz)	25	tr	5	–	–
puree	1 cup	119	2	26	–	–
FENNEL						
fresh bulb	1 (8.2 oz)	73	tr	17	–	7
fresh sliced	1 cup	27	tr	6	–	3
leaves	1 oz	7	tr	1	–	1
seed	1 tsp	7	tr	1	–	1
stir fried	1 cup	85	6	9	5	3
Ocean Mist						
Fennel Sweet Anise Sliced Fresh	1 cup	27	1	6	0	3
FENUGREEK						
seed	1 tsp	12	tr	2	–	1
FIBER						
Fiber Supreme						
Fiber	1 round tbsp (0.5 oz)	36	tr	12	0	7
ND Labs						
Apple Fiber	1 round tbsp (7 g)	15	tr	7	0	4
Liquid Fiber Flow	1 tbsp (0.5 oz)	42	0	11	0	7
FIDDLEHEAD FERNS						
fresh	3.5 oz	34	tr	6	–	–
FIG JUICE						
Smart Juice						
Organic 100% Juice	8 oz	131	0	35	29	1
FIGS						
calimyrna	3 (5.4 oz)	120	0	28	11	4
canned in heavy syrup	½ cup	114	tr	30	27	3
canned in light syrup	½ cup	87	tr	23	20	2

FOOD	PORTION	CAL	FAT	CARB	SUGAR	FIBER
canned water pack	½ cup	66	tr	17	15	3
dried california	½ cup (3.5 oz)	200	1	58	–	17
dried cooked	½ cup	139	1	36	30	5
dried small	1 (1.4 oz)	30	tr	8	7	1
dried whole	1 (8 g)	21	tr	5	4	1
fresh large	1 (2.2 oz)	47	tr	12	10	2
California Fresh						
fresh	3 (5.4 oz)	120	0	31	25	4
Hermes						
Organic Adriatic Fig Spread	1 tbsp	60	0	15	14	0
Nuta Figs						
Mission	¼ cup (1.4 oz)	110	0	26	20	5
Orchard Choice						
Mission	4–5 (1.4 oz)	110	0	26	20	5
Sun-Maid						
California Mission	4 (1.5 oz)	120	0	28	21	5
Calimyrna	3 (1.5 oz)	120	0	28	21	5
FIREWEED						
leaves chopped	1 cup (0.8 oz)	24	1	4	–	2
FISH (see also individual names, SUSHI)						
FROZEN						
breaded fillet	1 (2 oz)	155	7	14	–	–
sticks	1 stick (1 oz)	76	3	7	–	–
Dr. Praeger's						
Breaded Fillets	1 (2.1 oz)	100	4	12	1	0
Fishies	3 (1.5 oz)	90	4	9	1	0
Gorton's						
Classic Crispy Battered Fillets	2	230	10	22	3	5

FOOD	PORTION	CAL	FAT	CARB	SUGAR	FIBER
Classic Crunchy Golden Fillets	2	140	12	23	5	–
Fillets Beer Battered	2 (3.6 oz)	250	17	17	4	1
Fillets Breaded Lemon Herb	2 (3.6 oz)	240	13	21	4	–
Fillets Potato Crunch	2 (3.6 oz)	240	14	20	3	2
Fish Sticks Classic Breaded	6	290	18	19	2	1
Grilled Fillets Cajun Blackened	1 (3.8 oz)	100	3	1	0	0
Grilled Fillets Lemon Pepper	1 (3.7 oz)	100	3	1	0	0
Tenders Original Batter	3 pieces (3.6 oz)	230	12	23	3	2
TAKE-OUT						
fish cake	1 (4.7 oz)	166	7	6	–	–
jamaican brown fish stew	1 serv	426	22	9	–	2
kedgeree	5.6 oz	242	11	15	–	1
mousse	1 serv (3.5 oz)	185	14	3	tr	tr
stew	1 cup (7.9 oz)	157	4	10	–	–
taramasalata	2 tbsp	124	14	1	–	–
FISH OIL						
cod liver	1 tbsp	123	14	0	0	0
herring	1 tbsp	123	14	0	0	0
menhaden	1 tbsp	123	14	0	0	0
salmon	1 tbsp	123	14	0	0	0
sardine	1 tbsp	123	14	0	0	0
shark	1 oz	270	29	0	0	0
whale beluga	1 oz	256	29	0	0	0
whale bowhead	1 oz	252	28	0	0	0

FOOD	PORTION	CAL	FAT	CARB	SUGAR	FIBER
Nordic Naturals						
Omega-3 Effervescent as prep	1 pkg (9.7 g)	39	2	3	–	–
FISH PASTE						
fish paste	2 tsp	15	1	tr	–	0
FLAXSEED						
Flax USA						
Flax Sprinkles	2 tbsp (0.5 oz)	70	5	4	0	3
Natural Ovens						
Flax Complete Supplement	1 tbsp (0.4 oz)	60	4	4	1	2
Tree Of Life						
Flax Seed	3 tbsp (1 oz)	140	10	11	0	6
FLOUNDER						
FRESH						
cooked	3 oz	99	1	0	0	0
cooked	1 fillet (4.5 oz)	148	2	0	0	0
TAKE-OUT						
breaded & fried	3.2 oz	211	11	15	–	–
stuffed w/ crab	1 piece (7.6 oz)	332	11	14	2	1
FLOUR						
all-purpose self-rising	½ cup (2.2 oz)	221	1	46	tr	2
all-purpose unbleached	½ cup (2.2 oz)	228	1	48	tr	2
arrowroot	½ cup (2.2 oz)	228	tr	56	–	2
bread flour	½ cup (2.4 oz)	247	1	50	tr	2

FOOD	PORTION	CAL	FAT	CARB	SUGAR	FIBER
buckwheat whole groat	½ cup (2.1 oz)	201	2	42	2	6
cake	½ cup (2.4 oz)	248	1	53	tr	1
carob	½ cup (1.8 oz)	114	tr	46	25	21
carob	1 tbsp (0.2 oz)	13	tr	5	3	2
chickpea besan	½ cup (1.6 oz)	178	3	27	5	5
peanut low fat	½ cup (1.1 oz)	128	7	9	–	5
potato	½ cup (2.8 oz)	286	tr	66	3	5
rice brown	½ cup (2.8 oz)	287	2	60	1	4
rice white	½ cup (2.8 oz)	289	1	63	tr	2
rye dark	½ cup (2.2 oz)	207	2	44	1	15
rye light	½ cup (1.8 oz)	187	1	41	1	7
soy lowfat	½ cup (1.5 oz)	165	4	15	5	7
triticale whole grain	½ cup (2.3 oz)	220	1	48	–	10
white all-purpose enriched bleached	½ cup (2.2 oz)	228	1	48	tr	2
whole wheat	½ cup (2.1 oz)	203	1	44	tr	7

Gold Medal

FOOD	PORTION	CAL	FAT	CARB	SUGAR	FIBER
All Purpose	¼ cup (1 oz)	100	0	22	tr	tr
Self Rising	¼ cup (1 oz)	100	0	23	–	tr
Whole Wheat	¼ cup (1 oz)	100	1	21	–	3
Wondra	¼ cup (1 oz)	100	0	23	–	tr

FOOD COLORS

FOOD	PORTION	CAL	FAT	CARB	SUGAR	FIBER
blue	1 tsp	0	0	0	0	0
orange	1 tsp	0	0	0	0	0
yellow	1 tsp	tr	0	0	0	0

FOOD	PORTION	CAL	FAT	CARB	SUGAR	FIBER
FRENCH BEANS						
dried cooked	1 cup	228	1	43	–	17
FRENCH FRIES (see POTATOES)						
FRENCH TOAST						
french toast frzn	1 slice (2 oz)	126	4	19	–	2
TAKE-OUT						
plain	1 slice	151	7	16	–	–
sticks	5 (4.9 oz)	513	29	58	–	3
w/ butter	2 slices	356	19	36	–	–
FROG LEGS						
TAKE-OUT						
as prep w/ seasoned flour & fried	1 (0.8)	70	5	15	–	–
FRUCTOSE						
liquid	1 oz	84	0	23	23	0
powder	¼ cup (1.7 oz)	180	0	49	45	0
powder	1 tsp (4.2 g)	15	0	4	4	0
Tree Of Life						
Fructose	1 tsp (4 g)	15	0	4	4	0
FRUIT DRINKS (see also individual names, SMOOTHIES, YOGURT DRINKS)						
FROZEN						
Chiquita						
Banana Colada as prep	8 oz	125	2	25	24	1
Mixed Berry as prep	8 oz	120	0	28	27	–
Peach Mango as prep	8 oz	120	0	28	27	–
MIX						
South Beach						
Tide Me Over Strawberry Banana	1 pkg	30	0	6	0	5
Tide Me Over Tropical Breeze	1 pkg	30	0	6	0	5

FOOD	PORTION	CAL	FAT	CARB	SUGAR	FIBER
READY-TO-DRINK						
fruit punch	6 oz	87	tr	22	–	–
Back To Nature						
100% Juice Berry	1 pkg (6 oz)	90	0	21	17	–
Brazsoy						
Fruit Juice w/ Soy	8 oz	94	1	21	19	–
Drenchers						
Super Fruit Endurance Grape Apple	8 oz	120	0	29	27	1
Super Juice Fit N' Lean Heart Healthy Tropical Passion	8 oz	10	0	2	1	0
Super Juice Fit N' Lean Power Protein Orange Cream	8 oz	20	0	2	0	0
Super Juice Immunity Fruit & Veggie Berry	8 oz	110	0	26	22	1
GoodBelly						
Black Currant Probiotic Drink	8 oz	120	0	31	27	0
Blueberry Acai Probiotic Drink	1 bottle (2.7 oz)	50	0	12	9	tr
Cranberry Watermelon Probiotic Drink	8 oz	100	0	24	21	1
Peach Mango Probiotic Drink	1 bottle (2.7 oz)	50	0	13	9	tr
Strawberry Rosehips Probiotic Drink	1 bottle (2.7 oz)	50	0	12	9	tr
Land O Lakes						
Juice Cranberry Apple	1 cup (8 oz)	120	0	30	26	0
Mott's						
Apple Blueberry	8 oz	130	0	15	14	–

FOOD	PORTION	CAL	FAT	CARB	SUGAR	FIBER
Fruit Medley	1 bottle (14 oz)	230	0	54	54	0
Nantucket Nectars						
100% Juice Peach Orange	8 oz	130	0	32	32	0
100% Juice Pomegranate Cherry	8 oz	120	0	29	27	0
Kiwi Berry	8 oz	120	0	29	28	0
Organic Banana Mango Carrot	8 oz	140	0	32	30	0
Pineapple Orange Guava	8 oz	120	0	29	29	0
Northland						
100% Juice Cranberry Pomegranate	8 oz	140	0	34	30	–
Ocean Spray						
100% Juice Cranberry & Concord Grape	8 oz	150	0	37	37	–
Cran.Apple	8 oz	130	0	32	32	–
Cran.Raspberry	8 oz	110	0	28	28	0
Old Orchard						
Healthy Balance Apple Kiwi Strawberry	8 oz	31	0	6	6	–
Santa Cruz						
Organic Cranberry Goji	8 oz	120	0	30	28	0
Snapple						
100% Juiced Fruit Punch	8 oz	170	0	42	40	–
Juice Drink Acai Blackberry	8 oz	110	0	27	27	–
Juice Drink Cranberry Raspberry	8 oz	100	0	26	26	–
Tropical Grove						
Fruit Punch	8 oz	110	0	26	26	–

FOOD	PORTION	CAL	FAT	CARB	SUGAR	FIBER
Tropicana						
Organic Orchard Medley	8 oz	120	0	29	25	0
V8						
V-Fusion Acai Mixed Berry	8 oz	110	0	27	26	0
V-Fusion Light Peach Mango	8 oz	50	0	13	10	–
Welch's						
Light Strawberry Mango	8 oz	50	0	13	12	–

FRUIT MIXED (see also individual names)
CANNED

FOOD	PORTION	CAL	FAT	CARB	SUGAR	FIBER
fruit cocktail in heavy syrup	½ cup	93	tr	24	–	–
fruit cocktail juice pack	½ cup	56	tr	15	–	–
fruit cocktail water pack	½ cup	40	tr	10	–	–
fruit salad in heavy syrup	½ cup	94	tr	24	–	–
fruit salad in light syrup	½ cup	73	tr	19	–	–
fruit salad juice pack	½ cup	62	tr	16	–	–
fruit salad water pack	½ cup	37	tr	10	–	–
mixed fruit in heavy syrup	½ cup	92	tr	24	–	–
tropical fruit salad in heavy syrup	½ cup	110	tr	29	–	–
Dole						
Mixed Fruit Light Syrup	½ cup (4.3 oz)	80	0	21	20	tr
Homemade Harvey's						
Crushed Fruit Apple Pear & Spices	1 pkg (4.5 oz)	60	0	17	13	2
Crushed Fruit Mango Pinapple Banana & Passion Fruit	1 pkg (4.5 oz)	90	0	22	19	2

FOOD	PORTION	CAL	FAT	CARB	SUGAR	FIBER
Crushed Fruit Strawberries Bananas & Kiwis	1 pkg (4.5 oz)	100	1	23	19	2
Mott's						
Healthy Harvest Pomegranate	1 pkg (3.9 oz)	50	0	13	11	1
Polar						
Mixed Fruit Light Syrup	½ cup (4.9 oz)	50	0	12	11	2
S&W						
Chunky Mixed In Sweetened Juice	½ cup (4.3 oz)	80	0	19	16	3
Fruit Cocktail	½ cup (4.4 oz)	80	0	20	18	2
DRIED						
mixed	11 oz pkg	712	1	188	–	–
Brothers-All-Natural						
Crisps Strawberry Banana	1 pkg (0.42 oz)	45	0	10	6	2
Elizabeth's Natural						
Fancy Mixed	5 pieces	80	0	20	7	2
Fruitaceuticals						
PomaCrans	¼ cup	100	0	24	18	1
Fun-Yums						
Fresh Crispy Mixed Fruit	1 serv (0.9 oz)	25	5	18	2	1
Sun-Maid						
Fruit Bits	¼ cup (1.4 oz)	120	0	29	24	2
Mixed	¼ cup (1.4 oz)	100	0	26	21	3
FRESH						
Chiquita						
Apple & Grape Bites	1 pkg (2.5 oz)	40	0	10	8	1
FROZEN						
mixed fruit sweetened	1 cup	245	tr	61	–	–
FRUIT SNACKS						
fruit leather	1 bar (0.8 oz)	81	1	18	–	–

FOOD	PORTION	CAL	FAT	CARB	SUGAR	FIBER
fruit leather pieces	1 oz	97	2	22	–	–
fruit leather pieces	1 pkg (0.9 oz)	92	2	21	–	–
fruit leather rolls	1 sm (0.5 oz)	49	tr	12	–	–
fruit leather rolls	1 lg (0.7 oz)	73	1	18	–	–
Clif						
Twisted Fruit Grape	1 piece (0.7 oz)	70	0	16	9	1
Twisted Fruit Pineapple	1 piece (0.7 oz)	70	0	16	9	1
Twisted Fruit Tropical Twist	1 pices (0.7 oz)	70	0	16	9	1
Jelly Belly						
Fruit Snacks	1 pkg (2.5 oz)	220	0	58	37	1
Revolution Foods						
Organic Mashups Berry	1 pkg (3.2 oz)	40	0	10	8	1
Organic Mashups Tropical	1 pkg (3.2 oz)	60	0	13	11	1
Tahitian Noni						
Soft Chews Raspberry	1 pkg (2 oz)	240	3	50	44	0
Welch's						
Fruit'N Yogurt Strawberry	1 pkg (0.9 oz)	90	2	17	14	–
Mixed Fruit	1 pkg (0.9 oz)	80	0	19	15	–
GARLIC						
clove	1	4	tr	1	tr	tr
fresh chopped	1 tbsp	18	tr	4	tr	tr
powder	1 tsp	9	tr	2	1	tr
McSweet						
Pickled	8 pieces (1 oz)	40	0	5	tr	0
Spice World						
Ajo Garlic Clove	1 (3 g)	5	0	1	–	–
GEFILTE FISH						
sweet	1 piece (1.5 oz)	35	1	3	–	–

FOOD	PORTION	CAL	FAT	CARB	SUGAR	FIBER
Mrs. Adler's						
Gefilte Fish	1 piece (1.8 oz)	50	2	3	1	1
Ungar's						
Gefilte Fish	2 slices (1.8 oz)	83	5	5	3	0
Lite	2 slices (2.4 oz)	80	3	5	3	2
No Sugar	2 slices (1.8 oz)	70	4	3	tr	0
GELATIN						
READY-TO-EAT						
Jell-O						
Sugar Free Lemon Lime	1 serv (3.2 oz)	10	0	0	0	0
GIBLETS						
capon simmered	1 cup (5 oz)	238	8	0	0	0
chicken fried	1 cup (5 oz)	402	20	6	–	0
chicken simmered	1 cup (5 oz)	289	17	1	0	0
turkey simmered	1 cup (5 oz)	243	7	3	–	–
GINGER						
ground	1 tsp	6	tr	1	tr	tr
pickled	0.5 oz	5	0	1	–	tr
preserved	1.5 oz	34	0	8	7	1
root fresh	5 slices	9	tr	2	tr	tr
root fresh sliced	¼ cup	19	tr	4	tr	1
Tree Of Life						
Crystallized Pieces	7 (1.4 oz)	150	0	37	33	1
GINKGO NUTS						
canned	1 oz	32	tr	6	–	–
dried	1 oz	99	tr	21	–	–
raw	1 oz	52	tr	11	–	–
GINSENG						
dried	1 oz	90	tr	20	–	2
fresh	1 oz	28	tr	6	–	tr

FOOD	PORTION	CAL	FAT	CARB	SUGAR	FIBER
GIZZARDS						
chicken simmered	1 cup (5 oz)	212	4	0	0	0
turkey simmered	1 (3 oz)	103	3	tr	0	0
Perdue						
Fresh Chicken	3 oz	130	3	1	0	–
GNOCCHI						
Racconto						
Potato Whole Wheat as prep w/o salt	1 cup (5.8 oz)	248	0	60	tr	8
GOAT						
roasted	3 oz	122	3	0	0	0
GOJI BERRIES						
dried	1 oz	106	3	19	–	2
Kopali						
Organic Dark Chocolate Covered	½ pkg (1 oz)	120	6	18	13	2
Tree Of Life						
Organic	1 oz	110	0	25	15	<5
GOJI JUICE						
Arthur's						
Goji Plus	1 bottle (11 oz)	210	tr	49	38	2
GOOSE						
boneless roasted	2.7 oz	231	17	0	0	0
meat only raw	6.5 oz	298	13	0	0	0
w/ skin & bone roasted	1 serv (6.6 oz)	573	41	0	0	0
wild boneless roasted diced	1 cup (4.9 oz)	426	31	0	0	0

FOOD	PORTION	CAL	FAT	CARB	SUGAR	FIBER
GOOSEBERRIES						
canned in light syrup	1 cup	184	1	47	–	6
fresh	1 cup	66	1	15	–	7
Kopali						
Organic Goldenberry	1 pkg (1.8 oz)	150	0	31	4	18
GRAINS						
Kashi						
7 Whole Grain Pilaf Fiery Fiesta	1 cup (4.9 oz)	210	5	40	3	7
7 Whole Grain Pilaf Moroccan Curry	1 cup (4.9 oz)	220	5	42	3	7
7 Whole Grain Pilaf Original	1 cup (4.9 oz)	220	4	45	1	7
GRAPE JUICE						
bottled unsweetened	1 cup	154	tr	38	38	tr
Cascadian Farm						
Organic frzn as prep	8 oz	150	0	38	37	–
First Blush						
All Flavors	8 oz	154	0	38	38	0
Kedem						
100% Juice	8 oz	150	0	37	37	–
Mott's						
100% Juice Grape Medley	1 bottle (14 oz)	230	0	55	55	0
Nantucket Nectars						
Grapeade	8 oz	140	0	33	33	0
Organic Concord Grape	8 oz	130	0	31	31	0
Santa Cruz						
Organic Concord Grape	8 oz	160	0	40	39	0
Snapple						
100% Juiced Grape	8 oz	170	0	43	41	–
Grapeade	8 oz	100	0	26	26	–

FOOD	PORTION	CAL	FAT	CARB	SUGAR	FIBER
GRAPE LEAVES						
canned	1 (4 g)	3	tr	tr	–	–
fresh raw	1 (3 g)	3	tr	1	tr	tr
TAKE-OUT						
dolmas w/ beef & rice	1 (0.7 oz)	50	4	2	1	1
dolmas w/ lamb & rice	1 (0.7 oz)	56	4	3	1	1
dolmas w/ rice	1 (2 oz)	92	6	8	2	2
GRAPEFRUIT						
CANNED						
sections juice pack	½ cup (4.4 oz)	46	tr	11	11	1
sections light syrup	½ cup (4.5 oz)	76	tr	20	19	1
sections water pack	½ cup (4.3 oz)	44	tr	11	11	1
FRESH						
pink or red	½ (4.6 oz)	52	tr	13	8	2
sections pink or red	1 cup (8.1 oz)	97	tr	25	16	4
sections white	1 cup (8.1 oz)	76	tr	19	17	3
white	½ (4.1 oz)	39	tr	10	9	1
Ocean Spray						
Sweet Ruby Red	½ med (5.4 oz)	60	0	16	10	6
GRAPEFRUIT JUICE						
canned sweetened	1 cup (8.8 oz)	115	tr	28	28	tr
canned unsweetened	1 cup (8.7 oz)	94	tr	22	22	tr
pink fresh	1 cup (8.7 oz)	96	tr	23	–	–
white fresh	1 cup (8.7 oz)	96	tr	23	22	tr
Izze						
Sparkling Fortified Grapefruit	1 can (8.4 oz)	90	0	23	21	–
GRAPES						
muscadine	10–12 (3.5 oz)	76	0	14	–	3
scuppernongs	10–12 (3.5 oz)	68	0	12	–	3
seedless red or green	20	69	tr	18	15	1

FOOD	PORTION	CAL	FAT	CARB	SUGAR	FIBER
seedless red or green	1 cup	110	tr	29	24	1
thompson seedless in heavy syrup	½ cup	93	tr	25	24	1
thompson seedless water pack	½ cup	49	tr	13	12	1
with seeds red or green	1 cup	106	tr	28	24	1
with seeds red or green	20	80	tr	21	18	1
Chiquita						
Grapes	1 cup (3.2 oz)	62	0	16	15	1
Revolution Foods						
Organic Mashups Grape	1 pkg (3.2 oz)	60	0	14	12	0

GRAVY
CANNED

FOOD	PORTION	CAL	FAT	CARB	SUGAR	FIBER
beef	1 can (10 oz)	155	7	14	–	–
beef	1 cup	124	6	11	–	–
chicken	1 cup	189	14	13	–	–
mushroom	1 cup	120	6	13	–	–
turkey	1 cup	122	5	12	–	–
Heinz						
Classic Chicken Fat Free	¼ cup	15	0	3	0	0
HomeStyle Classic Chicken	¼ cup	25	1	4	0	0
Roasted Turkey Fat Free	¼ cup (2.1 oz)	20	0	3	0	0

MIX

FOOD	PORTION	CAL	FAT	CARB	SUGAR	FIBER
au jus as prep w/ water	1 cup	32	1	4	–	–
brown as prep w/ water	1 cup	75	2	13	–	–
chicken as prep	1 cup	83	2	14	–	–
mushroom as prep	1 cup	70	1	14	–	–
onion as prep w/ water	1 cup	77	1	16	–	–
pork as prep	1 cup	76	2	13	–	–
turkey as prep	1 cup	87	2	15	–	–
Bournvita						
Extract	2 heaping tsp	34	1	7	–	–

FOOD	PORTION	CAL	FAT	CARB	SUGAR	FIBER
Bovril						
Extract	1 heaping tsp	9	0	tr	–	0
Butterball						
Turkey	¼ cup (2 oz)	30	0	6	0	0
Marmite						
Extract	1 heaping tsp	9	0	tr	–	–
TAKE-OUT						
au jus	1 cup	62	6	1	tr	tr
giblet gravy	¼ cup	45	3	3	tr	tr

GREAT NORTHERN BEANS

FOOD	PORTION	CAL	FAT	CARB	SUGAR	FIBER
canned	1 cup	299	1	55	–	13
dried cooked	1 cup	209	1	37	–	12
HamBeens						
Great Northerns as prep	½ cup	120	1	22	1	11

GREEN BEANS

FOOD	PORTION	CAL	FAT	CARB	SUGAR	FIBER
CANNED						
drained	1 cup	27	tr	6	1	3
Allens						
No Salt	½ cup	15	0	3	1	2
Green Giant						
50% Less Sodium Cut	½ cup	20	0	4	2	1
McSweet						
Dilly Beans Whole	5 (1 oz)	30	0	7	6	tr
S&W						
Cut	½ cup (4.2 oz)	20	0	4	2	2
Dilled	1 oz	20	0	5	3	1
FRESH						
cooked w/o salt	1 cup	44	tr	10	2	4
raw	1 cup	34	tr	8	2	4
raw whole beans	10	17	tr	4	1	2
FROZEN						
cooked	1 cup	38	tr	9	2	4

FOOD	PORTION	CAL	FAT	CARB	SUGAR	FIBER
Birds Eye						
Steamfresh Whole	1 cup (2.9 oz)	35	0	5	2	2
Cascadian Farm						
Organic Petite Whole	1 cup	25	0	5	1	2
TAKE-OUT						
casserole w/ mushroom sauce	1 cup	108	6	11	3	3
pickled	½ cup	19	tr	4	1	2

GREENS
Allens
Seasoned Mixed	½ cup	45	1	6	2	1

GROUNDCHERRIES
fresh	½ cup	37	tr	8	–	–

GROUPER
cooked	3 oz	100	1	0	0	0
cooked	1 fillet (7.1 oz)	238	3	0	0	0
raw	3 oz	78	1	0	0	0

GUAVA
fresh	1	45	1	11	–	–
guava sauce	½ cup	43	tr	11	–	–

GUAVA JUICE
OKF
Sparkling Fresh Guava	1 bottle (8.3 oz)	20	0	13	1	3

GUINEA HEN
boneless w/o skin raw	½ hen (9.3 oz)	290	7	0	0	0
w/ skin raw	½ hen (12 oz)	545	22	0	0	0
Grimaud Farms						
Guinea Fowl	1 serv (3.7 oz)	130	4	tr	–	–

FOOD	PORTION	CAL	FAT	CARB	SUGAR	FIBER
HADDOCK						
fresh broiled	4 oz	127	1	0	0	0
roe raw	1 oz	37	tr	tr	–	–
smoked	1 oz	33	tr	0	0	0
TAKE-OUT						
breaded & fried	4 oz	229	10	10	1	1
HAGGIS						
scottish haggis	1 serv (6.4 oz)	473	32	31	3	5
Caledonian Kitchen						
Highland Beef	3 oz	173	10	12	2	2
Vegetarian	3 oz	190	13	12	0	3
House of Kenton						
Vegetarian	1 serv (3.5 oz)	249	20	14	–	–
MacSween						
Traditional	1 (8 oz)	260	16	18	0	–
Vegetarian	1 (8 oz)	238	12	22	1	–
HALIBUT						
atlantic & pacific cooked	½ fillet (5.6 oz)	223	5	0	0	0
atlantic & pacific cooked	3 oz	119	2	0	0	0
atlantic & pacific raw	3 oz	93	2	0	0	0
greenland baked	5.6 oz	380	28	0	0	0
greenland baked	3 oz	203	15	0	0	0
HAM						
boneless extra lean roasted	3 oz	123	5	1	0	0
boneless roasted	3 oz	151	8	0	0	0
canned extra lean roasted	3 oz	116	4	tr	–	0
canned lean roasted	3 oz	142	7	tr	–	0

FOOD	PORTION	CAL	FAT	CARB	SUGAR	FIBER
center slice lean & fat roasted	3 oz	173	11	tr	–	0
deviled	¼ cup	188	17	1	0	0
ham salad spread	2 tbsp	65	5	3	0	0
patty grilled	1 patty (2 oz)	205	19	1	0	0
prosciutto	4 slices (1.3 oz)	72	3	tr	0	0
sliced	3 slices (2.9 oz)	137	7	3	0	1
sliced extra lean	3 slices (2.2 oz)	69	2	2	0	0
westphalian smoked	1 oz	105	10	0	0	0
whole roasted	3 oz	207	14	0	0	0
Applegate Farms						
Organic Uncured	2 oz	70	2	1	0	0
Carl Buddig						
Ham Sliced	2 oz	85	5	1	–	–
Honey Ham Sliced	2 oz	90	5	2	–	–
Healthy Ones						
Honey 97% Fat Free	7 slices (2 oz)	90	2	2	2	–
Hormel						
Chunk Ham canned	2 oz	90	6	0	0	0
Deli Cooked	4 slices (2 oz)	70	2	1	1	0
Deli Honey	4 slices (2 oz)	70	2	3	3	0
Deli Smoked	4 slices (2 oz)	60	2	1	1	0
Dinner	2 oz	70	2	2	1	0
Oscar Mayer						
Ham Brown Sugar Thin Sliced	⅓ pkg (2 oz)	70	2	4	4	–
Virginia Shaved	2 oz	50	1	1	0	0
TAKE-OUT						
croquette	1 (2.2 oz)	149	9	8	2	tr
salad	½ cup	287	23	5	–	tr

FOOD	PORTION	CAL	FAT	CARB	SUGAR	FIBER
spam musubi	1 serv (6 oz)	253	6	42	–	1
thick slice fried	1 (2.2 oz)	140	9	tr	0	0

HAMBURGER
Applegate Farms
Organic Beef Cooked	1 (3 oz)	195	12	0	0	0
Organic Turkey Burger	1 (4 oz)	190	11	0	0	0

Hot Pockets
Cheeseburger	1 (4.5 oz)	310	13	37	9	2

Lean Pockets
Cheeseburger	1 (4.5 oz)	280	7	40	12	3

TAKE-OUT
cheeseburger + condiments	1 reg (4.5 oz)	347	17	28	5	1
double hamburger + condiments	1 reg (5.8 oz)	384	19	30	7	2
single patty + condiments	1 reg (4 oz)	299	11	35	8	2

HAMBURGER SUBSTITUTES (see also MEAT SUBSTITUTES)
Amy's
All American Burger	1 (2.5 oz)	120	3	15	2	3
Cheddar Veggie Burger	1 (2.5 oz)	160	5	20	2	3
Texas Burger	1 (2.5 oz)	120	3	14	2	3

Dr. Praeger's
Veggie Burger Bombay	1 (2.78 oz)	110	5	13	2	5
Veggie Burger California	1 (2.75 oz)	110	5	13	1	4
Veggie Burger California Gluten Free	1 (2.75 oz)	120	6	13	3	4

Sunshine Burgers
Garden	1 (2.6 oz)	190	13	14	3	3
Original	1 (2.6 oz)	190	13	14	3	3

FOOD	PORTION	CAL	FAT	CARB	SUGAR	FIBER
HAZELNUTS						
chocolate hazelnut spread	2 tbsp (1.3 oz)	200	11	23	20	2
chopped	¼ cup (1 oz)	181	17	5	1	3
ground	¼ cup (0.7 oz)	118	11	3	1	1
whole	¼ cup (1.2 oz)	212	21	6	1	3
whole nuts	21 (1 oz)	178	17	5	1	3
Chukar Cherries						
Chocolate Covered Spiced	3 tbsp (1.4 oz)	228	17	21	16	2
Fisher						
Chopped	¼ cup (1 oz)	180	17	5	1	3
HEART						
beef simmered	3 oz	140	4	tr	0	0
chicken cooked	1 (3 g)	5	tr	0	0	0
chicken diced simmered	½ cup	134	6	tr	–	0
lamb braised	3 oz	157	7	2	–	0
pork braised	1 (4.5 oz)	191	7	1	–	0
turkey simmered	½ cup	94	3	tr	0	0
veal braised	3 oz	158	6	tr	–	0
Rumba						
Beef	4 oz	130	4	3	0	0
HEARTS OF PALM						
canned	1 (1.2 oz)	9	tr	2	–	1
canned	½ cup	20	tr	3	–	2
HERBAL TEA (see TEA/HERBAL TEA)						
HERBS/SPICES (see also individual names)						
cajun seasoning	1 tbsp	19	1	3	–	1
chinese five spice	1 tsp	7	tr	2	–	tr
garam masala	1 tsp	8	tr	1	–	–
poultry seasoning	1 tsp	5	tr	1	tr	tr

FOOD	PORTION	CAL	FAT	CARB	SUGAR	FIBER
pumpkin pie spice	1 tsp	6	tr	1	tr	tr
Bragg						
Herb & Spice Seasoning	¼ tsp	0	0	0	0	0
Dave's Gourmet						
Insanity Spice	¼ tsp (1 g)	5	0	0	0	0
Mrs. Dash						
Grilling Blend Steak	¼ tsp (0.7 g)	0	0	0	0	0
Original Blend	¼ tsp (0.7 g)	0	0	0	0	0
Seasoning Blends Caribbean Citrus	¼ tsp (0.7 g)	0	0	0	0	0
Seasoning Blends Garlic & Herb	¼ tsp (0.7 g)	0	0	0	0	0
Seasoning Blends Italian Medley	¼ tsp (0.7 g)	0	0	0	0	0
Seasoning Blends Table Blend	¼ tsp (0.7 g)	0	0	0	0	0
Ribber City						
Rib-A-Dub-Rub Dry Rub Seasoning	¼ tsp (0.8 oz)	3	0	1	0	0
HERRING						
atlantic baked	4 oz	230	13	0	0	0
dried salted	1 fillet (1.4 oz)	161	9	0	0	0
pickled	1 oz	74	5	3	–	0
pickled in cream sauce	1 oz	72	5	2	tr	0
roe	1 tbsp	39	2	tr	0	0
smoked kippered	1 oz	62	4	0	0	0
TAKE-OUT						
breaded fried	1 serv (4 oz)	225	14	9	1	1
HIBISCUS						
flowers dried sweetened	⅓ cup	100	0	23	21	2
Santa Cruz						
Organic Hibiscus Cooler	8 oz	100	0	24	24	0

FOOD	PORTION	CAL	FAT	CARB	SUGAR	FIBER
HICKORY NUTS						
dried	1 oz	187	18	5	–	–
HOMINY						
white canned	1 cup	119	1	24	3	4
yellow canned	½ cup	115	1	23	–	4
Allens						
White	½ cup	100	1	22	1	4
Bush's						
Golden	½ cup	60	0	13	0	3
HONEY						
honey	¼ cup (3 oz)	258	0	70	70	tr
honey	1 tbsp (0.7 oz)	64	0	17	17	–
orange blossom	1 tbsp	60	0	17	16	0
wild honey	1 tbsp	60	0	17	16	–
Comfort Care						
Raw Clover	1 tbsp (0.7 oz)	60	0	17	16	–
Dutch Gold						
Clover	1 tbsp	60	0	17	16	0
Tree Of Life						
Alfalfa Honey Raw Unfiltered	1 tbsp	60	0	17	16	–
Avocado Honey Raw Unfiltered	1 tbsp (0.7 oz)	60	0	17	16	0
Buckwheat Honey Raw Unfiltered	1 tbsp	60	0	17	16	–
Tupelo Honey Raw Unfiltered	1 tbsp	60	0	17	16	–
Wholesome Sweeteners						
Organic Fair Trade Amber	1 tbsp	60	0	17	16	0
Organic Fair Trade Raw	1 tbsp (0.7 oz)	60	0	17	16	0

FOOD	PORTION	CAL	FAT	CARB	SUGAR	FIBER
HONEYDEW						
balls frzn	1 cup (8 oz)	83	tr	21	19	2
fresh cut up	1 cup	61	tr	15	14	1
fresh wedge	⅛ melon (4.5 oz)	45	tr	11	10	1
whole fresh	1 (35 oz)	360	1	91	81	8
Chiquita						
Fresh Cut Up	1 cup (6.2 oz)	64	0	16	14	1
HORSE						
roasted	3 oz	149	5	0	0	0
HORSERADISH						
japanese wasabi	¼ tsp	1	–	tr	–	0
sauce	1 tbsp	7	tr	2	1	1
wasabi root raw	1 (5.9 oz)	184	1	40	–	13
wasabi root raw sliced	½ cup (2.3 oz)	71	tr	15	–	5
Gold's						
Horse Radish	1 tsp (5 g)	0	0	0	0	0
Zatarain's						
Prepared	1 tbsp	15	0	2	–	–
HOT CHOCOLATE						
mix not prep	1 pkg (1 oz)	111	1	23	18	1
mix w/ no calorie sweetener as prep w/ water	8 oz	72	1	14	7	2
mix w/ sugar as prep w/ nonfat milk	8 oz	209	1	30	29	1
mix w/ sugar as prep w/ water	8 oz	138	1	29	23	1
Hershey's						
Goodnight Hugs	1 pkg (1.2 oz)	140	3	27	26	–

FOOD	PORTION	CAL	FAT	CARB	SUGAR	FIBER
Nestle						
Hot Cocoa Milk Chocolate	1 pkg (1 oz)	80	3	15	13	tr
Hot Cocoa Rich Chocolate as prep w/ water	1 pkg	80	3	15	12	tr
Silhouette Solution						
Down East not prep	1 pkg (0.88 oz)	90	2	5	1	1
Starbucks						
Hot Cocoa Mix	1 pkg	130	2	28	24	2
Swiss Miss						
Cocoa Caramel as prep	1 pkg	120	3	22	17	tr
Cocoa No Sugar Added as prep	1 pkg	60	1	10	7	1
Cocoa Rich Creamy as prep	1 pkg	110	2	22	16	tr
Cocoa w/ Marshmallows as prep	1 pkg	120	2	24	16	1
Cocoa w/ Marshmallows Fat Free as prep	1 pkg	140	3	29	21	1
French Vanilla as prep	1 pkg	110	2	24	18	tr
Milk Chocolate as prep	1 pkg	120	3	23	17	1
TAKE-OUT						
chocolate caliente w/ lowfat milk	1 serv (8.4 oz)	221	9	27	25	1
chocolate caliente w/ whole milk	1 serv (8.4 oz)	276	17	25	23	1
hot chocolate	1 cup (8.7 oz)	192	6	30	24	3
mexican hot chocolate	1 cup	173	6	20	–	1

HOT DOG (see also HOT DOG SUBSTITUTES)

FOOD	PORTION	CAL	FAT	CARB	SUGAR	FIBER
beef	1 (1.5 oz)	149	13	2	2	0
beef & pork	1 (1.5 oz)	137	12	1	0	1
beef low fat	1 (2 oz)	133	11	1	0	0

FOOD	PORTION	CAL	FAT	CARB	SUGAR	FIBER
chicken	1 (1.5 oz)	116	9	3	0	0
fat free	1 (2 oz)	62	1	6	0	0
low fat	1 (2 oz)	88	6	3	0	0
low sodium	1 (2 oz)	180	16	1	0	0
pork and beef cheese smokie	1 (1.5 oz)	141	12	1	1	0
turkey	1 (1.5 oz)	102	8	1	0	0
Applegate Farms						
Natural Beef	1 (1.5 oz)	80	6	0	0	0
Organic Chicken	1 (1.5 oz)	70	5	0	0	0
Healthy Ones						
Beef	1 (1.8 oz)	70	3	7	2	0
Franks	1 (1.8 oz)	70	3	6	2	0
Oscar Mayer						
Beef	1 (1.6 oz)	140	13	1	1	0
Beef Light	1 (1.6 oz)	90	6	2	1	–
Cheese Dogs	1 (1.6 oz)	140	13	1	0	0
Corn Dogs	1	210	12	21	6	1
Smokies	1 (1.8 oz)	150	13	1	1	0
TAKE-OUT						
corndog	1	460	19	56	–	–
w/ bun chili	1	297	13	31	–	–
w/ bun plain	1	242	15	18	–	–

HOT DOG SUBSTITUTES

Health Is Wealth

Vegetarian Cocktail Franks	3 (2.4 oz)	220	16	16	0	3

HUMMUS

Athenos

Original	2 tbsp	80	5	5	0	1
Roasted Garlic	2 tbsp	80	5	5	0	1
Roasted Red Pepper	2 tbsp	80	6	5	0	1

FOOD	PORTION	CAL	FAT	CARB	SUGAR	FIBER
Emerald Valley						
Organic Greek Olive & Roasted Garlic	2 tbsp (1 oz)	60	3	6	1	2
Organic Original	2 tbsp (1 oz)	50	2	7	1	2
Organic Spinach Feta	2 tbsp (1 oz)	50	2	6	1	2
Guiltless Gourmet						
Original	2 tbsp (1.1 oz)	50	2	8	1	2
Tribe						
40 Spices	2 tbsp	50	4	3	0	1
French Onion	2 tbsp	50	4	4	0	1
Organic Classic	2 tbsp	50	4	4	0	1
Organic Roasted Red Peppers	2 tbsp	40	3	3	0	1
Roasted Eggplant	2 tbsp	35	3	3	0	1
Scallion	2 tbsp	50	4	4	0	1
Zesty Lemon	2 tbsp	50	3	4	0	1
Wholesome Valley						
Organic Classic	2 tbsp (1 oz)	60	4	5	tr	1
TAKE-OUT						
hummus	¼ cup (2.2 oz)	109	5	12	tr	3

HYACINTH BEANS

FOOD	PORTION	CAL	FAT	CARB	SUGAR	FIBER
dried cooked	1 cup	228	1	40	–	–

ICE CREAM AND FROZEN DESSERTS (*see also* ICES AND ICE POPS, SHERBET, YOGURT FROZEN)

FOOD	PORTION	CAL	FAT	CARB	SUGAR	FIBER
chocolate	½ cup (4 fl oz)	143	7	19	13	–
dixie cup chocolate	1 (3.5 fl oz)	125	6	16	11	–
dixie cup strawberry	1 (3.5 fl oz)	112	5	16	9	–
dixie cup vanilla	1 (3.5 fl oz)	116	6	14	9	–
freeze dried ice cream chocolate strawberry & vanilla	1 pkg (0.75 oz)	158	5	24	10	1
strawberry	½ cup (4 fl oz)	127	6	18	10	–

FOOD	PORTION	CAL	FAT	CARB	SUGAR	FIBER
vanilla	½ cup (4 fl oz)	132	7	16	10	–
vanilla soft serve	½ cup	111	2	19	–	–
Breyers						
Butter Pecan	½ cup	150	10	14	14	0
Carb Smart Chocolate	½ cup	90	6	13	4	4
Carb Smart Fudge Bar	1 (3.5 oz)	100	7	9	3	1
Carb Smart Vanilla	½ cup	90	6	13	4	4
Carb Smart Vanilla Bar Chocolate Coated	1 (3 oz)	170	15	9	5	2
Cherry Vanilla	½ cup	130	6	08	17	0
Chocolate Crackle	½ cup	160	10	15	15	0
Chocolate Extra Creamy	½ cup	140	7	17	15	1
Coffee	½ cup	130	7	15	15	0
Cookies & Cream	½ cup	150	7	19	16	0
Double Churn ½ Fat Chocolate Mocha Silk	½ cup	130	5	19	15	1
Double Churn ½ Fat Creamy Vanilla	½ cup	100	3	17	13	0
Double Churn ½ Fat Mint Chocolate Chip	½ cup	130	5	19	15	1
Double Churn ½ Fat Rocky Road	½ cup	130	5	22	16	1
Double Churn Fat Free Chocolate Fudge Brownie	½ cup	110	0	25	15	4
Double Churn Fat Free Creamy Vanilla	½ cup	90	0	21	12	3
Double Churn Fat Free French Chocolate	½ cup	90	0	22	13	4
Double Churn No Sugar Added Vanilla	½ cup	80	4	14	4	4
Dulce De Leche	½ cup	150	6	21	19	0
French Vanilla	½ cup	140	7	14	14	0
Heath English Toffee	½ cup	160	6	25	20	0

FOOD	PORTION	CAL	FAT	CARB	SUGAR	FIBER
Overload Very Chocolate Cherry	½ cup	120	3	21	16	1
Overload Waffle Cone	½ cup	130	3	22	16	0
Peach	½ cup	120	5	17	16	0
Sandwich Mrs. Fields Brownie	1 (6 oz)	450	19	64	39	2
Sandwich Mrs. Fields Cookie	1 (3 oz)	190	8	29	17	0
Sandwich Oreo	1 (3 oz)	170	6	26	13	1
Snicker	½ cup	170	8	20	16	0
Strawberry	½ cup	120	5	15	15	0
Strawberry Cheesecake Sara Lee	½ cup	150	6	20	17	0
Vanilla Fudge Brownie	½ cup	150	7	20	17	1
Vanilla Lactose Free	½ cup	130	7	14	14	0
Ciao Bella						
Gelato Chocolate	1 pkg (3.5 oz)	210	13	22	18	1
Gelato Hazelnut	1 pkg (3.5 oz)	210	13	21	17	1
Gelato Vanilla	1 pkg (3.5 oz)	184	11	19	16	0
Dippin' Dots						
Banana Split	½ cup	170	10	16	14	0
Chocolate	½ cup	165	10	15	14	0
Fudge Fat Free No Sugar Added	½ cup	92	0	18	7	0
Horchata	½ cup	170	10	16	14	0
Java Delight	½ cup	170	10	16	14	0
Root Beer Float	½ cup	111	3	20	16	0
Vanilla	½ cup	170	10	16	14	0
Good Humor						
Bar Chocolate Eclair	1 (3 oz)	160	8	21	11	1
Bar Cookies & Cream	1 (3 oz)	190	11	21	14	1
Bar King Heath	1 (4 oz)	310	20	31	26	1

FOOD	PORTION	CAL	FAT	CARB	SUGAR	FIBER
Bar Vanilla Chocolate Coated	1 (4 oz)	260	17	24	20	1
Cone King Giant	1 (8 oz)	390	21	44	30	2
Cone King Vanilla	1 (4.6 oz)	250	13	30	19	1
Cone Sundae	1 (4.3 oz)	260	15	29	18	1
Sandwich Oreo	1 (4.5 oz)	240	10	36	19	2
Sandwich Vanilla	1 (3 oz)	130	2	26	12	2
Sandwich Giant Vanilla	1 (6 oz)	220	4	43	23	1
Swirlwind	1 (6 oz)	160	3	31	23	0
Haagen-Dazs						
Bailey's Irish Cream	½ cup (3.6 oz)	260	17	21	21	0
Bar Chocolate & Dark Chocolate	1 (3 oz)	290	20	24	20	2
Bar Vanilla & Almonds	1 (3 oz)	310	22	22	20	tr
Bar Vanilla & Milk Chocolate	1 (3 oz)	290	21	22	21	0
Butter Pecan	½ cup (3.7 oz)	310	23	21	18	tr
Caramel Cone	½ cup (4 oz)	320	19	32	27	0
Cherry Vanilla	½ cup (3.5 oz)	240	15	23	22	0
Chocolate Chip Cookie Dough	½ cup (3.6 oz)	310	20	29	24	0
Chocolate Peanut Butter	½ cup (3.8 oz)	360	24	27	24	2
Cookies & Cream	½ cup (3.6 oz)	270	17	23	21	0
Dulce De Leche	½ cup (3.7 oz)	290	17	28	28	0
Five Coffee	½ cup (3.6 oz)	220	12	23	21	0

FOOD	PORTION	CAL	FAT	CARB	SUGAR	FIBER
Five Milk Chocolate	½ cup (3.6 oz)	220	12	22	20	tr
Five Mint	½ cup (3.6 oz)	220	12	24	23	0
Five Passion Fruit	½ cup (3.6 oz)	220	11	25	24	0
Five Vanilla	½ cup (3.7 oz)	270	18	21	21	0
Green Tea	½ cup (3.6 oz)	250	17	20	19	0
Mango	½ cup (3.7 oz)	250	14	28	27	tr
Reserve Amazon Valley Chocolate	½ cup (3.7 oz)	290	19	25	21	0
Reserve Caramelized Hazelnut Gianduja	½ cup (3.5 oz)	290	18	27	24	0
Reserve Fleur De Sel Caramel	½ cup (3.7 oz)	280	17	28	28	0
Reserve Hawaiian Lehua Honey & Sweet Cream	½ cup (3.8 oz)	270	17	26	24	0
Rocky Road	½ cup (3.6 oz)	300	18	29	24	1
Strawberry	½ cup (3.7 oz)	250	16	23	22	tr
Vanilla Honey Bee	½ cup (3.6 oz)	270	17	23	20	1
Hershey's						
Banana Split	½ cup (2.5 oz)	160	9	18	16	0
Chocolate	½ cup (2.5 oz)	140	8	15	13	tr

FOOD	PORTION	CAL	FAT	CARB	SUGAR	FIBER
Cookies And Cream	½ cup (2.5 oz)	160	9	16	15	0
Fudge Royale	½ cup (2.5 oz)	180	9	19	18	0
Mint Moose Tracks	½ cup (2.5 oz)	200	14	21	19	tr
Raspberry	½ cup (2.5 oz)	170	9	21	18	0
Tally-Ho Low Fat Butter Pecan	½ cup (2.5 oz)	90	2	14	14	0
Vanilla	½ cup (2.5 oz)	150	9	14	14	0
Klondike						
Bar Caramel Pretzel	1 (4 oz)	260	14	30	21	1
Bar Original Vanilla	1 (4.5 oz)	250	17	22	18	0
Bar Reese's	1 (4 oz)	260	16	26	21	1
Bar Whitehouse Cherry	1 (4.5 oz)	250	17	24	20	0
Cone Crunchy Vanilla	1 (4.3 oz)	280	16	30	20	1
Slim A Bear 100 Calorie Sandwich Vanilla	1 (3 oz)	100	2	21	10	2
Slim A Bear Bar Vanilla	1 (4 oz)	170	9	21	7	4
Land O Lakes						
Vanilla	½ cup (2.4 oz)	150	8	17	16	0
Vanilla Light	½ cup (2.3 oz)	100	3	17	13	0
Molli Coolz						
Cup Banana Cream Pie	1	120	9	9	8	1
Cup Chocolate Fusion	1	140	10	10	7	1
Cup Chocolate Peanut Butter	1	160	12	12	10	0
Ionz Cotton Candy	1 cup	100	7	8	5	0
Ionz S'mores	1 cup	110	9	7	5	1

FOOD	PORTION	CAL	FAT	CARB	SUGAR	FIBER
Rocks Cherry Blue Raz & Lemon	1 cup	80	2	15	8	0
Rocks Lemon Lime	1 cup	80	2	15	8	0
Shakers Chocolate	1 (10.2 oz)	250	11	35	17	5
Popsicle						
Creamsicle	1 (2.5 oz)	100	2	20	12	0
Purely Decadent						
Dairy Free Bar Chocolate Coated Vanilla	1 (2.7 oz)	200	9	26	22	3
Dairy Free Bar Chocolate Coated Vanilla Almond	1 (2.7 oz)	210	10	28	22	4
Organic Coconut Milk Chocolate	½ cup	150	9	20	12	6
Organic Coconut Milk Vanilla Bean	½ cup	150	8	19	12	6
Organic Dairy Free Belgian Chocolate	½ cup	180	7	30	25	4
Organic Dairy Free Chocolate Obsession	½ cup	210	9	36	20	5
Organic Dairy Free Gluten Free Cookie Dough	½ cup	230	8	36	27	5
Organic Dairy Free Mocha Almond Fudge	½ cup	200	9	32	22	6
Organic Dairy Free Snickerdoodle	½ cup	190	6	34	20	5
Organic Dairy Free Vanilla	½ cup	170	8	29	18	6
Sheer Bliss						
Bar Pomegranate	1 (3.1 oz)	260	16	24	22	tr
Blissbites	2 (1.1 oz)	100	7	9	8	0

FOOD	PORTION	CAL	FAT	CARB	SUGAR	FIBER
Blisswich	1 (3.3 oz)	270	10	39	21	tr
Freedom	½ cup (4 oz)	290	16	32	29	0
Mediterranean Coffee	½ cup (4 oz)	260	18	25	23	0
Pomegranate	½ cup (4 oz)	290	16	32	29	0
Vanilla	½ cup (4 oz)	300	19	29	27	0
Skinny Cow						
Bar Dippers Vanilla & Caramel	1	80	3	11	7	2
Bar Truffle Caramel	1	100	2	19	12	3
Bar Truffle French Vanilla	1	100	2	18	12	3
Cone Chocolate w/ Fudge	1	150	3	29	17	3
Cone Vanilla w/ Caramel	1	150	3	29	18	3
Fudge Bar	1	100	1	22	13	4
Sandwich Chocolate Peanut Butter	1	150	2	30	15	3
Sandwich Cookies 'N Cream	1	150	2	31	15	3
Sandwich Vanilla	1	140	2	30	15	3
Sandwich Vanilla No Sugar Added	1	140	2	30	5	5
SoDelicious						
Dairy Free Sandwich Minis Pomegranate	1 (1.4 oz)	90	2	18	8	1
Dairy Free Sandwich Mint	1 (2.2 oz)	150	3	28	13	2
Dairy Free Sandwich Vanilla	1 (2 oz)	150	3	28	13	2
Dairy Free Sugar Free Chocolate Coated Vanilla Bar	1 (2.2 oz)	150	14	15	0	6

FOOD	PORTION	CAL	FAT	CARB	SUGAR	FIBER
Dairy Free Sugar Free Fudge Bar	1 (2 oz)	80	5	12	0	6
Organic Dairy Free Sandwich Neapolitan	1 (2.2 oz)	150	3	28	13	2
Starbucks						
Caramel Macchiato	½ cup (3.6 oz)	240	13	27	21	0
Coffee	½ cup (3.5 oz)	210	13	21	19	0
Java Chip Frappuccino	½ cup (3.5 oz)	250	15	25	22	0
Mocha Frappuccino	½ cup (3.5 oz)	220	13	23	20	tr
Mocha Bar	1	280	19	26	23	1
Straus						
Organic Coffee	4 oz	240	15	19	19	0
Organic Vanilla Bean	4 oz	240	15	19	19	0
The Greek Gods						
Pagoto Ice Krema Baklava	½ cup (4 oz)	240	12	29	27	1
Pagoto Ice Krema Chocolate Fig	½ cup (4 oz)	240	11	32	30	0
Pagoto Ice Krema Honey Pomegranate	½ cup (4 oz)	230	11	31	30	0
Turkey Hill						
Banana Split	½ cup	150	7	19	15	1
Choco Mint Chip	½ cup	160	9	17	13	1
Chocolate All Natural	½ cup	150	8	18	17	0
Chocolate Marshmallow	½ cup	160	6	24	18	1
Coconut Cream Pie	½ cup	170	9	20	20	0
Cookies 'N Cream	½ cup	150	8	19	13	0
Duetto Cherry	½ cup	120	3	21	19	0
Duetto Lemon	½ cup	120	4	21	19	0

FOOD	PORTION	CAL	FAT	CARB	SUGAR	FIBER
Duetto Root Beer	½ cup	120	3	21	19	0
French Vanilla	½ cup	140	7	16	12	0
Light Banana Split	½ cup	110	3	19	15	1
Light Dulce De Chocolate	½ cup	120	3	22	17	1
Light Moose Tracks	½ cup	140	6	20	15	1
Light Vanilla Bean	½ cup	100	2	17	13	1
No Sugar Added Cherry Fudge Ripple	½ cup	80	0	22	5	4
No Sugar Added Vanilla Bean	½ cup	70	0	19	6	5
Original Vanilla	½ cup	140	7	16	12	0
Peanut Butter Ripple	½ cup	170	11	16	11	1
Rocky Road	½ cup	170	8	23	17	1
Sandwich Chocolate Chunk	1 (3.2 oz)	320	15	44	29	1
Sandwich Vanilla Bean	1 (2.5 oz)	190	7	29	15	1
Sandwich Light Vanilla Bean	1 (2.5 oz)	160	3	32	15	3
Sundae Cone Vanilla Fudge	1 (3.3 oz)	320	18	35	20	2
Tin Roof Sundae	½ cup	150	8	19	15	0
TAKE-OUT						
cone vanilla light soft serve	1 (4.6 oz)	164	6	24	–	–
gelato chocolate hazelnut	½ cup (5.3 oz)	370	29	26	21	2
gelato vanilla	½ cup (3 oz)	211	15	18	18	0
ice cream pie no crust	1 slice (3.4 oz)	218	14	21	18	1
mud pie	⅛ pie (8 oz)	698	32	96	64	3
sundae caramel	1 (5.4 oz)	303	9	49	–	–
sundae hot fudge	1 (5.4 oz)	284	9	48	–	–
sundae strawberry	1 (5.4 oz)	269	8	45	–	–

FOOD	PORTION	CAL	FAT	CARB	SUGAR	FIBER
ICE CREAM CONES AND CUPS						
brown sugar cone	1 (10 g)	40	tr	8	3	tr
wafer cone	1	17	tr	3	tr	tr
waffle cone	1 lg	121	2	23	2	1
Keebler						
Cone Sugar	1	50	1	10	4	0
Ice Creme Cone	1	15	0	4	0	0
Waffle Bowl	1	50	1	10	4	0
Waffle Cone	1	50	1	10	4	0
ICE CREAM TOPPINGS						
butterscotch	2 tbsp (1.4 oz)	103	tr	27	–	–
caramel	2 tbsp (1.4 oz)	103	tr	27	–	–
marshmallow cream	1 oz	88	tr	23	–	–
marshmallow cream	1 jar (7 oz)	615	tr	157	–	–
nuts in syrup	2 tbsp	184	9	24	15	1
pineapple	2 tbsp (1.5 oz)	106	0	28	–	–
pineapple	1 cup (11.5 oz)	861	–	226	–	–
strawberry	2 tbsp (1.5 oz)	107	tr	28	–	–
strawberry	1 cup (11.5 oz)	863	1	225	–	–
Hershey's						
Sundae Syrup Caramel	2 tbsp (1.4 oz)	100	0	25	20	0
ICED TEA						
READY-TO-DRINK						
Delta Blues						
Tea Punch Black Tea Sumptuous Spearmint	8 oz	90	0	21	20	0
Tea Punch Green Tea Peach & Delectable Lemongrass	8 oz	90	0	22	21	–

FOOD	PORTION	CAL	FAT	CARB	SUGAR	FIBER
Tea Punch Green Tea Peach Apricot Pineapple Quince	8 oz	100	0	24	21	–
Fuze						
Antioxidant Tea	8 oz	60	0	15	15	–
Green Tea	8 oz	60	0	16	16	–
White Tea	8 oz	60	0	15	15	–
Gold Peak Tea						
Green Tea Sweetened	1 bottle (16.9 oz)	170	0	45	44	–
Hawaiian						
Iced Tea	1 can (11.5 oz)	120	0	35	35	0
Kombucha						
Wonder Drink Asian Pear Ginger	1 bottle (8.5 oz)	65	0	16	8	–
Wonder Drink Rooibus Red Peach	1 bottle (8.5 oz)	60	0	15	13	–
Nantucket Nectars						
Half & Half	8 oz	90	0	22	22	0
Original Lemon	8 oz	80	0	22	21	0
Osteo						
Fruit Tea All Flavors	1 can (12 oz)	120	0	32	32	0
Pixie						
Black Tea Mate Lemon Ginger	8 oz	35	0	8	6	0
Yerba Mate Authentic	8 oz	30	0	7	7	0
Santa Cruz						
Organic Lemon	8 oz	60	0	15	14	0
Organic Peppermint	8 oz	60	0	15	14	0
Organic TeaZer Passionfruit	1 bottle (12 oz)	90	0	22	21	0
Organic TeaZer Pear	1 bottle (12 oz)	90	0	21	21	0

FOOD	PORTION	CAL	FAT	CARB	SUGAR	FIBER
Snapple						
Black Tea Lemon	8 oz	80	0	21	21	–
Diet Lemon Tea	8 oz	10	0	0	0	–
Diet Lemonade Iced Tea	8 oz	10	0	2	2	–
Diet Peach	8 oz	0	0	0	0	–
Diet Plum-A-Granate	8 oz	5	0	0	0	0
Green Tea Mango Metabolism	8 oz	60	0	15	15	–
Peach	8 oz	90	0	23	23	–
Red Tea Pomegranate Raspberry	8 oz	80	0	21	21	–
White Tea Apple Plum	8 oz	80	0	21	21	–
Sweet Leaf						
Diet Mint & Honey Green Tea	8 oz	0	0	tr	0	0
Lemon & Lime Unsweet	8 oz	0	0	0	0	0
Original Sweet	8 oz	70	0	18	17	–
Pomegranate Green Tea	8 oz	60	0	16	14	–
Swiss Tea						
Diet	8 oz	0	0	1	0	0
Diet Decafe	8 oz	0	0	0	0	0
Green Tea w/ Ginseng & Honey	8 oz	80	0	20	20	0
Sweet Tea Southern Style	8 oz	90	0	23	23	0
W/ Lemon	8 oz	100	0	24	23	0
White Tea Sweetened w/ Raspberry	8 oz	90	0	24	23	0
True Brew						
Cranberry Orange	8 oz	72	0	18	18	0
Green Tea	8 oz	64	0	16	16	0
Sweet Tea	8 oz	76	0	19	19	0

FOOD	PORTION	CAL	FAT	CARB	SUGAR	FIBER
Turkey Hill						
Decaffeinated	8 oz	80	0	20	20	–
Diet Decaffeinated	8 oz	0	0	0	0	0
Nature's Accents Blueberry Oolong	8 oz	100	0	24	24	–
Nature's Accents Chai Spiced Zero Calorie	8 oz	0	0	1	0	–
Nature's Accents Green Tea	8 oz	70	0	17	17	–
Southern Brew Extra Sweet	8 oz	90	0	21	19	–

ICES AND ICE POPS
Breyers

FOOD	PORTION	CAL	FAT	CARB	SUGAR	FIBER
Pure Fruit Pop Lemon Lime	1 (1.75 oz)	40	0	10	9	–
Pure Fruit Pop Pomegranate Blends	1 (1.75 oz)	40	0	10	9	–
Dippin' Dots						
Cherry Berry	½ cup	90	0	23	12	0
Watermelon	½ cup	90	0	23	12	0
Haagen-Dazs						
Fat Free Sorbet Mango	½ cup (4 oz)	120	0	37	36	0
Fat Free Sorbet Raspberry	½ cup (3.7 oz)	120	0	30	26	2
Fat Free Sorbet Zesty Lemon	½ cup (4 oz)	110	0	29	28	tr
Lowfat Sorbet Chocolate	½ cup (3.7 oz)	130	1	28	20	2
Mr. J						
All Flavors	1 bar (2.25 oz)	50	tr	12	5	–
PickleSickle						
Pop	1 (2 oz)	3	0	1	0	0

FOOD	PORTION	CAL	FAT	CARB	SUGAR	FIBER
Popsicle						
Creamsicle Pop No Sugar Added	2 (1.65 oz)	45	1	10	3	2
Creamsicle Pop Sugar Free	2 (1.65 oz)	40	2	10	0	6
Diet Soda Pops	1 (1.6 oz)	15	0	3	0	–
Firecracker	1 (1.6 oz)	35	0	9	6	–
Fudgsicle Bar	1 (2.5 oz)	100	2	17	14	1
Fudgsicle Pops No Sugar Added	1 (1.65 oz)	40	1	10	2	2
Lifesavers Pop	1 (3.5 oz)	90	0	22	15	–
Pop Ups Orange Burst	1 (2.75 oz)	90	1	18	10	0
Rainbow Pops	1 (1.65 oz)	40	0	10	7	–
Snow Cone	1 (7 oz)	30	0	7	5	–
SoDelicious						
Dairy Free Creamy Orange Bar	1 (2.2 oz)	80	2	18	12	2
Sweet Nothings						
Bar Mango Raspberry	1 (2.6 oz)	100	0	23	12	0
Turkey Hill						
Venice Mango	½ cup	100	0	23	22	0
Venice Pomegranate Blueberry w/	½ cup	100	0	25	23	0
JACKFRUIT						
fresh	3.5 oz	70	tr	4	–	–
JALAPENO (see PEPPERS)						
JAM/JELLY/PRESERVES						
apple butter	1 tbsp (0.6 oz)	31	tr	8	6	tr
jam all flavors	1 pkg (0.5 oz)	39	tr	10	7	tr
jam all flavors	1 tbsp (0.7 oz)	56	tr	14	10	tr
jam apricot	1 tbsp (0.7 oz)	48	tr	13	9	tr
jam diet all flavors	1 tbsp (0.5 oz)	18	tr	8	5	tr

FOOD	PORTION	CAL	FAT	CARB	SUGAR	FIBER
jelly all flavors	1 tbsp (0.7 oz)	51	0	13	10	tr
jelly reduced sugar all flavors	1 tbsp (0.7 oz)	34	tr	9	9	tr
jelly diet all flavors	1 tbsp (0.7 oz)	25	tr	10	7	1
orange marmalade	1 tbsp (0.7 oz)	49	0	13	12	tr
preserves all flavors	1 tbsp (0.7 oz)	56	tr	14	10	tr
Cascadian Farm						
Organic Fruit Spread Blackberry	1 tbsp	45	0	11	10	–
Organic Fruit Spread Raspberry	1 tbsp	45	0	11	10	–
Organic Sweet Orange Marmalade	1 tbsp	45	0	11	10	–
Chukar Cherries						
Preserve Red Sour Cherry	1 tbsp	40	0	10	8	tr
Preserves No Sugar Added Cherry Amaretto	1 tbsp	24	0	18	1	tr
Preserves Vanilla Peach	1 tbsp	28	0	19	6	tr
Columia Empire Farms						
Marionberry Seedless Perserves	1 tbsp	60	0	14	9	–
Comfort Care						
Country Apple Butter	1 tbsp (1 oz)	40	0	11	10	1
Delicia						
Fruit Spread Black Cherry	1 tbsp (0.7 oz)	40	0	10	10	–
Gedney						
State Fair Preserves Strawberry Rhubarb	1 tbsp	50	0	12	11	0
Hero						
Swiss Preserves Black Cherry	1 tbsp (0.7 oz)	50	0	13	10	2

FOOD	PORTION	CAL	FAT	CARB	SUGAR	FIBER
Polaner						
All Fruit w/ Fiber Grape	1 tbsp (0.6 oz)	30	0	9	6	3
Revolution Foods						
Organic Jelly Grape	1 tbsp (0.7 oz)	60	0	14	14	0
Organic Preserves Strawberry	1 tbsp (0.7 oz)	60	0	14	13	0
Trappist						
Jelly Pomegranate	1 tbsp (0.7 oz)	50	0	14	11	–
Tree Of Life						
Organic Fruit Spread Grape	1 tbsp (0.6 oz)	30	0	8	7	0
Organic Fruit Spread Peach	1 tbsp (0.6 oz)	30	0	8	7	0
Welch's						
Grape Jelly	1 tbsp	50	0	13	13	–

JAPANESE FOOD (*see* ASIAN FOOD, SUSHI)

JELLY (*see* JAM/JELLY/PRESERVES)

JELLYFISH

FOOD	PORTION	CAL	FAT	CARB	SUGAR	FIBER
pickled	½ cup (1 oz)	10	tr	0	0	0

JERKY

FOOD	PORTION	CAL	FAT	CARB	SUGAR	FIBER
beef	1 piece (0.7 oz)	82	5	2	2	tr
pork	1 strip (0.5 oz)	62	4	2	1	tr
venison	1 strip (0.5 oz)	55	3	2	2	0
Applegate Farms						
Natural Joy Stick	1 (1 oz)	100	7	0	tr	tr
Dakota Gourmet						
Fruit Jerky Strawberry Kiwi	1	70	0	16	12	1
Frank's RedHot						
Chile'N Lime Steak Strips	1 oz	80	4	2	1	0
Original Beef	1 oz	80	1	5	4	0

FOOD	PORTION	CAL	FAT	CARB	SUGAR	FIBER
Gary West						
Beef Strips Hickory Smoked	1 oz	70	1	5	5	0
Buffalo Strips	½ pkg (1 oz)	60	0	3	2	0
Elk Strips	½ pkg (1 oz)	70	1	4	2	0
Outpost						
Beef	1 oz	70	1	4	3	0
Beef Steak	1 pkg (0.9 oz)	60	3	2	tr	0
Beef Stick	1 (0.4 oz)	60	5	2	1	0
Primal						
Mealtless Vegan Hickory Smoke	1 pkg (1 oz)	99	3	8	3	1
Meatless Vegan Mesquite Lime	1 pkg (1 oz)	74	2	7	4	0
Meatless Vegan Texas BBQ	1 pkg (1 oz)	81	1	11	5	1
Meatless Vegan Thai Peanut	1 pkg (1 oz)	74	2	8	4	1
Slim Jim						
Beef	7 pieces	130	8	3	tr	0
Beef Jerky Hickory Smoked	1 oz	80	2	4	3	0
Classic Handipack	1 box	210	19	3	tr	tr
Giant Caddy Pepperoni	1 pkg	150	13	3	tr	0
Twin Pack Cheese & Pepperoni	1 pkg	150	12	2	0	1
Tony's Smokehouse						
Salmon	1 pkg (0.5 oz)	40	1	2	1	1
JICAMA						
fresh	1 sm (12.8 oz)	139	tr	32	7	18
raw sliced	1 cup	46	tr	11	2	6

FOOD	PORTION	CAL	FAT	CARB	SUGAR	FIBER
JUJUBE						
dried	1 oz	82	tr	21	–	–
JUTE						
cooked	1 cup	32	tr	6	1	2
KALE						
chopped cooked w/o salt	1 cup	36	1	7	2	3
fresh cooked w/ fat	1 cup	69	4	7	2	2
scotch chopped cooked w/o salt	1 cup	36	1	7	–	2
Allens						
Seasoned	½ cup	35	1	5	1	1
KEFIR						
kefir	8 oz	98	2	12	12	0
Evolve						
Plain	8 oz	120	3	15	10	5
Strawberry	8 oz	180	2	31	27	5
Nancy's						
Organic Lowfat Blackberry	1 cup	180	3	34	32	2
Organic Lowfat Plain	1 cup	110	3	14	13	1
Organic Lowfat Raspberry	1 cup	180	3	35	32	3
KETCHUP						
banana	1 tsp	10	0	2	2	0
ketchup	1 pkg (0.2 oz)	6	tr	2	–	tr
ketchup	1 tbsp	15	tr	4	3	0
low sodium	1 tbsp	15	tr	4	3	0
Heinz						
Ketchup	1 tbsp	15	0	4	4	0

FOOD	PORTION	CAL	FAT	CARB	SUGAR	FIBER
Muir Glen						
Organic	1 tbsp	20	0	4	3	0
OrganicVille						
No Added Sugar	1 tbsp (0.6 oz)	20	0	4	3	0
Texas Sassy						
Tequila Ketchup	1 tbsp (0.5 oz)	20	0	5	5	–
Tree Of Life						
Organic	1 tbsp (0.6 oz)	20	0	4	4	0
Wholemato						
Organic Agave	1 tbsp	15	0	3	3	0
KIDNEY						
beef simmered	3 oz	134	4	0	0	0
lamb braised	3 oz	116	3	1	–	0
pork braised	3 oz	128	4	0	0	0
veal braised	3 oz	139	5	0	0	0
Rumba						
Beef	4 oz	120	4	2	0	0
KIDNEY BEANS						
canned	½ cup	108	1	19	2	6
dried cooked w/o salt	½ cup	112	tr	20	tr	6
B&M						
Red Kidney Baked Beans	½ cup (4.6 oz)	200	3	36	10	6
Progresso						
Cannellini	½ cup (4.6 oz)	110	0	20	2	6
Van Camp's						
New Orleans	½ cup	90	0	19	1	6
KIWI						
fresh	1 lg (3.2 oz)	56	tr	13	8	3
fresh	1 med (2.6 oz)	46	tr	11	7	2
Chiquita						
fresh	1 (2.7 oz)	46	0	11	7	2

FOOD	PORTION	CAL	FAT	CARB	SUGAR	FIBER
KNISH						
TAKE-OUT						
cheese	1 (2.1 oz)	205	12	19	tr	1
meat	1 (1.8 oz)	174	11	13	tr	1
potato	1 (2.1 oz)	212	12	21	tr	1
potato	1 lg (7 oz)	332	12	49	5	1
KOHLRABI						
raw sliced	1 cup	36	tr	8	4	4
sliced cooked w/o salt	1 cup	48	tr	11	5	2
TAKE-OUT						
creamed	1 cup	150	9	14	6	1
KRILL						
fresh	1 oz	22	1	tr	–	0
KUMQUATS						
canned in syrup	1	13	tr	3	3	1
fresh	1	13	tr	3	2	1
LAMB						
cubed lean & fat braised	4 oz	253	10	0	0	0
cubed lean broiled	4 oz	211	8	0	0	0
ground broiled	4 oz	321	22	0	0	0
leg roasted	4 oz	213	15	0	0	0
loin chop lean & fat broiled	1 chop (4 oz)	222	16	0	0	0
rib chop lean & fat broiled	1 chop (1.6 oz)	165	14	0	0	0
rib roast baked	4 oz	386	31	0	0	0
shank lean & fat braised	4 oz	360	20	0	0	0
shoulder chop lean & fat cooked	1 chop (5.5 oz)	274	20	0	0	0
shoulder w/ bone braised	4 oz	231	17	0	0	0

FOOD	PORTION	CAL	FAT	CARB	SUGAR	FIBER
LAMB DISHES						
TAKE-OUT						
keema w/ coconut milk	1 serv (8 oz)	380	28	18	9	6
moussaka	4 in sq (16 oz)	659	43	32	10	8
shepherd's pie	1 (21.3 oz)	742	31	76	9	9
stew w/ potatoes & vegetables	1 cup	260	6	29	3	4
LAMBSQUARTERS						
chopped cooked w/ salt	1 cup	58	1	9	–	4
LECITHIN						
lecithin	1 tbsp	104	14	0	0	0
Tree Of Life						
Granules	1 tbsp (0.3 oz)	55	4	1	0	0
LEEKS						
chopped cooked w/o salt	¼ cup	8	tr	2	–	tr
cooked	1 (4.4 oz)	38	tr	9	–	1
freeze dried	1 tbsp	1	0	tr	–	0
LEMON						
fresh	1 med (4 oz)	22	tr	12	–	5
peel	1 tbsp	3	tr	1	tr	1
peel	1 tsp	1	0	tr	tr	tr
wedge	1 (7 g)	2	tr	1	tr	tr
True Lemon						
Crystallized Lemon	1 pkg (1 g)	0	0	tr	–	–
LEMON CURD						
lemon curd made w/ egg	2 tsp	29	1	4	–	0
LEMON GRASS						
fresh	1 tbsp	5	tr	1	–	–

FOOD	PORTION	CAL	FAT	CARB	SUGAR	FIBER
LEMON JUICE						
bottled	1 oz	6	tr	2	1	tr
bottled	1 tbsp	3	tr	1	tr	tr
fresh	1 oz	8	0	3	1	tr
from 1 lemon	1.6 oz	12	0	4	1	tr
from wedge	6 g	1	0	1	tr	0
Canarino						
Italian Hot Lemon Beverage as prep	1 cup	0	0	0	0	0
Natalie's Orchid Island Juice						
100% Juice	1 tsp	1	0	0	0	0
Santa Cruz						
Organic 100% Juice	1 tsp	0	0	0	0	0
LEMONADE						
READY-TO-DRINK						
Mike's						
Hard Lemonade	1 bottle (12 oz)	220	0	32	–	–
Nantucket Nectars						
Lemonade	8 oz	110	0	28	28	0
Natalie's Orchid Island Juice						
Lemonade	8 oz	130	0	33	33	0
Santa Cruz						
Organic Sparkling	8 oz	110	0	27	27	0
Sweet Leaf						
Half & Half Lemonade Tea	8 oz	85	0	20	19	–
Original	8 oz	90	0	24	22	–
Turkey Hill						
Lemonade	8 oz	120	0	29	29	–
LENTILS						
dried cooked	1 cup	230	1	40	4	16

FOOD	PORTION	CAL	FAT	CARB	SUGAR	FIBER
Near East						
Lentil Pilaf as prep	1 cup	200	3	36	3	8
TastyBite						
Madras Lentils	½ pkg (5 oz)	120	5	14	3	5
TruRoots						
Organic Sprouted Green not prep	¼ cup (1.4 oz)	140	1	25	1	7
TAKE-OUT						
lentil loaf	1 slice (1.6 oz)	83	4	10	1	3
yemiser selatta ethiopian lentil salad	1 serv (3 oz)	115	7	11	1	2

LETTUCE (*see also* SALAD)

FOOD	PORTION	CAL	FAT	CARB	SUGAR	FIBER
arugula	6 leaves (0.4 oz)	3	tr	tr	tr	tr
arugula shredded	1 cup	5	tr	1	tr	tr
boston	1 head (5.7 oz)	21	tr	4	2	2
boston chopped	6 leaves	7	tr	1	1	1
cornsalad field salad	1 cup (1.9 oz)	7	tr	1	–	1
iceberg	1 lg head (26.5 oz)	106	1	22	15	9
iceberg	6 med leaves	7	tr	1	1	1
iceberg shredded	1 cup	10	tr	2	1	1
looseleaf outer leaves	6 (5 oz)	22	tr	4	1	2
looseleaf shredded	1 cup	5	tr	1	tr	1
red leaf	6 leaves (3.6 oz)	16	tr	2	tr	1
red leaf shredded	1 cup	4	tr	1	tr	tr
romaine	3 leaves (3 oz)	14	tr	3	1	2
romaine heart	6 leaves (1.3 oz)	6	tr	1	tr	1
romaine shredded	1 cup	8	tr	2	1	1
Fresh Express						
5 Lettuce Mix	3 cups	15	0	1	1	1
Lettuce Trio	2½ cups	15	0	3	1	1
Organic Baby Arugula	3 cups	20	1	3	2	1

FOOD	PORTION	CAL	FAT	CARB	SUGAR	FIBER
Organic Hearts Of Romaine	1½ cups	15	0	2	0	1
Premium Romaine	2 cups	15	0	3	1	2
Shreds Iceberg	1½ cups	15	0	3	2	1
Sweet Butter	2½ cups	10	0	2	1	1
Mann's						
Romaine Hearts	6 leaves (3 oz)	15	1	3	2	1
Ocean Mist						
Butter Leaf Shredded	1 cup (2 oz)	7	0	1	1	1
Green Or Green Leaf Shredded	1 cup (1.3 oz)	5	0	1	0	0
Iceberg	⅙ head (3 oz)	15	0	3	2	1
LILY ROOT						
dried	1 oz	89	1	21	–	tr
fresh	1 oz	32	tr	8	–	tr
LIMA BEANS						
CANNED						
lima beans	½ cup	95	tr	18	–	6
Allens						
Baby Butter Beans	½ cup	120	1	22	2	6
Medium Green	½ cup	140	1	26	0	7
East Texas Fair						
Green	½ cup	120	0	23	0	8
DRIED						
cooked	½ cup	150	tr	20	1	5
FROZEN						
Green Giant						
Baby & Butter Sauce as prep	⅔ cup	100	2	18	1	5
LIME						
fresh	1 (2.4 oz)	20	tr	7	1	1
wedge	1 (8 g)	2	tr	1	tr	tr

FOOD	PORTION	CAL	FAT	CARB	SUGAR	FIBER
True Lime						
Crystallized Lime	1 pkg	0	0	0	0	0
LIME JUICE						
bottled	1 oz	6	tr	2	tr	tr
fresh	1 oz	8	tr	3	1	tr
from 1 lime	1.1 oz	11	tr	4	1	tr
Angostura						
Lime Mixer	1 tsp	5	0	2	2	0
Natalie's Orchid Island Juice						
100% Juice	1 tsp	0	0	0	0	0
Santa Cruz						
Organic 100% Juice	1 tsp	0	0	0	0	0
Sweet Leaf						
Limeade Cherry	8 oz	90	0	24	22	–
Turkey Hill						
Limonade	8 oz	120	0	29	27	–
LING						
blue raw	3.5 oz	83	1	0	0	0
fresh baked	3 oz	95	1	0	0	0
fresh fillet baked	5.3 oz	168	1	0	0	0
LINGCOD						
baked	3 oz	93	1	0	0	0
fillet baked	5.3 oz	164	2	0	0	0
LIQUOR/LIQUEUR (*see also* BEER AND ALE, CHAMPAGNE, MALT, WINE)						
7&7	1 serv	178	0	19	–	0
alabama slammer	1 serv	103	tr	7	–	tr
amaretto sour	1 serv	295	tr	57	–	4
angel's kiss	1 serv	85	1	5	–	0
anisette	1 oz	111	0	11	–	0
antifreeze	1 serv	177	tr	31	–	tr
apricot brandy	1 oz	96	0	9	–	0

FOOD	PORTION	CAL	FAT	CARB	SUGAR	FIBER
apricot sour	1 serv	164	tr	8	–	tr
aquavit	1 oz	65	0	0	0	0
b 52	1 serv	247	4	25	–	0
b&b	1 serv	75	0	0	0	0
bahama breeze	1 serv	70	tr	9	–	tr
bahama mama	1 serv	153	tr	23	–	tr
bailey's & amaretto	1 serv	184	5	16	–	0
banana colada	1 serv	376	1	64	–	3
bay breeze	1 serv	173	tr	18	–	tr
bend me over	1 serv	242	tr	32	–	tr
benedictine	1 oz	104	0	11	–	0
betsy ross	1 serv	206	0	5	–	0
black devil	1 serv	220	tr	1	–	tr
black russian	1 serv	184	tr	12	–	0
bloody mary	1 serv	150	tr	5	–	1
blue whale	1 serv	222	tr	23	–	0
bourbon & soda	1 serv (4 oz)	105	0	0	0	0
bourbon sour	1 serv	166	tr	8	–	tr
brandy alexander	1 serv	266	6	12	–	0
brandy sour	1 serv	164	tr	8	–	tr
bushwacker	1 serv	286	5	27	–	tr
coffee liqueur	1 serv (1.5 oz)	175	tr	24	24	0
cognac	1 oz	67	0	tr	0	0
cosmopolitan martini	1 serv	126	tr	7	–	tr
creme de menthe	1 serv (1.5 oz)	186	tr	21	21	0
curacao liqueur	1 oz	81	0	9	–	0
daiquiri	1 serv (2 oz)	112	tr	4	3	tr
daiquiri banana	1 serv	277	tr	32	–	1
dark & stormy	1 serv	64	0	0	0	0
doctor pepper	1 serv	95	0	12	–	0
frozen daiquiri pineapple	1 serv	186	tr	28	–	2

FOOD	PORTION	CAL	FAT	CARB	SUGAR	FIBER
frozen tequila screwdriver	1 serv	159	tr	17	–	1
fuzzy navel	1 serv	247	tr	10	–	tr
gin	1 serv (1.5 oz)	110	0	0	0	0
gin & tonic	1 serv (7.5 oz)	171	0	16	–	–
gin ricky	1 serv	114	tr	1	–	tr
grasshopper	1 serv	275	5	26	–	0
happy hawaiian	1 serv	434	8	60	–	tr
harvey wallbanger	1 serv	198	tr	16	–	tr
head banger	1 serv	165	0	4	–	0
hot buttered rum	1 serv (8.8 oz)	316	12	4	4	tr
hot toddy	1 serv	188	1	13	–	5
hurricane	1 serv	205	tr	19	–	tr
kamikaze	1 serv	136	0	2	–	0
long island iced tea	1 serv	292	tr	7	–	0
lynchburg lemonade	1 serv	465	tr	85	–	1
mai tai	1 serv	165	tr	17	–	tr
manhattan	1 serv	171	tr	3	–	tr
margarita	1 serv	173	0	11	–	0
margarita strawberry	1 serv	106	tr	11	–	1
martini	1 serv (3 oz)	206	0	2	tr	0
martini apple	1 serv	147	tr	4	–	tr
martini rum	1 serv	131	0	tr	–	tr
mellow yellow	1 serv	95	0	4	–	0
mexican grasshopper	1 serv	638	19	52	–	0
mint julep	1 serv	136	tr	17	–	tr
mississippi mud	1 serv	496	12	46	–	0
mudslide	1 serv	566	10	46	–	0
narragansett	1 serv	168	0	2	–	0
nutcracker	1 serv	730	10	64	–	0
old fashioned	1 serv	223	tr	4	–	tr
orange crush	1 serv	461	tr	65	–	tr
pain killer	1 serv	277	tr	20	–	tr

FOOD	PORTION	CAL	FAT	CARB	SUGAR	FIBER
peppermint pattie	1 serv	344	tr	37	–	0
pina colada	1 serv (4.5 oz)	245	3	32	31	tr
planter's cocktail	1 serv	105	0	3	–	tr
planter's punch	1 serv	233	tr	34	–	4
presbyterian	1 serv	170	0	8	–	tr
purple passion	1 serv	215	tr	22	–	0
rob roy	1 serv	171	0	3	–	tr
rum	1 serv (1.5 oz)	97	0	0	0	0
rum boogie	1 serv	134	tr	12	–	tr
rum cola	1 serv	209	tr	21	–	tr
rum highball	1 serv	170	0	11	–	0
rum punch	1 serv	448	1	88	–	1
rum screwdriver	1 serv	166	tr	16	–	tr
rum sour	1 serv	156	tr	8	–	tr
rum swizzle	1 serv	187	0	15	–	0
rusty nail	1 serv	159	0	6	–	0
sake	1 serv (1 oz)	39	0	1	0	0
salty dog	1 serv	210	tr	19	–	tr
scotch & soda	1 serv	104	0	tr	–	tr
sea breeze	1 serv	207	tr	19	–	tr
sex on the beach	1 serv	190	tr	18	–	tr
slippery nipple	1 serv	142	2	11	–	0
sloe gin fizz	1 serv (2.5 oz)	132	0	4	–	0
snake bite	1 serv	362	0	22	–	0
tequila gimlet	1 serv	150	tr	6	–	1
tequila sour	1 serv	156	tr	8	–	tr
tequila stinger	1 serv	221	tr	14	–	0
tequila sunrise	1 serv (6.8 oz)	232	tr	24	–	0
tom collins	1 serv (7.5 oz)	121	0	3	–	–
vermouth cassis	1 serv	97	tr	5	–	tr
vodka	1 serv (1.5 oz)	97	0	0	0	0
vodka gimlet	1 serv	150	tr	6	–	1

FOOD	PORTION	CAL	FAT	CARB	SUGAR	FIBER
vodka sour	1 serv	138	tr	3	–	tr
vodka stinger	1 serv	378	tr	28	–	0
whiskey	1 serv (1.5 oz)	105	0	tr	–	0
whiskey sour	1 serv (3.5 oz)	162	tr	14	14	0
white russian	1 serv	290	8	17	–	0
zombie	1 serv	235	tr	10	–	tr
Absolut						
Vodka	1 shot (1.5 oz)	98	0	0	–	–
Barcardi						
Gold Rum	1 shot (1.5 oz)	98	0	0	–	–
Capt. Morgan's						
Original Spiced Rum	1 shot (1.5 oz)	86	0	0	–	–
Crown Royal						
Canadian Whiskey	1 shot (1.5 oz)	96	0	0	–	–
Jack Daniel's						
Old No.7 Tennessee Whiskey	1 shot (1.5 oz)	98	0	0	–	–
Jose Cuervo						
Gold Tequila	1 shot (1.5 oz)	96	0	0	–	–
Seagram's						
Gin	1 shot (1.5 oz)	120	0	0	–	–
Smirnoff						
Vodka	1 shot (1.5 oz)	96	0	0	–	–
LIVER (see also PATE)						
beef braised	1 slice (2.4 oz)	130	4	3	0	0
beef pan-fried	1 slice (2.8 oz)	142	4	4	0	0
chicken fried	3 oz	146	5	1	0	0
chicken simmered	3 oz	142	6	1	0	0
duck raw	1 (1.5 oz)	60	2	2	–	0
goose raw	1 (3.3 oz)	125	4	6	–	0
lamb braised	3 oz	187	7	2	–	0
lamb fried	3 oz	202	11	3	–	0
moose braised	3 oz	132	4	3	–	–

FOOD	PORTION	CAL	FAT	CARB	SUGAR	FIBER
pork braised	3 oz	140	4	3	–	0
turkey simmered	1 liver (2.9 oz)	227	17	1	0	0
veal braised	1 slice (2.8 oz)	154	5	3	0	0
veal pan fried	1 slice (2.4 oz)	129	4	3	0	0
Perdue						
Chicken Fresh	4 oz	130	6	0	0	0
Rumba						
Beef	4 oz	160	5	7	0	0
TAKE-OUT						
calves liver w/ onions	1 serv (5 oz)	177	4	10	2	1
LOBSTER						
northern cooked	3 oz	83	1	1	–	–
northern cooked	1 cup	142	1	2	–	–
northern raw	1 lobster (5.3 oz)	136	1	1	–	–
northern raw	3 oz	77	1	tr	–	–
spiny steamed	3 oz	122	2	3	–	–
spiny steamed	1 (5.7 oz)	233	3	5	–	–
TAKE-OUT						
newburg	1 cup	485	27	13	–	–
LOGANBERRIES						
fresh	½ cup (2.5 oz)	40	tr	9	6	4
frzn thawed	½ cup (2.6 oz)	40	tr	10	6	4
LONGANS						
fresh	1	2	0	tr	–	–
LOQUATS						
fresh	1 lg (0.7 oz)	9	tr	2	–	tr
fresh	1 sm (0.5 oz)	6	tr	2	–	tr
fresh cubed	½ cup (2.6 oz)	35	tr	9	–	1

FOOD	PORTION	CAL	FAT	CARB	SUGAR	FIBER
LOTUS						
root raw sliced	10 slices	45	tr	14	–	–
root sliced cooked	10 slices	59	tr	14	–	–
seeds dried	1 oz	94	1	18	–	–
LOX (see SALMON)						
LUPINES						
dried cooked	1 cup	197	5	16	–	–
LYCHEES						
canned in syrup	1 (0.7 oz)	19	tr	5	5	tr
canned in syrup	½ cup (4.4 oz)	114	tr	29	28	1
dried	1 (2.5 g)	7	tr	2	2	tr
fresh	1 (0.3 oz)	6	tr	2	1	tr
fresh cut up	½ cup (3.3 oz)	63	tr	16	14	1
Polar						
Lychee	1	110	0	27	26	1
MACADAMIA NUTS						
dry roasted w/ salt	11 nuts (1 oz)	200	22	4	2	1
oil roasted	1 oz	204	22	4	–	–
Chukar Cherries						
Extra Dark Chocolate Covered	3 tbsp (1.4 oz)	216	20	14	9	3
Emily's						
Milk Chocolate Covered	4 (1.5 oz)	260	19	21	18	2
Fisher						
Macadamia Nuts	¼ cup (1 oz)	200	21	4	1	3
Mauna Loa						
Dry Roasted Salted	¼ cup (1 oz)	230	24	4	1	2
Dry Roasted Unsalted	¼ cup (1 oz)	230	24	4	1	2
Honey Roasted	¼ cup (1 oz)	200	19	9	6	2
Kona Coffee	¼ cup (1 oz)	180	15	12	8	1

FOOD	PORTION	CAL	FAT	CARB	SUGAR	FIBER
MACE						
ground	1 tsp	8	1	1	–	tr
MACKEREL						
CANNED						
jack	1 can (12.7 oz)	563	23	0	0	0
jack	1 cup	296	12	0	0	0
Polar						
Jack	⅓ cup	90	4	0	0	0
FRESH						
atlantic cooked	3 oz	223	15	0	0	0
atlantic raw	3 oz	174	12	0	0	0
jack baked	3 oz	171	9	0	0	0
jack fillet baked	6.2 oz	354	18	0	0	0
king baked	3 oz	114	2	0	0	0
king fillet baked	5.4 oz	207	4	0	0	0
pacific baked	3 oz	171	9	0	0	0
pacific fillet baked	6.2 oz	354	18	0	0	0
spanish cooked	1 fillet (5.1 oz)	230	9	0	0	0
spanish cooked	3 oz	134	5	0	0	0
spanish raw	3 oz	118	5	0	0	0
SMOKED						
atlantic	3.5 oz	296	24	0	0	0
MAHI MAHI						
fresh baked	4 oz	192	13	1	tr	0
MALANGA						
dasheen mashed	1 cup	226	tr	53	1	8
dasheen pieces boiled	1 cup	212	tr	50	1	8
pieces fried	1 cup	304	11	52	1	8
root raw	1 (10.7 oz)	299	1	72	–	5

FOOD	PORTION	CAL	FAT	CARB	SUGAR	FIBER
MALT						
malt liquor	1 bottle (12 oz)	148	0	13	tr	tr
nonalcoholic	1 bottle (12 oz)	133	tr	29	29	0
MALTED MILK						
chocolate as prep w/ milk	1 cup	179	5	27	15	1
chocolate flavor powder	3 heaping tsp (0.7 oz)	79	1	18	5	1
natural flavor as prep w/ milk	1 cup	186	6	24	22	tr
natural flavor powder	3 heaping tsp (0.7 oz)	87	2	16	12	tr
MAMMY-APPLE						
fresh	1	431	4	106	–	–
MANGO						
dried	½ cup (1.8 oz)	74	tr	41	38	3
dried	1 slice (5 g)	16	tr	4	4	tr
fresh	1 (7.3 oz)	135	1	35	31	4
fresh sliced	½ cup (3 oz)	54	tr	14	12	2
pickled	1 slice (1 oz)	38	tr	10	9	tr
Kopali						
Organic Dried	1 pkg (1.8 oz)	140	0	38	34	4
Polar						
Sliced	3 pieces (5 oz)	100	0	24	21	2
MANGO JUICE						
nectar canned	1 cup (8.8 oz)	128	tr	33	31	1
GoodBelly						
Mango Probiotic Drink	8 oz	100	0	25	21	1

FOOD	PORTION	CAL	FAT	CARB	SUGAR	FIBER
Snapple						
Juice Drinks Mango Madness	8 oz	100	0	26	25	–
MANGOSTEEN						
canned in syrup	½ cup (3.4 oz)	72	1	18	–	2
MARGARINE						
margarine butter blend	1 tbsp (0.5 oz)	101	11	tr	0	0
squeeze	1 pkg (0.2 oz)	36	4	0	0	0
squeeze liquid	1 tbsp (0.5 oz)	102	11	0	0	0
stick	1 tbsp (0.5 oz)	100	11	tr	0	0
stick	1 stick (4 oz)	810	91	1	0	0
tub diet	1 tbsp (0.5 oz)	26	3	tr	0	0
tub fat free	1 tbsp (0.5 oz)	27	tr	1	0	0
tub light	1 tbsp (0.5 oz)	59	7	tr	–	0
tub salted	1 tbsp (0.5 oz)	101	11	tr	0	0
whipped salted	1 tbsp (0.3 oz)	67	8	tr	0	0
Brummel & Brown						
Spread w/ Natural Yogurt	1 tbsp (0.5 oz)	45	5	0	0	0
Country Crock						
Light	1 tbsp (0.5 oz)	50	5	0	0	0
Regular	1 tbsp (0.5 oz)	90	7	0	0	0
Spread w/ Calcium + Vitamin D	1 tbsp (0.5 oz)	50	5	0	0	0
Earth Balance						
Butter Blend Salted	1 tbsp	100	11	0	0	0
Buttery Spread Original	1 tbsp	100	11	0	0	0
Buttery Spread Soy Garden	1 tbsp	100	11	0	0	0
Buttery Sticks Vegan	1 tbsp	100	11	0	0	0

FOOD	PORTION	CAL	FAT	CARB	SUGAR	FIBER
Land O Lakes						
Soft	1 tbsp (0.5 oz)	100	11	0	0	0
Stick	1 tbsp (0.5 oz)	100	11	0	0	0
Move Over Butter						
Spread	1 tbsp	50	6	0	0	0
Promise						
Buttery Spread	1 tbsp	80	8	0	0	0
Buttery Spread Activ	1 tbsp	70	8	0	0	0
Fat Free	1 tbsp	5	0	0	0	0
Light	1 tbsp	45	5	0	0	0
Light Activ	1 tbsp	45	5	0	0	0
MARINADE (see SAUCE)						
MARJORAM						
dried	1 tsp	2	tr	tr	tr	tr
MARLIN						
raw	3 oz	110	3	0	0	0
MARSHMALLOW						
chocolate coated	1 (0.4 oz)	41	1	8	6	tr
cocunut coated	1 (0.4 oz)	33	1	7	5	tr
marshmallow regular	1 (0.3 oz)	23	tr	6	4	0
miniatures	10 (0.3 oz)	22	tr	6	4	0
miniatures	1 cup (1.8 oz)	159	tr	41	29	tr
MATZO						
brie	1 piece (0.5 oz)	54	3	5	3	tr
egg	1 (1 oz)	109	1	22	–	1
matzo ball	1 med (1.2 oz)	48	2	6	tr	tr
plain	1 (1 oz)	111	tr	23	–	1
whole wheat	1 (1 oz)	98	tr	22	–	3

FOOD	PORTION	CAL	FAT	CARB	SUGAR	FIBER
Holiday Candies						
Dark Chocolate Coated	1 oz	130	5	20	9	1
Manischewitz						
Egg & Onion	1 (1 oz)	100	1	23	2	2
Matzo Ball Mix	2 tbsp	50	0	11	0	1
Yehuda						
Organic	1 (1 oz)	110	1	23	0	3
MAYONNAISE						
diet	1 tbsp	36	3	3	1	0
imitation	1 tbsp	35	3	2	1	0
mayonnaise	1 tbsp	99	11	1	tr	0
Hellman's						
W/ Extra Virgin Olive Oil	1 tbsp	50	5	tr	–	–
Kraft						
Mayo W/ Olive Oil	1 tbsp	45	4	2	tr	0
NatureNaise						
Organic Spread	1 tbsp (0.5 oz)	40	3	2	–	–
Vegenaise						
Grapeseed Oil	1 tbsp (0.5 oz)	90	9	0	0	0
Organic	1 tbsp (0.5 oz)	90	9	0	0	0
Original	1 tbsp (0.5 oz)	90	9	0	0	0

MEAT SUBSTITUTES (*see also* BACON SUBSTITUTES, CANADIAN BACON SUBSTITUTES, CHICKEN SUBSTITUTES, HAMBURGER SUBSTITUTES, MEATBALL SUBSTITUTES, SAUSAGE SUBSTITUTES, TURKEY SUBSTITUTES)

FOOD	PORTION	CAL	FAT	CARB	SUGAR	FIBER
Amy's						
Veggie Loaf w/ Mashed Potatoes & Vegetables	1 pkg (10 oz)	290	8	47	6	7
Veat						
Gourmet Bites	1 serv (2.5 oz)	90	3	8	2	1
Vegetarian Fillet	1 (1.8 oz)	170	5	19	1	1

MEATBALL SUBSTITUTES

FOOD	PORTION	CAL	FAT	CARB	SUGAR	FIBER
meatless	2 (1.3 oz)	71	3	3	tr	2

FOOD	PORTION	CAL	FAT	CARB	SUGAR	FIBER
MEATBALLS						
beef cocktail	1 (0.2 oz)	18	1	0	0	0
beef lg	1 (1.5 oz)	111	7	0	0	0
beef med	1 (1 oz)	74	5	0	0	0
chicken cocktail	1 (0.2 oz)	12	tr	1	tr	0
chicken lg	1 (1.5 oz)	71	3	3	1	tr
chicken med	1 (1 oz)	47	2	2	1	tr
turkey med	1 (1 oz)	47	2	2	1	tr
Butterball						
Seasoned Italian frzn	6 (3 oz)	170	6	6	1	1
DelGrosso						
Italian Style	3 (3 oz)	180	12	5	0	0
Organic Classics						
Italian Beef	3 (3 oz)	180	11	5	1	1
Perdue						
Turkey Italian Style	4 (3 oz)	180	10	5	0	–
TAKE-OUT						
albondigas w/ sauce	3 + sauce (5.3 oz)	372	27	11	3	1
porcupine + tomato sauce	3 + sauce	160	7	14	3	1
swedish w/ cream sauce	3 + sauce (4.7 oz)	215	12	9	2	tr
sweet & sour	3 + sauce (4.5 oz)	188	11	8	1	1
MELON						
sprite	1 (10.6 oz)	110	0	29	27	1
MEXICAN FOOD (see SALSA, SPANISH FOOD, TORTILLA)						
MILK						
CANNED						
condensed sweetened	1 cup (10.7 oz)	982	27	166	166	0

FOOD	PORTION	CAL	FAT	CARB	SUGAR	FIBER
condensed sweetened	1 tbsp (0.7 oz)	61	2	10	10	0
evaporated nonfat	1 cup (9 oz)	200	1	29	29	0
evaporated nonfat	1 tbsp (0.5 oz)	12	tr	2	2	1
Borden						
Sweetened Condensed Low Fat	2 tbsp	120	2	23	23	0
Carnation						
Evaporated Fat Free	2 tbsp (1 oz)	25	0	4	4	–
Evaporated Lowfat 2%	2 tbsp (1 oz)	25	1	3	3	–
DRIED						
buttermilk	¼ cup (1 oz)	111	2	14	14	0
buttermilk	1 tbsp (0.2 oz)	25	tr	3	3	0
nonfat instant	1 tbsp (0.6 oz)	61	tr	9	9	0
nonfat instant	1 pkg (3.2 oz)	326	1	47	47	0
whole milk	¼ cup (1.1 oz)	159	9	12	12	0
Carnation						
Instant Nonfat as prep	1 cup	80	0	12	12	0
Sanalac						
Powder	¼ cup (0.8 oz)	80	0	13	12	0
REFRIGERATED						
1%	1 cup (8.6 oz)	102	3	12	13	0
2%	1 cup (8.6 oz)	122	5	11	12	0
buffalo	7 oz	224	16	10	–	–
buttermilk lowfat	1 cup (8.6 oz)	98	2	12	12	0
camel	7 oz	160	8	10	–	–
donkey	7 oz	86	2	12	–	–
fat free	1 cup (8.6 oz)	83	tr	12	12	0
goat	1 cup (8.6 oz)	168	10	11	11	0
human	1 cup (8.6 oz)	172	11	17	07	0
indian buffalo	1 cup (8.6 oz)	237	17	13	–	0
mare	7 oz	98	4	12	–	–
sheep	1 cup (8.6 oz)	265	17	13	–	0
whole	1 cup (8.6 oz)	146	8	11	14	0

FOOD	PORTION	CAL	FAT	CARB	SUGAR	FIBER
Dairy Ease						
Fat Free Lactose Free	1 cup (8 oz)	90	0	12	12	0
Reduced Fat 2% Lactose Free	1 cup (8 oz)	130	5	12	12	0
Whole Lactose Free	1 cup (8 oz)	160	9	11	11	0
Friendship						
Buttermilk Lowfat	1 cup	120	4	12	12	0
Land O Lakes						
1%	1 cup (8 oz)	100	3	13	13	0
2%	1 cup (8 oz)	120	5	12	12	0
Skim	1 cup (8 oz)	90	0	13	13	0
Whole	1 cup (8 oz)	150	8	12	12	0
Straus						
Organic Reduced Fat 2% Cream Top	8 oz	130	5	13	13	0
Turkey Hill						
Cool Moos Whole Milk	8 oz	160	3	27	26	0
Valio						
100% Lactose Free 0% Fat	8 oz	80	0	7	7	0
100% Lactose Free 2% Fat	8 oz	120	5	7	7	0

MILK DRINKS

FOOD	PORTION	CAL	FAT	CARB	SUGAR	FIBER
chocolate milk	1 cup (8.8 oz)	208	8	26	24	2
chocolate milk lowfat	1 cup (8.8 oz)	158	3	26	25	1
Cocio						
Chocolate Milk	8 oz	140	4	20	17	0
Land O Lakes						
2% Swiss Chocolate	1 cup (8.4 oz)	190	5	26	26	tr
Chocolate Skim	1 cup (8 oz)	160	0	31	28	tr
Strawberry	1 cup (8 oz)	190	8	22	22	0

FOOD	PORTION	CAL	FAT	CARB	SUGAR	FIBER
Nesquik						
Chocolate Powder No Sugar Added as prep w/ lowfat milk	1 cup (8 oz)	160	5	18	3	1
Chocolate Powder as prep w/ lowfat milk	1 cup (8 oz)	180	5	27	13	tr
Ready-To-Drink Banana	1 cup (8 oz)	200	5	30	29	0
Ready-To-Drink Chocolate	1 cup (8 oz)	200	5	32	30	tr
Ready-To-Drink Strawberry	1 cup (8 oz)	200	5	33	31	0
Ready-To-Drink Vanilla	1 cup (8 oz)	200	5	30	29	0
Strawberry Powder as prep w/ lowfat milk	1 cup (8 oz)	190	4	27	15	0
Strawberry Powder not prep	2 tbsp (0.6 oz)	60	0	15	15	0
Turkey Hill						
Cool Moos 2% Reduced Fat	8 oz	120	5	12	12	0
Cool Moos Chocolate	8 oz	180	3	32	30	0
MILK SUBSTITUTES						
soy milk	1 cup	79	5	4	–	–
Brazsoy						
Condensed Soy Milk	1 serv (0.7 oz)	54	1	10	9	0
Soy Cream	1 tbsp (0.5 oz)	27	3	0	0	0
Silk						
Chocolate	1 cup (8 oz)	140	4	23	19	2
Plain	8 oz	100	4	8	6	1
Soy Heart Health	1 cup	80	2	10	7	1
Soy Plain Light	1 cup	70	2	8	6	1
Soy Plus DHA Omega-3	1 cup	110	5	8	6	1
Soy Pumpkin Spice	1 cup	170	4	28	24	0
Soy Unsweetened	1 cup	80	4	4	1	1
Vanilla	1 cup (8 oz)	100	4	10	7	1

FOOD	PORTION	CAL	FAT	CARB	SUGAR	FIBER
SoyZen						
Soy Milk Cappuccino	8 oz	150	4	22	17	1
WildWood						
Organic Probiotic Soymilk Blueberry	8 oz	190	3	33	19	4
Organic Probiotic Soymilk Pomegranate	8 oz	180	3	31	17	4
ZenSoy						
Soy Milk Chocolate	8 oz	170	4	27	23	2
Soy Milk Plain	8 oz	90	4	9	6	1
Soy Milk Vanilla	8 oz	110	4	14	12	1
Soy On The Go Vanilla w/ Omega 3	1 pkg (8.25 oz)	110	4	14	12	1
MILKFISH (AWA)						
baked	4 oz	215	10	0	0	0
MILKSHAKE						
chocolate	1 serv (10.6 oz)	357	8	63	63	1
malted milk shake	1 serv (10 oz)	402	14	62	58	1
vanilla	1 (11 oz)	351	9	56	56	0
Buffy's Cool Cow						
Chocolate	1 pkg (8 oz)	150	3	23	17	tr
Vanilla	1 pkg (8 oz)	150	3	24	18	0
Lean Body						
Hi-Protein Chocolate Ice Cream	1 (17 oz)	260	9	9	0	5
Molli Coolz						
Shakers Vanilla as prep w/ skim milk	1 (10.2 oz)	240	10	30	17	5
Nesquik						
Ready-To-Drink Chocolate	1 cup (8 oz)	170	5	26	23	tr

FOOD	PORTION	CAL	FAT	CARB	SUGAR	FIBER
Silhouette Solution						
Colassal Chocolate not prep	1 pkg (1.05 oz)	110	3	8	4	2
Vanilla Creme not prep	1 pkg (1.02 oz)	100	2	8	5	2
MILLET						
cooked	1 cup (6.1 oz)	207	2	41	–	2
MINERAL WATER (see WATER)						
MISO						
dried	1 oz	86	3	10	–	1
miso	½ cup	284	8	39	–	7
MOLASSES						
blackstrap	1 tbsp (0.7 oz)	47	0	12	–	–
molasses	¼ cup (3 oz)	244	tr	63	47	0
molasses	1 tbsp (0.7 oz)	58	tr	15	11	0
Tree Of Life						
Blackstrap Unsulphured	1 tbsp	45	0	11	8	–
MONKFISH						
baked	3 oz	82	2	0	0	0
MOOSE						
roasted	4 oz	142	1	0	0	0
MOTH BEANS						
dried cooked	1 cup	207	1	37	–	–
MOUSSE						
TAKE-OUT						
chocolate	½ cup	454	32	32	30	1
fish timbale	1 cup	329	25	3	1	0

FOOD	PORTION	CAL	FAT	CARB	SUGAR	FIBER
MUFFIN						
MIX						
blueberry as prep	1 (1¾ oz)	149	4	24	–	–
corn as prep	1 (1.75 oz)	160	5	25	–	–
wheat bran as prep	1 (1¾ oz)	138	5	23	–	–
Betty Crocker						
Banana Nut as prep	1	120	3	22	10	0
Blueberry as prep	1	120	3	23	11	–
Cornbread Muffin as prep	1	160	6	24	5	tr
Fiber One Banana Nut as prep	1	170	7	27	12	5
Fiber One Blueberry as prep	1	160	6	30	13	5
Lemon Poppyseed as prep	1	200	8	29	17	–
Duncan Hines						
Blueberry Struesel as prep	1	210	8	32	19	3
Cinnamon Swirl 100% Whole Grain as prep	1	220	8	34	21	3
Triple Chocolate Chunk 100% Whole Grain as prep	1	240	11	35	23	3
Martha White						
Whole Grain Apple Cinnamon not prep	¼ cup (1.2 oz)	140	4	24	13	1
Whole Grain Blueberry not prep	¼ cup (1.2 oz)	140	4	24	13	1
Yellow Corn not prep	¼ cup (1.2 oz)	140	3	26	6	1
READY-TO-EAT						
blueberry	1 (2 oz)	158	4	27	–	2
oat bran wheat free	1 (2 oz)	154	4	28	–	4

FOOD	PORTION	CAL	FAT	CARB	SUGAR	FIBER
toaster type blueberry	1	103	3	18	–	–
toaster type corn	1	114	4	19	–	–
toaster type wheat bran w/ raisins	1 (1.3 oz)	106	3	19	–	–
Hostess						
100 Calorie Pack Mini Banana Streusel	1 pkg (1.2 oz)	100	4	19	7	4
100 Calorie Pack Mini Blueberry Streusel	1 pkg (1.2 oz)	100	3	20	7	4
VitaMuffin						
VitaTops Banana Nut	1 (2 oz)	100	2	19	3	5
TAKE-OUT						
corn	1 lg (2.5 oz)	214	7	32	5	2
raisin bran lowfat	1 (4 oz)	270	1	61	35	5
MULBERRIES						
fresh	20 (1 oz)	13	tr	3	2	1
fresh	½ cup (2.5 oz)	30	tr	7	6	1
Kopali						
Organic Dark Chocolate Covered	½ pkg (1 oz)	140	6	20	15	2
Organic Dried	1 pkg (1.7 oz)	240	1	38	22	6
MULLET						
striped cooked	3 oz	127	4	0	0	0
striped raw	3 oz	99	3	0	0	0
MUNG BEANS						
dried cooked	1 cup	213	1	39	–	–
TruRoots						
Organic Sprouted not prep	¼ cup (1.4 oz)	140	1	30	1	7
MUNGO BEANS						
dried cooked	1 cup	190	1	33	–	–

FOOD	PORTION	CAL	FAT	CARB	SUGAR	FIBER
MUSHROOMS						
CANNED						
caps	8 (1.6 oz)	12	tr	2	1	1
caps pickled	6 (0.8 oz)	5	tr	1	tr	tr
chanterelle	3.5 oz	12	1	tr	–	6
pickled	1 cup	33	tr	5	2	1
pieces	½ cup	20	tr	2	1	1
straw	1 cup	58	1	8	–	5
Green Giant						
Pieces & Stems	½ cup	25	0	4	1	1
Polar						
Straw	½ cup	20	0	4	0	2
Whole Button	½ cup	30	0	4	1	2
Whole Shiitake	½ cup	30	1	4	0	tr
DRIED						
chanterelle	1 oz	25	tr	tr	–	17
shiitake	1 (3.6 g)	11	tr	3	tr	tr
tree ear	½ cup (0.4 oz)	36	tr	10	–	–
wood ear mok yee	½ cup (0.4 oz)	25	tr	8	–	4
Ocean Spring						
Fresh Crispy Mixed Mushrooms	1 serv (0.9 oz)	113	4	18	2	1
FRESH						
brown italian or crimini sliced	1 cup	19	tr	3	1	tr
brown italian or crimini whole	1 (0.7 oz)	5	tr	1	tr	tr
chanterelle	3.5 oz	11	tr	tr	–	6
enoki raw	1 lg (5 g)	2	tr	tr	tr	tr
enoki sliced	1 cup	29	tr	5	tr	2
enoki whole	1 cup	28	tr	5	tr	2
maitake diced	1 cup	26	tr	5	1	2
maitake whole	1 (6.6 g)	2	tr	tr	tr	tr

FOOD	PORTION	CAL	FAT	CARB	SUGAR	FIBER
morel	3.5 oz	9	tr	0	–	7
oyster	1 sm (0.5 oz)	5	tr	1	tr	tr
oyster sliced	1 cup	30	tr	6	1	2
portabella raw	1 cap (3 oz)	22	tr	4	2	1
portabella sliced grilled	1 cup (4.2 oz)	42	1	6	0	3
raw sliced	½ cup	8	tr	1	1	tr
shiitake cooked	4 (2.5 oz)	40	tr	10	3	2
shiitake pieces cooked	1 cup	81	tr	21	5	3
white	1 (0.6 oz)	4	tr	1	tr	tr
white sliced cooked	1 cup	28	tr	4	0	2
Giorgio						
Mushrooms	3 oz	20	0	3	1	1
Golden Gourmet						
Beech Brown	4 oz	20	1	7	–	–
Beech White	4 oz	13	1	6	–	–
King Trumpet	4 oz	20	0	7	–	–
Maitake	4 oz	20	1	8	–	–
Hokto						
Organic Bunashimeji Beech Mushrooms	1 pkg (3.5 oz)	30	1	3	–	3
Organic Maitake Hen Of The Wood	1 pkg (3.5 oz)	30	1	4	–	3
TAKE-OUT						
battered fried	1 lg (0.6 oz)	39	3	3	1	tr
creamed	1 cup	171	11	15	7	3
stuffed	1 (0.8 oz)	67	4	6	1	1
MUSKRAT						
roasted	3 oz	199	10	0	0	0
MUSSELS						
blue raw	1 cup	129	3	6	–	–
blue raw	3 oz	73	2	3	–	–
fresh blue cooked	3 oz	147	4	6	–	–

FOOD	PORTION	CAL	FAT	CARB	SUGAR	FIBER
Polar						
Mussels	2 oz	60	3	tr	0	0
MUSTARD						
dry mustard	1 tsp	15	1	1	–	–
hot chinese	1 tsp	3	tr	tr	tr	tr
organic yellow	1 tsp	5	0	0	0	0
seed	1 tsp	15	1	1	tr	1
yellow prepared	1 tbsp	3	tr	tr	tr	tr
Dave's Gourmet						
Insanity	1 tsp (5 g)	5	0	1	–	–
D'Oni						
Bold As Love Honey Habanero	1 tsp	5	0	2	1	–
Texas Sassy						
Mustard Sauce	2 tbsp (1 oz)	15	0	3	3	–
Vivi's						
Classic	1 tbsp (0.5 oz)	15	0	4	3	0
Sizzlin' Chipotle	1 tbsp (0.5 oz)	15	0	4	3	0
MUSTARD GREENS						
canned	1 cup	23	tr	3	tr	3
fresh as prep w/ fat	1 cup	50	3	3	tr	3
fresh chopped boiled w/o salt	1 cup	21	tr	3	tr	3
fresh raw chopped	1 cup	15	tr	3	1	2
frozen chopped boiled w/o salt	1 cup	28	tr	5	tr	4
Allen's						
Seasoned	½ cup	45	1	6	2	1
Sylvia's						
Specially Seasoned	½ cup	30	0	5	2	2
NATTO						
natto	½ cup	187	10	13	–	–

FOOD	PORTION	CAL	FAT	CARB	SUGAR	FIBER
House						
Natto	2 oz	120	6	5	0	0
NAVY BEANS						
canned	1 cup	296	1	54	–	–
dried cooked	1 cup	259	1	48	–	–
NECTARINE						
fresh	1 sm (4.5 oz)	57	tr	14	10	2
fresh	1 lg (5.5 oz)	69	1	16	12	3
fresh sliced	1 cup (5 oz)	63	tr	15	11	2
Chiquita						
fresh	1 (5 oz)	63	0	15	11	2
NEUFCHATEL						
neufchatel	1 pkg (3 oz)	221	20	3	–	–
neufchatel	1 oz	74	7	1	–	–
NONI JUICE						
Snapple						
Juice Drink Low Calorie Metabolism Noni Berry	8 oz	15	0	2	1	–
Tree Of Life						
100% Juice Concentrate	2 tbsp	15	0	4	3	0
NOODLES						
cellophane	1 cup	492	tr	121	–	–
chow mein	1 cup (1.6 oz)	237	14	25	–	2
egg	1 cup (38 g)	145	2	27	–	–
egg cooked	1 cup (5.6 oz)	213	2	40	–	2
japanese soba cooked	1 cup (4 oz)	113	tr	24	–	–
japanese somen cooked	1 cup (6.2 oz)	231	tr	48	–	–
korean acorn noodles not prep	2 oz	195	tr	41	–	tr
rice cooked	1 cup (6.2 oz)	192	tr	44	–	2
spinach/egg cooked	1 cup (5.6 oz)	211	3	39	–	4

FOOD	PORTION	CAL	FAT	CARB	SUGAR	FIBER
Gluten Free Cafe						
Asian Noodles	1 pkg (9.2 oz)	340	10	53	11	5
House						
Shirataki Tofu Noodles	2 oz	20	1	3	0	2
Shirataki Yam Noodles	2 oz	5	0	1	0	0
Krasdale						
Egg Wide not prep	1 cup (2 oz)	210	2	41	2	2
La Choy						
Chow Mein Noodles	½ cup (1 oz)	130	5	19	0	tr
Rice	½ cup	130	4	21	1	tr
No Yolks						
Dumplings	2 oz	210	1	41	3	3
Ronzoni						
Healthy Harvest Whole Grain Extra Wide not prep	2 oz	180	1	41	0	6
Thai Kitchen						
Stir-Fry Rice Linguini not prep	2 oz	210	1	46	0	0
NUTMEG						
ground	1 tsp	12	1	1	1	1
nutmeg butter	1 tbsp	120	14	0	0	0

NUTRITION SUPPLEMENTS (*see also* CEREAL BARS, ENERGY BARS, ENERGY DRINKS)

FOOD	PORTION	CAL	FAT	CARB	SUGAR	FIBER
Clif						
Shot Bloks Black Cherry	3 (1 oz)	100	0	24	12	0
Shot Bloks Cola	3 (1 oz)	100	0	24	12	0
Shot Bloks Margarita	3 (1 oz)	90	0	24	12	0
Shot Bloks Orange	3 (1 oz)	100	0	24	12	0
Glowelle						
Beauty Drink All Flavors	1 bottle	100	0	24	13	–

FOOD	PORTION	CAL	FAT	CARB	SUGAR	FIBER
Jelly Belly						
Sport Beans Lemon Lime	1 pkg (1 oz)	100	0	25	19	–
Joint Juice						
Tropical Fruit	1 can (8 oz)	25	0	6	3	–
Luna						
Electrolyte Splash	1 pkg	80	0	20	20	–
Moons Energy Chews Watermelon	6 (1 oz)	100	0	24	12	0
Recovery Smoothie	1 pkg	120	0	21	14	1
Oxylent						
Oxygenating Multivitamin Drink	1 pkg	10	0	2	2	–
S/7						
Prenatal Vitamin Drink Berry	1 pkg (0.5 oz)	45	1	9	8	–
To Go						
Extreme Berries	½ pkg (3.15 g)	12	tr	3	1	tr
NUTS MIXED (see also individual names)						
dry roasted w/ peanuts salted	¼ cup	203	18	9	–	3
dry roasted w/ peanuts w/o salt	¼ cup	203	18	9	–	3
mixed nuts chocolate covered	¼ cup (1.5 oz)	240	17	20	17	2
oil roasted w/o peanuts salted	¼ cup	221	20	8	2	2
oil roasted w/o peanuts w/o salt	¼ cup	221	20	8	–	2
Back To Nature						
Tuscan Herb Roast	1 oz	170	15	7	2	2
Dave's Gourmet						
Burning Nuts	1 oz	200	17	7	1	3

FOOD	PORTION	CAL	FAT	CARB	SUGAR	FIBER
Emily's						
Roasted Mixed Nuts	¼ cup (1.3 oz)	230	20	8	2	2
Mauna Loa						
Mixed Nuts	¼ cup (1 oz)	180	16	6	1	2
NuttZo						
Multi-Nut Butter Organic	2 tbsp (1.1 oz)	180	16	7	1	3
Planters						
Mixed	30 nuts (1 oz)	170	15	6	1	2
True North						
Clusters Pecan Almond Peanut	8 (1 oz)	170	13	13	5	2
OCTOPUS						
dried boiled	3 oz	144	2	4	0	0
fresh steamed	3 oz	139	2	4	0	0
smoked	1 oz	40	1	1	0	0
TAKE-OUT						
ensalada de pulpo	1 cup	299	21	10	4	2
OHELOBERRIES						
fresh	1 cup	39	tr	10	–	–
OIL						
almond	1 cup	1927	218	0	0	0
almond	1 tbsp	120	14	0	0	0
apricot kernel	1 cup	1927	218	0	0	0
apricot kernel	1 tbsp	120	14	0	0	0
avocado	1 cup	1927	218	0	0	0
avocado	1 tbsp	124	14	0	0	0
babassu palm	1 tbsp	120	14	0	0	0
butter oil	1 tbsp	112	13	0	0	0
butter oil	1 cup	1795	204	0	0	0
canola	1 tbsp	124	14	0	0	0

FOOD	PORTION	CAL	FAT	CARB	SUGAR	FIBER
canola	1 cup	1927	218	0	0	0
coconut	1 tbsp	117	14	0	0	0
corn	1 tbsp	120	14	0	0	0
corn	1 cup	1927	218	0	0	0
cottonseed	1 tbsp	120	14	0	0	0
cottonseed	1 cup	1927	218	0	0	0
cupu assu	1 tbsp	120	14	0	0	0
garlic oil	1 tbsp	150	17	0	0	0
grapeseed	1 tbsp	120	14	0	0	0
hazelnut	1 tbsp	120	14	0	0	0
hazelnut	1 cup	1927	218	0	0	0
mustard	1 tbsp	124	14	0	0	0
mustard	1 cup	1927	218	0	0	0
oat	1 tbsp	120	14	0	0	0
olive	1 cup	1909	216	0	0	0
olive	1 tbsp	119	14	0	0	0
palm	1 cup	1927	218	0	0	0
palm	1 tbsp	120	14	0	0	0
palm kernel	1 tbsp	117	14	0	0	0
palm kernel	1 cup	1879	218	0	0	0
peanut	1 cup	1909	216	0	0	0
peanut	1 tbsp	119	14	0	0	0
peppermint	1 tsp	42	4	0	0	0
poppyseed	1 tbsp	120	14	0	0	0
pumpkin seed	1 oz	217	29	0	0	0
rice bran	1 tbsp	120	14	0	0	0
safflower	1 cup	1927	218	0	0	0
safflower	1 tbsp	120	14	0	0	0
sesame	1 tbsp	120	14	0	0	0
sheanut	1 tbsp	120	14	0	0	0
soybean	1 cup	1927	218	0	0	0
soybean	1 tbsp	120	14	0	0	0
sunflower	1 cup	1927	218	0	0	0

FOOD	PORTION	CAL	FAT	CARB	SUGAR	FIBER
sunflower	1 tbsp	120	14	0	0	0
teaseed	1 tbsp	120	14	0	0	0
tomatoseed	1 tbsp	120	14	0	0	0
vegetable	1 cup	1927	218	0	0	0
vegetable	1 tbsp	120	14	0	0	0
walnut	1 tbsp	120	14	0	0	0
walnut	1 cup	1927	218	0	0	0
wheat germ	1 tbsp	120	14	0	0	0
Bell Plantation						
Extra Virgin Roasted Peanut	1 tbsp	120	14	0	0	0
Bragg						
Olive Extra Virgin	1 tbsp	120	14	2	2	0
Colavita						
Olive Extra Virgin	1 tbsp (0.5 oz)	120	14	0	0	0
Crisco						
Cooking Spray Original	1/3 sec spray	0	0	0	0	0
Frying Oil Blend	1 tbsp	130	14	0	0	0
Light Olive	1 tbsp	120	14	0	0	0
Peanut	1 tbsp	120	14	0	0	0
Pure Vegetable	1 tbsp	120	14	0	0	0
Gaea						
Olive Carbon Neutral	1 tbsp (0.5 oz)	130	14	0	0	0
Gourme Mist						
Extra Virgin Olive Cold Pressed	1 sec spray	4	tr	0	0	0
LouAna						
Canola	1 tbsp (0.5 oz)	120	14	0	0	0
Lucini						
Extra Virgin Premium Select	1 tbsp (0.5 oz)	120	14	0	0	0

FOOD	PORTION	CAL	FAT	CARB	SUGAR	FIBER
Martinis						
Kalamata Olive Extra Virgin Cold Pressed	1 tbsp (0.5 oz)	120	15	0	0	0
Monini						
Grapeseed	1 tbsp (0.5 oz)	120	14	0	0	0
Navitas Naturals						
Organic Virgin Coconut	1 tbsp (0.5 oz)	120	14	0	0	0
Tree Of Life						
Almond Expeller Pressed	1 tbsp (0.5 oz)	120	14	0	0	0
Avocado Expeller Pressed	1 tbsp (0.5 oz)	120	14	0	0	0
Macadamia Nut Expeller Pressed	1 tbsp (0.5 oz)	120	14	0	0	0
Organic Coconut Expeller Pressed	1 tbsp	120	14	0	0	0
Walnut Expeller Pressed	1 tbsp (0.5 oz)	120	14	0	0	0
Wesson						
Canola	1 tbsp	120	14	0	0	0
OKRA						
CANNED						
pickled	6 pods (2.3 oz)	18	tr	4	1	2
Allens						
Cut	½ cup	30	0	6	1	3
Trappey's						
Creole Gumbo	½ cup	35	0	6	1	3
FRESH						
cooked w/ salt	8 pods	19	tr	4	2	2
luffa chinese okra cooked	1 cup	39	tr	8	4	4
sliced cooked w/ salt	½ cup	18	tr	4	2	2

FOOD	PORTION	CAL	FAT	CARB	SUGAR	FIBER
TAKE-OUT						
batter dipped fried	10 pieces (2.6 oz)	142	10	12	3	2
OLIVES						
black	2 med (0.3 oz)	8	1	tr	0	tr
greek	1 (0.5 oz)	16	1	1	0	tr
green	2 med (0.2 oz)	10	1	tr	tr	tr
green	2 lg (0.3 oz)	11	1	tr	tr	tr
green	2 extra lg (0.5 oz)	19	2	1	tr	tr
green	1 sm (0.2 oz)	8	1	tr	tr	tr
green chopped	¼ cup (1.2 oz)	48	5	1	tr	1
green olive tapenade	1 tbsp	25	3	1	1	0
green stuffed	2 sm (0.2 oz)	9	1	tr	tr	tr
green stuffed	2 med (0.3 oz)	10	1	tr	tr	tr
green stuffed	¼ cup (1.3 oz)	47	5	1	tr	1
green stuffed	2 lg ((0.3 oz)	12	1	tr	tr	tr
ripe	2 sm (0.2 oz)	7	1	tr	0	tr
ripe	2 lg (0.3 oz)	10	1	1	0	tr
ripe	2 extra lg (0.4 oz)	12	1	1	0	tr
ripe sliced	¼ cup (1.2 oz)	35	3	2	0	1
spanish stuffed	5 (0.5 oz)	15	1	1	0	0
Dave's Gourmet						
Olives In Pain	⅛ jar (0.5 oz)	15	2	0	0	0
ONION						
CANNED						
cocktail	½ cup	41	tr	9	4	2
McSweet						
Pickled Onions	4 (1 oz)	10	0	2	tr	0

FOOD	PORTION	CAL	FAT	CARB	SUGAR	FIBER
The Gracious Gourmet						
Balsamic Four Onion Spread	1 tbsp (0.5 oz)	20	0	6	4	0
DRIED						
flakes	1 tbsp	17	tr	4	2	1
powder	1 tsp	7	tr	2	1	tr
shallots	1 tbsp	3	0	1	–	–
FRESH						
cooked w/o salt	1 med (3.3 oz)	41	tr	10	4	1
cooked w/o salt	1 sm (2 oz)	26	tr	6	3	1
cooked w/o salt	1 lg (4.5 oz)	56	tr	13	6	2
cooked w/o salt chopped	1 tbsp	7	tr	2	1	tr
raw chopped	½ cup	32	tr	7	3	1
raw chopped	1 tbsp	4	tr	1	tr	tr
raw slice	1 (0.5 oz)	6	tr	1	1	tr
raw sliced	½ cup	23	tr	5	2	1
scallions raw	1 med (0.5 oz)	5	tr	1	tr	tr
scallions raw chopped	¼ cup	8	tr	2	1	1
shallots raw chopped	¼ cup	29	tr	7	–	–
sweet whole raw	1 (11.6 oz)	106	tr	25	17	3
whole raw	1 sm (2.5 oz)	28	tr	7	3	1
whole raw	1 lg (5.3 oz)	60	tr	14	6	3
whole raw	1 med (4 oz)	44	tr	10	5	2
Bland Farms						
Vidalia Sweet	1 (5 oz)	60	0	14	5	3
Ocean Mist						
Green Onions Chopped	¼ cup	10	0	2	1	1
TAKE-OUT						
creamed	1 cup	187	9	22	10	2
fried	½ cup	57	5	3	tr	1
rings breaded & fried	8 to 9 (3 oz)	276	16	31	–	–

FOOD	PORTION	CAL	FAT	CARB	SUGAR	FIBER
OPOSSUM						
roasted	3 oz	188	9	0	0	0
ORANGE						
FRESH						
california valencia	1 (4.2 oz)	59	tr	14	–	3
california valencia	½ cup (3.2 oz)	44	tr	11	–	2
florida	1 (5.3 oz)	69	tr	17	14	4
florida sections	½ cup (3.2 oz)	43	tr	11	8	2
navel	1 (4.9 oz)	69	tr	18	12	3
navel sections	1 cup (5.8 oz)	81	tr	21	14	4
peel	1 tbsp (0.2 oz)	3	tr	1	tr	1
Darling						
Mandarine	1 med (3.8 oz)	50	0	13	9	3
ORANGE JUICE						
chilled	1 cup (8.7 oz)	112	1	26	21	1
fresh	1 cup (8.7 oz)	112	1	26	21	1
mandarin orange	7 oz	94	tr	20	–	–
Florida's Natural						
Calcium & Vitamin D	8 oz	110	0	26	22	0
Izze						
Sparkling Esque Mandarin Orange	1 bottle (12 oz)	50	0	12	11	–
Land O Lakes						
Juice	1 cup (8 oz)	110	0	25	23	0
Juice w/ Calcium	1 cup (8 oz)	120	0	29	28	0
Mott's						
100% Juice Sunkist Orange Sensation	1 bottle (14 oz)	210	0	50	49	0
Mr. J						
100% Juice Calcium Fortified	1 pkg (4 oz)	60	0	19	14	–

FOOD	PORTION	CAL	FAT	CARB	SUGAR	FIBER
Snapple						
Orangeade	8 oz	100	0	26	26	–
Tropicana						
Organic	8 oz	120	0	28	22	0
Trop50' Orange Juice Beverage	8 oz	50	0	13	10	0
TAKE-OUT						
orange julius	1 cup (9.2 oz)	212	tr	39	35	tr
OREGANO						
crumbled	1 tsp	3	tr	1	tr	tr
ground	1 tsp	6	tr	1	tr	1

ORGAN MEATS (*see* BRAINS, GIBLETS, GIZZARDS, HEART, KIDNEY, LIVER, SWEETBREAD)

FOOD	PORTION	CAL	FAT	CARB	SUGAR	FIBER
OSTRICH						
cooked	4 oz	195	8	0	0	0
cooked diced	1 cup (4.7 oz)	215	9	0	0	0
Natural Frontier Foods						
Filets	1 (4 oz)	130	3	0	0	0
Ground Lean	4 oz	130	3	0	0	0
OYSTERS						
canned eastern	1 cup	112	4	6	0	0
eastern baked	6 med	47	1	4	–	0
eastern raw	6 med	50	1	5	–	0
eastern sauteed	6 med	76	5	3	0	0
smoked	6	33	1	2	0	0
Polar						
Whole	¼ cup	70	3	4	0	0
Whole Smoked	⅓ cup	95	5	4	0	0
TAKE-OUT						
breaded & fried	6	368	18	40	–	–
fritter	1 (1.4 oz)	121	6	12	tr	tr

FOOD	PORTION	CAL	FAT	CARB	SUGAR	FIBER
oysters rockefeller	1 cup	302	17	22	2	4
stew	1 cup	208	13	11	9	0

PANCAKE/WAFFLE SYRUP

lite	¼ cup	98	0	27	20	0
pancake syrup	¼ cup	209	tr	55	50	0
pancake syrup	1 pkg (2 oz)	156	tr	41	38	0
Aunt Jemima						
Butter Lite	¼ cup (2.1 oz)	100	0	26	25	1
Naturally Fresh						
Maple Mountain Sugar Free	2 tbsp	0	0	0	0	0
Wholesome Sweeteners						
Organic	¼ cup	240	0	60	60	0

PANCAKES
FROZEN
Dr. Praeger's

Broccoli	1 (2 oz)	80	4	9	1	2
Potato	1 (2.2 oz)	100	4	13	1	3
Golden						
Zucchini	1 (1.3 oz)	70	3	8	tr	1
Jimmy Dean						
Breakfast Bowls Pancake & Sausage Links	1 pkg	710	31	93	34	3
Griddle Cake Sandwich Sausage Egg & Cheese	1 (4 oz)	370	23	32	13	1
Original Pancakes & Sausage On A Stick	1 (2.5 oz)	110	13	21	8	0
Pillsbury						
Blueberry	3 (4 oz)	230	4	46	14	2
Buttermilk	3 (4 oz)	240	4	47	13	2
Original	3 (4 oz)	250	4	49	14	2

FOOD	PORTION	CAL	FAT	CARB	SUGAR	FIBER
Ratner's						
Potato Latkes	1 (1.5 oz)	80	2	15	tr	tr
MIX						
Batter Blaster						
Organic Original Pancake & Waffle Batter not prep	¼ cup (2 oz)	112	1	23	7	2
Bisquick						
Shake 'N Pour Buttermilk as prep	3	220	3	42	7	1
TAKE-OUT						
buckwheat	1 (7 in)	142	5	19	4	2
norwegian lefse	1 (9 in) (2.7 oz)	163	5	27	2	2
plain	1 (7 in)	183	3	35	10	1
potato	1 (1.3 oz)	70	4	8	tr	1
w/ butter & syrup	2 (8.1 oz)	520	14	91	–	–
whole wheat	1 (7 in)	183	8	23	5	3

PANCREAS (see SWEETBREAD)

PANINI (see SANDWICHES)

PAPAYA

canned in syrup	½ cup (2.3 oz)	50	tr	13	11	1
dried	1 strip (0.8 oz)	59	tr	15	9	3
fresh	1 sm (5.3 oz)	59	tr	15	9	3
fresh	1 lg (13.3 oz)	148	1	37	22	7
fresh cubed	1 cup (4.9 oz)	55	tr	14	8	3
green cooked	½ cup (2.3 oz)	18	tr	5	3	1

PAPAYA JUICE

nectar	1 cup (8.8 oz)	142	tr	36	35	2

PAPRIKA

dried	1 tsp	1	tr	tr	re	tr

FOOD	PORTION	CAL	FAT	CARB	SUGAR	FIBER
PARSLEY						
dried	1 tbsp	4	tr	1	tr	1
freeze dried	1 tbsp	1	tr	tr	–	tr
fresh chopped	¼ cup	5	tr	1	tr	1
fresh chopped	1 tbsp	1	tr	tr	tr	tr
fresh sprigs	5 (1.8 oz)	18	tr	3	tr	2
PARSNIPS						
fresh sliced cooked w/o salt	½ cup (2.7 oz)	55	tr	13	4	3
whole cooked	1 (5.6 oz)	114	tr	27	8	6
TAKE-OUT						
creamed	1 cup (8 oz)	237	11	31	10	5
PASSION FRUIT						
fresh	1 (0.6 oz)	17	tr	4	2	2
fresh cut up	½ cup (4.1 oz)	114	1	28	13	12
PASSION FRUIT JUICE						
nectar	1 cup (8.8 oz)	168	tr	44	43	tr
yellow lilikoi	1 cup (8.7 oz)	138	tr	35	34	1
Santa Cruz						
Organic 100% Juice Nectar	8 oz	150	0	40	36	0

PASTA (*see also* NOODLES, PASTA DINNERS, PASTA SALAD)

DRY

FOOD	PORTION	CAL	FAT	CARB	SUGAR	FIBER
corn cooked	1 cup (4.9 oz)	176	1	39	–	7
elbows not prep	1 cup	389	2	78	–	–
elbows cooked	1 cup (4.9 oz)	197	1	40	–	2
shells small cooked	1 cup (4 oz)	162	1	33	–	2
spaghetti cooked	1 cup (4.9 oz)	197	1	40	–	2
spinach spaghetti cooked	1 cup (4.9 oz)	182	1	37	–	–
spirals cooked	1 cup (4.7 oz)	189	tr	38	–	2

FOOD	PORTION	CAL	FAT	CARB	SUGAR	FIBER
vegetable cooked	1 cup (4.7 oz)	172	tr	36	–	6
whole wheat all shapes cooked	1 cup	174	tr	37	–	4
Amish Natural						
Fettuccine Fiber Rich not prep	2 oz	200	1	42	3	11
Fettuccine not prep	2 oz	201	1	41	5	2
Fettuccine Whole Wheat not prep	2 oz	210	2	41	2	7
DeBoles						
Organic Angel Hair Whole Wheat not prep	¼ pkg (2 oz)	210	2	42	2	5
Gillian's						
Penne Brown Rice Pasta Wheat Gluten Egg Free not prep	2 oz	200	2	43	0	2
Ronzoni						
Elbows not prep	½ cup (2 oz)	210	1	42	2	2
Garden Delight Radiatore not prep	2 oz	190	1	40	2	4
Garden Delight Spaghetti not prep	2 oz	190	1	40	2	4
Wacky Mac						
Veggie All Shapes not prep	2 oz	200	1	41	0	1
FRESH						
cooked	2 oz	75	1	14	–	–
spinach cooked	2 oz	74	1	14	–	–
Monterey Gourmet						
Whole Wheat Ravioli Vegetable & Cheese	1 cup (3.5 oz)	240	6	35	1	4
Whole Wheat Tortellini Italian Cheese	1 cup (3.5 oz)	290	6	48	1	5

FOOD	PORTION	CAL	FAT	CARB	SUGAR	FIBER
PASTA DINNERS (see also PASTA SALAD)						
CANNED						
Chef Boyardee						
Mini Ravioli	1 cup	250	9	35	5	3
Mini-Bites Spaghetti & Meatballs	1 cup	250	10	30	7	3
Hormel						
Kid's Kitchen Microwave Meals Cheezy Mac 'N Beef	1 pkg (7.5 oz)	250	6	34	8	1
Kid's Kitchen Microwave Meals Cheezy Mac 'N Cheese	1 pkg (7.5 oz)	270	14	24	3	1
Kid's Kitchen Microwave Meals Mini Beef Ravioli	1 pkg (7.5 oz)	240	6	38	6	1
Kid's Kitchen Microwave Meals Spaghetti Rings & Franks	1 pkg (7.5 oz)	240	8	32	11	1
Lasagna w/ Meat Sauce	1 pkg (7.5 oz)	210	5	31	14	3
Spaghetti w/ Meat Sauce	1 pkg (7.5 oz)	210	5	31	14	3
FROZEN						
4Real						
Mac+Cheese	1 pkg (8 oz)	230	5	33	1	2
Meat Sauce w/ Beef Ravioli	1 pkg (8 oz)	190	4	32	5	2
Spaghetti Rings	1 pkg (8 oz)	180	1	37	5	2
Amy's						
Bowls Baked Ziti	1 pkg	390	12	62	8	6
Bowls Stuffed Pasta Shells	1 pkg	310	13	30	7	5
Lasagna Cheese	1 pkg (10.2 oz)	380	14	44	8	4
Lasagna Tofu Vegetable	1 pkg (9.4 oz)	310	11	41	6	6

FOOD	PORTION	CAL	FAT	CARB	SUGAR	FIBER
Macaroni & Cheese	1 pkg (8.9 oz)	410	16	47	6	3
Macaroni & Cheese Light In Sodium	1 pkg (8.9 oz)	400	16	47	6	3
Macaroni & Soy Cheese	1 pkg (8.9 oz)	370	15	42	2	4
Rice Mac & Cheese	1 pkg (9 oz)	400	16	47	6	1
Banquet						
Lasagna Family Entree	1 cup	510	16	63	7	3
Macaroni & Cheese	1 cup	200	6	30	7	3
Noodles & Beef	1 cup	160	4	20	0	2
Birds Eye						
Steamfresh Meals For Two Shrimp Alfredo	½ pkg (11.9 oz)	420	12	55	7	4
Steamfresh Meals For Two Shrimp Pasta Primavera	½ pkg (11.9 oz)	450	24	39	6	3
Blue Horizon Organic						
Penne Alfredo w/ Shrimp	½ pkg (9.9 oz)	430	22	39	0	2
Penne Alla Vodka w/ Shrimp	½ pkg (9.9 oz)	270	6	38	0	3
Pesto Farfalle w/ Shrimp	½ pkg (9.9 oz)	280	6	38	0	3
Scampi Rotini w/ Shrimp	½ pkg (9.9 oz)	410	19	44	0	4
Cedarlane						
Zone Chicken & Vegetables Pasta & Ginger	1 pkg (10 oz)	340	12	35	2	3
Zone Lasagna Vegetable	1 pkg (10.9 oz)	310	12	33	12	5
Gluten Free Cafe						
Fettuccini Alfredo	1 pkg (9.2 oz)	400	16	55	tr	2
Pasta Primavera	1 pkg (9.2 oz)	270	9	42	4	4

FOOD	PORTION	CAL	FAT	CARB	SUGAR	FIBER
Healthy Choice						
Creamy Garlic Shrimp w/ Bow Tie Pasta	1 pkg (11.5 oz)	280	5	44	16	5
Portabella Marsala Pasta	1 pkg (9 oz)	270	7	38	4	5
Tomato Basil Penne	1 pkg (10 oz)	280	6	39	6	7
Joy Of Cooking						
Al Dente Cavatappi Bolognese	1 cup (7.7 oz)	280	12	29	5	2
Best Loved Macaroni & Cheese	1 cup (5.4 oz)	280	18	36	4	1
Cheese Ravioli Pomodoro	1 cup (7.7 oz)	250	7	34	5	3
Creamy Fettuccine Carbonara	1 cup (7.5 oz)	330	16	31	3	3
Marie Callender's						
Fettucine Chicken & Broccoli	1 meal	630	37	43	5	6
Meat Lasagna	1 cup	240	9	24	9	2
Milton's						
Lasagna Vegetable w/ Multi-Grain Pasta	1 cup (8 oz)	340	16	30	7	5
Mon Cuisine						
Vegetarian Spaghetti & Meatballs	1 pkg (10 oz)	360	4	54	8	9
Moosewood						
Organic Vegetarian Broccoli & Pasta Parmesan	1 pkg (10 oz)	380	13	52	7	4
Organic Vegetarian Farfalle & Spinach Pesto Sauce	1 pkg (10 oz)	370	11	56	6	4
Organic Vegetarian Spicy Penne Puttanesca	1 pkg (10 oz)	300	10	45	5	2

FOOD	PORTION	CAL	FAT	CARB	SUGAR	FIBER
New York Ravioli						
Jolie Kid Shapes Ravioli Cheese	1 cup	330	9	47	5	4
Jolie Kid Shapes Ravioli Cheese & Broccoli	1 cup	340	8	53	2	2
Ravioli Four Cheese	1 cup	360	6	58	2	2
Ravioli Tomato Basil & Mozzarella	1 cup	340	5	64	3	2
Organic Bistro						
Pasta Puttanesca	1 pkg (12.15 oz)	330	6	57	6	9
Organic Classics						
Cajun Chicken Tetrazzine w/ Penne Pasta	1 pkg (10 oz)	370	10	43	4	3
Chicken Cacciatore w/ Penne Pasta	1 pkg (10 oz)	270	4	37	5	3
Macaroni & Meat Sauce	1 pkg (10 oz)	340	9	49	9	3
Plum Organics						
Bowtie Pasta	1 pkg (6.9 oz)	230	6	37	2	3
Cheese Filled Spinach Tortellini	1 pkg (6.9 oz)	190	2	37	6	3
Putney Pasta						
Ravioli Butternut Squash & Vermont Maple Syrup	1 cup	200	4	35	–	1
Ravioli Portobello & Grilled Onion	7 (5.2 oz)	240	5	39	–	3
Ravioli Whole Wheat Spinach & Cheese	9 (5 oz)	300	9	42	–	2
Skillet Meal Chicken Piccata	1 serv (9 oz)	300	11	35	–	2

FOOD	PORTION	CAL	FAT	CARB	SUGAR	FIBER
Skillet Meal Shrimp Pesto	1 serv (9 oz)	540	38	32	–	3
Tortellini Spinach Mozzarella & Walnuts	1 cup	360	8	51	–	2
Tortellini Tri-Color Three Cheese	1 cup	340	8	51	–	1
Taste Above						
Meatless Thai Peanut Coconut Sauce w/ Veggie Chicken & Vermicelli	1 pkg (10 oz)	320	19	22	3	8
Meatless Tuscan Marinara Sauce w/ Veggie Chicken & Penne Pasta	1 pkg (10 oz)	320	19	22	3	8
MIX						
Back To Nature						
Crazy Bugs Macaroni & Cheese as prep	1 cup	370	10	60	8	2
Harvest Wheat Elbows & Cheddar as prep	½ pkg	380	12	60	10	2
Organic Shells & Cheese as prep	½ pkg	380	12	60	10	2
Hamburger Helper						
Cheesy Jambalaya as prep	1 cup	330	13	30	2	1
La Bella Vita						
Chicken & Lemon Borsellini as prep	1 cup	270	6	39	1	2
Near East						
Basil & Herb as prep	1 cup	240	5	42	1	3
Spicy Tomato as prep	1 cup	230	5	38	2	3

FOOD	PORTION	CAL	FAT	CARB	SUGAR	FIBER
Thai Kitchen						
Stir-Fry Rice Noodles Thai Peanut as prep	½ pkg	310	6	54	13	1
REFRIGERATED						
Country Crock						
Elbow Macaroni & Cheese	1 cup (8 oz)	370	17	40	6	1
Four Cheese Pasta	1 cup (8 oz)	380	17	41	7	2
Rozzano						
Organic Ravioli Grilled Vegetable	1 cup (3.5 oz)	200	6	26	2	2
SHELF-STABLE						
Allergaroo						
Gluten Free Spaghetti	1 pkg (8 oz)	220	3	49	9	3
Gluten Free Spyglass Noodles	1 pkg (8 oz)	230	3	49	9	3
Betty Crocker						
Bowl Appetit! Cheddar Broccoli Pasta	1 bowl (2.8 oz)	330	11	49	7	2
Bowl Appetit! Garlic Parmesan Pasta	1 bowl (2.8 oz)	320	9	50	5	1
Healthy Choice						
Fresh Mixers Ziti & Meat Sauce	1 pkg (6.9 oz)	340	6	56	10	8
Hormel						
Compleats Microwave Meals Chicken & Noodles	1 pkg (9.9 oz)	240	8	27	3	2
TAKE-OUT						
bami goreng indonesian noodle dish	1 cup	170	3	25	4	4
lasagna meatless	1 piece (9 oz)	356	11	46	8	3
lasagna w/ meat	1 piece (8 oz)	362	14	37	6	3

FOOD	PORTION	CAL	FAT	CARB	SUGAR	FIBER
lasagna w/ vegetables	1 serv (9 oz)	315	10	41	8	4
macaroni & cheese w/ ham	1 cup	542	33	41	7	3
manicotti cheese filled w/ marinara sauce	1 (5 oz)	229	10	22	3	1
manicotti cheese filled w/ meat sauce	1 (5 oz)	239	11	20	1	3
pasta w/ pesto sauce	1 cup	370	25	27	1	2
ravioli cheese & spinach filled w/ cream sauce	1 cup	362	17	38	5	2
ravioli cheese w/ tomato sauce	1 cup	335	14	38	4	2
ravioli meat filled w/ marinara sauce	1 cup	372	16	36	5	3
rigatoni w/ sausage sauce	¾ cup	260	12	28	–	3
spaghetti w/ red clam sauce	1 cup	285	8	41	3	3
spaghetti w/ sauce & meatballs	2 cups	670	26	80	15	12
spaghetti w/ white clam sauce	1 cup	456	20	43	1	3
tortellini cheese w/ tomato sauce	1 cup	332	14	38	4	2
tortellini meat filled w/ marinara sauce	1 cup	281	10	33	3	2
tortellini spinach filled w/ marinara sauce	1 cup	238	8	32	3	2

PASTA SALAD
MIX
Suddenly Salad

FOOD	PORTION	CAL	FAT	CARB	SUGAR	FIBER
Caesar as prep	1 cup (1.8 oz)	310	14	38	3	1
Classic as prep	¾ cup	250	8	39	4	1

FOOD	PORTION	CAL	FAT	CARB	SUGAR	FIBER
Creamy Italian as prep	¾ cup	350	20	36	4	2
Creamy Parmesan as prep	¾ cup	370	22	33	2	1
TAKE-OUT						
pasta salad w/ crab vegetables mayonnaise	1 cup	317	16	33	2	2
tortellini salad cheese filled w/ vinaigrette dressing	1 cup	333	18	30	1	1
PATE						
chicken liver canned	1 tbsp	26	2	1	0	0
duck pate	1 oz	96	8	1	tr	–
fish pate	1 oz	76	7	1	–	–
liver w/ truffle	1 serv (2 oz)	183	16	4	–	–
mushroom pate	1 can (2.25 oz)	130	11	7	1	1
pate de foie gras smoked canned	1 tbsp	60	6	1	–	0
pork pate	1 oz	107	10	1	1	0
pork pate en croute	1 oz	91	7	3	tr	tr
rabbit pate	1 oz	66	5	1	–	–
shrimp	1 can (2.25 oz)	140	10	7	1	0
Patchwork						
All Flavors	2 oz	270	27	5	0	0
PEACH						
CANNED						
halves in light syrup	1 half (3.4 oz)	53	tr	14	13	1
halves juice pack	1 half (3.4 oz)	43	tr	11	10	1
in heavy syrup	½ cup (2.6 oz)	85	tr	22	20	2
peach sauce	½ cup	120	0	32	31	1

FOOD	PORTION	CAL	FAT	CARB	SUGAR	FIBER
pickled	½ cup (4.2 oz)	143	tr	35	34	1
pickled whole	1 (3.1 oz)	104	tr	26	25	1
slices juice pack	½ cup (4.4 oz)	55	tr	14	13	2
slices light syrup	½ cup (4.4 oz)	68	tr	18	17	2
slices water pack	½ cup (4.3 oz)	29	tr	7	6	2
spiced in heavy syrup	½ cup (4.2 oz)	91	tr	24	23	2
Polar						
White	½ cup	70	0	17	16	1
S&W						
Slices Natural Style	½ cup (4.4 oz)	80	0	19	18	1
DRIED						
halves	1 (0.5 oz)	31	tr	8	5	1
halves	½ cup (2.8 oz)	191	1	49	33	7
halves cooked w/o sugar	½ cup (4.5 oz)	99	tr	25	22	4
Mrs. May's						
Fruit Chips	1 pkg	35	0	8	7	1
Stoneridge Orchards						
Whole	⅓ cup (1.4 oz)	140	0	31	29	1
FRESH						
peach	1 lg (6.1 oz)	68	tr	17	15	3
peach	1 med (5.3 oz)	58	tr	14	13	2
sliced	½ cup (2.7 oz)	30	tr	8	6	1
PEACH JUICE						
nectar	1 cup (8.7 oz)	134	tr	35	33	2
Froose						
Playful Peach	1 box (4.2 oz)	80	0	19	7	3
Izze						
Sparkling Peach	1 bottle (12 oz)	130	0	32	30	–

FOOD	PORTION	CAL	FAT	CARB	SUGAR	FIBER
OKF						
Sparkling Fresh Peach	1 bottle (8.3 oz)	50	0	12	9	3
Santa Cruz						
Organic Nectar	8 oz	120	0	31	29	0
PEANUT BUTTER						
chunky	2 tbsp	188	16	7	–	2
chunky	1 cup	1520	129	56	–	17
chunky w/o salt	2 tbsp	188	16	7	–	2
chunky w/o salt	1 cup	1520	129	56	–	17
smooth	2 tbsp	188	16	7	–	2
smooth	1 cup	1517	128	53	–	15
smooth w/o salt	1 cup	1517	129	53	–	15
smooth w/o salt	2 tbsp	188	16	7	–	2
Barney Butter						
Crunchy	2 tbsp	180	16	7	3	3
Smooth	2 tbsp	180	15	8	3	3
Better'n Peanut Butter						
Creamy	2 tbsp (1.1 oz)	100	2	13	2	2
Low Sodium	2 tbsp (1.1 oz)	100	2	13	2	2
Chet's						
Chocolate	2 tbsp	180	14	10	4	2
Roasted Nut	2 tbsp	180	14	9	4	2
Earth Balance						
Creamy or Chunky	1 tbsp	190	17	7	2	3
Justin's						
Organic Cinnamon	2 tbsp (1.1 oz)	180	15	8	2	3
Organic Classic	2 tbsp (1.1 oz)	150	17	7	1	2
Naturally More						
Natural	2 tbsp	169	11	8	2	4
Organic	2 tbsp	170	11	8	2	4
PB2						
Powdered Chocolate	2 tbsp	52	13	6	4	1

FOOD	PORTION	CAL	FAT	CARB	SUGAR	FIBER
Powdered Chocolate Chip	2 tbsp	53	2	3	2	tr
Reese's						
Creamy	2 tbsp (1.1 oz)	190	16	7	3	3
Peanut Butter Chips	1 tbsp (0.5 oz)	80	5	8	6	tr
Revolution Foods						
Organic Creamy & Crunchy	1 tbsp (1.1 oz)	200	16	5	2	2
Santa Cruz						
Organic Creamy	2 tbsp (1.1 oz)	210	16	6	1	2
Wonder						
Peanut Spread	2 tbsp	100	3	13	2	0
Peanut Spread Low Sodium	2 tbsp	100	3	13	2	0

PEANUT BUTTER SUBSTITUTES
NoNuts

FOOD	PORTION	CAL	FAT	CARB	SUGAR	FIBER
Golden Peabutter	1 tbsp	93	7	6	–	1

PEANUTS

FOOD	PORTION	CAL	FAT	CARB	SUGAR	FIBER
chocolate coated	¼ cup	193	12	18	14	2
chocolate coated	1	21	1	2	2	tr
cooked w/ salt	½ cup	286	20	19	2	8
dry roasted w/ salt	28 (1 oz)	164	14	6	2	1
dry roasted w/ salt	1 oz	166	14	6	1	2
dry roasted w/o salt	28 (1 oz)	164	14	6	1	2
dry roasted w/o salt	¼ cup	214	18	8	2	3
honey roasted	¼ cup	191	16	8	5	3
sugar coated	¼ cup	203	13	18	16	2
yogurt coated	¼ cup	230	16	18	15	2
Fisher						
Butter Toffee	¼ cup (1 oz)	140	6	18	15	1
Honey Roasted	¼ cup (1 oz)	170	13	9	5	2

FOOD	PORTION	CAL	FAT	CARB	SUGAR	FIBER
Lance						
Salted	1 pkg (1.1 oz)	200	15	6	0	4
True North						
Clusters	6 (1 oz)	170	13	9	5	2
PEAR						
CANNED						
halves in heavy syrup	1 (1.7 oz)	36	tr	9	8	1
halves in heavy syrup	½ cup (3.5 oz)	74	tr	19	17	3
halves in light syrup	1 (2.7 oz)	43	tr	12	9	1
halves juice pack	1 (2.7 oz)	38	tr	10	7	1
halves juice pack	½ cup (4.4 oz)	62	tr	16	12	2
halves light syrup	½ cup (4.4 oz)	72	tr	19	15	2
halves water pack	1 (2.7 oz)	22	tr	6	5	1
Liberty Gold						
Bartlett In Heavy Syrup	½ cup (4.5 oz)	90	0	23	22	2
S&W						
Halves Light Syrup	½ cup (4.4 oz)	80	0	19	17	2
DRIED						
halves	½ cup (3.2 oz)	236	1	63	56	7
halves	1 (0.6 oz)	47	tr	13	11	1
halves	5 (3 oz)	229	1	61	54	7
halves cooked w/o sugar	½ cup (4.5 oz)	162	tr	43	35	8
Brothers-All-Natural						
Crisps Asian Pear	1 pkg (0.35 oz)	40	0	9	7	1
Crispy Green						
Pears	1 pkg (0.35 oz)	40	0	8	7	1
FRESH						
asian	1 lg (9.6 oz)	116	1	30	19	10
asian	1 med (4.3 oz)	51	tr	13	9	4
pear	1 med (6.2 oz)	103	tr	28	17	6

FOOD	PORTION	CAL	FAT	CARB	SUGAR	FIBER
pear	1 lg (8.1 oz)	133	tr	36	23	7
pear	1 sm (5.2 oz)	86	tr	23	15	5
sliced w/ skin	1 cup (4.9 oz)	81	tr	22	14	4
Chiquita						
Pear	1 (6.2 oz)	103	0	28	17	6
PEAR JUICE						
nectar canned	1 cup (8.8 oz)	150	tr	39	38	2
Froose						
Perfect Pear	1 box (4.2 oz)	80	0	18	5	3
Santa Cruz						
Organic Nectar	8 oz	120	0	30	25	0
PEAS						
CANNED						
green	½ cup	59	tr	11	–	–
green low sodium	½ cup	59	tr	11	–	–
Green Giant						
Young Tender Sweet	½ cup	60	0	12	5	3
S&W						
Petit Pois	½ cup (4.4 oz)	60	0	10	5	4
DRIED						
split cooked	1 cup	231	1	41	–	–
HamPeas						
Green Split Peas as prep	½ cup	120	1	21	1	4
Jack Rabbit						
Green Split	¼ cup (1.6 oz)	110	0	27	1	11
Tree Of Life						
Wasabi Peas	¼ cup (1.1 oz)	120	4	17	5	2
FRESH						
green cooked	½ cup	67	tr	13	–	–
green raw	½ cup	58	tr	11	–	–
snap peas cooked	½ cup	34	tr	6	–	2
snap peas raw	½ cup	30	tr	5	–	2

FOOD	PORTION	CAL	FAT	CARB	SUGAR	FIBER
Mann's						
Snow Peas	1 serv (3 oz)	35	0	6	3	2
FROZEN						
green cooked	½ cup	63	tr	11	–	–
snap peas cooked	½ cup	42	tr	7	–	–
Birds Eye						
Steamfresh Singles Sweet Peas	1 pkg (3.2 oz)	70	0	13	4	4
PECANS						
candied	1 oz	190	17	10	4	5
dry roasted	1 oz	187	18	6	–	–
dry roasted salted	1 oz	187	18	6	–	–
halves dry roasted w/ salt	20 (1 oz)	200	21	4	1	3
halves dried	1 cup	721	73	20	–	7
oil roasted	1 oz	195	20	5	–	–
oil roasted salted	1 oz	195	20	5	–	–
Emily's						
Roasted & Salted	¼ cup (1 oz)	210	22	4	1	3
Fisher						
Roasted & Salted	¼ cup (1 oz)	200	21	4	1	3
PECTIN						
liquid	1 oz	3	0	1	0	1
powder	1 pkg (1.75 oz)	162	tr	45	–	4
Sure Jell						
Fruit Pectin	1 pkg (1.75 oz)	0	0	0	0	0
PEPEAO						
dried	¼ cup	18	tr	5	–	–
raw sliced	1 cup	25	tr	7	–	–

FOOD	PORTION	CAL	FAT	CARB	SUGAR	FIBER
PEPPER						
black	1 tsp	5	tr	1	tr	1
cayenne	1 tsp	6	tr	1	tr	1
white	1 tsp	7	tr	2	–	1
PEPPERMINT						
fresh chopped	2 tbsp	2	tr	tr	–	tr
PEPPERS						
CANNED						
chili green	1 cup (5.5 oz)	29	tr	6	–	2
chili green hot chopped	½ cup	17	tr	4	–	–
chili pepper paste	1 tbsp	6	1	1	–	1
chili red hot	1 (2.6 oz)	18	tr	4	–	–
chili red hot chopped	½ cup	17	tr	4	–	–
green halves	½ cup	13	tr	3	–	–
jalapeno chopped	½ cup	17	tr	3	–	–
red halves	½ cup	13	tr	3	–	–
Gedney						
Hot & Sweet Jalapeno Peppers	¼ cup	30	0	5	5	0
Hot Banana Pepper Rings	¼ cup	10	0	1	0	0
DRIED						
ancho	1 tsp	3	tr	1	–	tr
ancho	1 (0.6 oz)	48	1	9	–	4
casabel	1 tsp	3	tr	1	–	tr
chipotle smoked	1 tsp	3	tr	1	–	tr
green	1 tbsp	1	tr	tr	–	–
guajillo	1 tsp	3	tr	1	–	tr
mulato	1 tsp	3	tr	1	–	tr
pasilla	1 tsp	3	tr	1	–	tr
pasilla	1 (7 g)	24	1	4	–	2
red	1 tbsp	1	tr	tr	–	–

FOOD	PORTION	CAL	FAT	CARB	SUGAR	FIBER
FRESH						
banana	1 (4 in) (1.2 oz)	9	tr	2	–	1
banana	1 cup (4.4 oz)	33	1	7	–	4
chili green hot	1	18	tr	4	–	–
chili green hot chopped	½ cup	30	tr	7	–	–
chili red chopped	½ cup	30	tr	7	–	–
chili red hot	1 (1.6 oz)	18	tr	4	–	–
green	1 (2.6 oz)	20	tr	5	–	1
green chopped	½ cup	13	tr	3	–	1
green chopped cooked	½ cup	19	tr	5	–	–
green cooked	1 (2.6 oz)	20	tr	5	–	–
habanero	1 tsp	9	tr	2	–	1
hungarian	1 (0.9 oz)	8	tr	2	–	0
jalapeno	1 (0.5 oz)	4	tr	1	–	tr
jalapeno sliced	1 cup (3.2 oz)	27	1	5	–	3
red	1 (2.6 oz)	20	tr	5	–	1
red chopped	½ cup	13	tr	3	–	1
red chopped cooked	½ cup	19	tr	5	–	–
red cooked	1 (2.6 oz)	20	tr	5	–	–
serrano	1 (6 g)	2	tr	tr	–	tr
serrano chopped	1 cup (3.7 oz)	34	tr	7	4	4
yellow	1 (6.5 oz)	50	tr	12	–	–
yellow	10 strips	14	tr	3	–	–
FROZEN						
green chopped	1 oz	6	tr	1	–	–
red chopped	1 oz	6	tr	1	–	–

PERCH
FRESH

FOOD	PORTION	CAL	FAT	CARB	SUGAR	FIBER
cooked	3 oz	99	1	0	0	0
cooked	1 fillet (1.6 oz)	54	1	0	0	0
ocean perch atlantic cooked	3 oz	103	2	0	0	0

FOOD	PORTION	CAL	FAT	CARB	SUGAR	FIBER
ocean perch atlantic cooked	1 fillet (1.8 oz)	60	1	0	0	0
ocean perch atlantic raw	3 oz	80	1	0	0	0
raw	3 oz	77	1	0	0	0
red raw	3.5 oz	114	4	0	0	0
FROZEN						
Bell						
Cajun Nuggets	12 (4.5 oz)	170	3	16	0	1
Fillets Breaded	1 piece (4.5 oz)	170	3	16	0	tr
Fillets Unbreaded	1 piece (3.5 oz)	80	1	0	0	0
PERSIMMONS						
dried japanese	1 (1.2 oz)	93	tr	25	–	5
fresh	1 (6 oz)	118	tr	31	21	6
PHEASANT						
breast boneless cooked	½ (4.4 oz)	312	15	0	0	0
cooked diced	1 cup	332	16	0	0	0
drumstick & thigh cooked	1 (2.6 oz)	184	9	0	0	0
PHYLLO						
sheet	1 (0.7 oz)	57	1	10	tr	tr
Ekizian						
Sheets	2 (4 oz)	433	9	76	2	3
Fillo Factory						
Kataifi Shredded Fillo	1 (2 oz)	180	2	35	1	4
Organic	2 sheets (1.5 oz)	130	1	27	0	1
Organic Whole Wheat	2 sheets (1.8 oz)	140	1	30	0	2
Shells Large	1 (0.7 oz)	80	2	13	0	0

FOOD	PORTION	CAL	FAT	CARB	SUGAR	FIBER
PICANTE (*see* SALSA)						
PICKLES						
bread & butter	6 slices	39	tr	9	4	1
dill	1 lg (4.7 oz)	24	tr	6	5	2
dill low sodium	1 med (2.3 oz)	12	tr	3	–	1
dill sliced	6 slices	7	tr	2	1	1
sweet gherkin	1 (1.2 oz)	41	tr	11	5	tr
tsukemono japanese pickles sliced	¼ cup	10	tr	2	1	1
Claussen						
Bread 'N Butter Chips	1 oz	20	0	4	3	–
Kosher Dills Halves	1 (1 oz)	5	0	1	0	0
Sweet Gerkins	1 (0.9 oz)	30	0	7	6	–
Gedney						
Baby Dills	3 (1 oz)	5	0	1	0	0
Organic Baby Dills	2 (1 oz)	5	0	1	0	0
Texas Sassy						
Pickle Chips	1 tbsp (0.5 oz)	30	0	7	7	–
Tree Of Life						
Organic Sweet Bread & Butter Chips	4 (1 oz)	30	0	8	7	0
PIE (*see also* PIE CRUST, PIE FILLING)						
READY-TO-EAT						
Lance						
Pecan	1 (3 oz)	350	17	46	35	3
TAKE-OUT						
apple one crust	1 slice (5.3 oz)	363	14	59	36	2
apple tart	1 (4.2 oz)	370	19	48	20	1
apple two crust	1 slice (5.3 oz)	356	17	51	23	2
apricot tart	1 (4.2 oz)	356	17	48	20	2

FOOD	PORTION	CAL	FAT	CARB	SUGAR	FIBER
apricot two crust	1 slice (5.3 oz)	417	19	59	28	3
banana cream	1 slice (5.1 oz)	387	20	47	17	1
blackberry one crust	1 slice (4.4 oz)	341	17	44	18	4
blackberry two crust	1 slice (5.3 oz)	394	19	54	24	5
blueberry one crust	1 slice (4.8 oz)	292	12	45	23	3
blueberry tart	1 (4.2 oz)	346	17	47	21	2
blueberry two crust	1 slice (5.3 oz)	348	15	52	15	2
cherry one crust	1 slice (4.8 oz)	312	12	50	30	2
cherry two crust	1 slice (5.3 oz)	390	17	60	21	1
chess	1 slice (3 oz)	365	18	48	37	1
chocolate cream	1 slice (5 oz)	380	18	50	29	2
coconut creme	1 slice (5 oz)	429	24	54	52	2
custard	1 slice (4.8 oz)	286	16	28	16	2
grasshopper	1 slice (3.5 oz)	341	19	33	23	1
key lime	1 slice (5 oz)	420	14	71	28	tr
lemon meringue	1 slice (4.8 oz)	367	12	65	33	2
lemon meringue tart	1 (4.1 oz)	298	14	41	22	1
mince two crust	1 slice (5.3 oz)	434	16	72	42	4
peach two crust	1 slice (5.3 oz)	334	15	49	9	1

FOOD	PORTION	CAL	FAT	CARB	SUGAR	FIBER
pear two crust	1 slice (5.3 oz)	400	18	57	27	3
pecan	1 slice (4 oz)	456	21	65	32	4
pineapple two crust	1 slice (5.3 oz)	394	18	55	23	2
plum two crust	1 slice (5.3 oz)	441	21	61	29	2
prune one crust	1 slice (5.3 oz)	450	14	77	55	2
pumpkin	1 slice (5.4 oz)	323	15	42	21	4
raisin tart	1 (4.2 oz)	348	16	49	21	2
raisin two crust	1 slice (5.3 oz)	376	16	55	26	2
raspberry one crust	1 slice (4.8 oz)	330	13	52	29	6
raspberry two crust	1 slice (5.3 oz)	422	20	58	25	5
rhubarb two crust	1 slice (5.3 oz)	444	23	55	16	2
shoo-fly	1 slice (4 oz)	404	13	69	39	1
strawberry rhubarb two crust	1 slice (5.3 oz)	422	21	53	18	2
strawberry two crust	1 slice (6 oz)	386	16	58	29	3
sweet potato	1 piece (5.4 oz)	276	14	32	13	2

PIE CRUST

FOOD	PORTION	CAL	FAT	CARB	SUGAR	FIBER
baked	1/6 crust (1 oz)	147	9	14	1	tr
chocolate wafer	1/8 crust (1.2 oz)	177	11	19	8	1
chocolate wafer tart shell	1 (0.8 oz)	111	7	12	5	tr

FOOD	PORTION	CAL	FAT	CARB	SUGAR	FIBER
deep dish frzn	⅛ crust (1.8 oz)	266	16	27	–	1
graham cracker	⅙ crust (1.2 oz)	172	9	23	13	1
graham cracker tart shell	1 (0.8 oz)	109	5	14	8	tr
puff pastry shell	1 (1.4 oz)	223	15	18	tr	1
tart shell	1 (1 oz)	149	10	14	1	tr
Honey Maid						
Graham Cracker Crumbs as prep	⅛ pie	160	9	18	4	0
Keebler						
Graham Reduced Fat	⅛ pie (0.7 oz)	100	4	15	6	tr
Ready Crust Chocolate	⅛ pie (0.7 oz)	100	5	14	6	tr
Ready Crust Graham	⅒ pie (0.9 oz)	130	6	18	7	tr
Ready Crust Shortbread	⅛ pie (0.7 oz)	110	5	14	6	0
Pillsbury						
Crusts Just Unroll	⅛ (1 oz)	110	7	12	0	0
Deep Dish frzn	⅛ (0.7 oz)	90	5	11	1	0
Pet Ritz Deep Dish frzn	⅛ (0.6 oz)	90	5	11	1	0

PIE FILLING

FOOD	PORTION	CAL	FAT	CARB	SUGAR	FIBER
apple	1 cup	155	tr	41	34	2
blueberry	1 cup	474	1	116	99	7
cherry	1 cup	317	2	76	66	2
lemon	1 cup	923	18	185	166	1
pumpkin pie mix	1 cup	281	tr	71	–	22
CANNED						
Chukar Cherries						
Triple Cherry	½ cup	190	1	47	39	2
Comstock						
Country Cherry Original	⅓ cup (3.1 oz)	90	0	23	19	1

FOOD	PORTION	CAL	FAT	CARB	SUGAR	FIBER
Farmer's Market						
Organic Pumpkin Pie Mix	½ cup	100	0	25	20	2
PIEROGI						
potato	1 (1.3 oz)	70	2	11	tr	1
Mrs. T's						
Mini Potato & Cheddar	7 (3 oz)	130	2	25	1	1
Potato & Cheddar	4 (4 oz)	170	3	32	1	1
Potato & Onion	3 (4 oz)	160	2	32	1	1
Potato Broccoli & Cheddar	3 (4 oz)	190	5	31	2	2
Sauerkraut	3 (4 oz)	140	2	28	1	3
Sour Cream & Chive	3 (4 oz)	190	5	32	1	1
PIGEON PEAS						
dried cooked	½ cup	102	tr	20	–	–
dried cooked	1 cup	204	1	39	–	–
PIGNOLIA (see PINE NUTS)						
PIG'S FEET						
cooked	1	201	14	0	0	0
pickled	1	177	14	tr	tr	0
Hormel						
Pigs Feet	2 oz	80	6	0	0	0
PIKE						
northern cooked	3 oz	96	1	0	0	0
northern cooked	½ fillet (5.4 oz)	176	1	0	0	0
northern raw	3 oz	75	1	0	0	0
roe raw	1 oz	37	tr	tr	–	–
walleye baked	3 oz	101	1	0	0	0
walleye fillet baked	4.4 oz	147	2	0	0	0

FOOD	PORTION	CAL	FAT	CARB	SUGAR	FIBER
PILLNUTS						
canarytree dried	1 oz	204	23	1	–	–
PIMIENTOS						
canned	1 slice	0	0	tr	–	–
canned	1 tbsp	3	tr	1	–	–
PINE NUTS						
pine nuts dried	¼ cup (1.2 oz)	277	23	4	1	1
pinyon dried	20 (2 g)	13	1	tr	–	tr
pinyon dried	1 oz	178	17	5	–	3
Fisher						
Pine Nuts	¼ cup (1 oz)	190	19	4	1	1
PINEAPPLE						
CANNED						
chunks in heavy syrup	1 cup	199	tr	52	–	–
chunks juice pack	1 cup	150	tr	39	–	–
crushed in heavy syrup	1 cup	199	tr	52	–	–
slices in heavy syrup	1 slice	45	tr	12	–	–
slices in light syrup	1 slice	30	tr	8	–	–
slices juice pack	1 slice	35	tr	9	–	–
slices water pack	1 slice	19	tr	5	–	–
tidbits in heavy syrup	1 cup	199	tr	52	–	–
tidbits in juice	1 cup	150	tr	19	–	–
tidbits in water	1 cup	79	tr	20	–	–
Gefen						
Chunks In Juice	½ cup (4.9 oz)	80	0	19	17	1
Liberty Gold						
Chunks In Natural Juice	½ cup (4.7 oz)	80	0	21	19	2
DRIED						
Brothers-All-Natural						
Crisps	1 pkg (0.53 oz)	60	0	14	11	1

FOOD	PORTION	CAL	FAT	CARB	SUGAR	FIBER
Crispy Green						
Freeze-Dried	1 pkg (0.35)	35	0	9	7	1
Kopali						
Organic	1 pkg (1.7 oz)	170	0	43	36	2
Mrs. May's						
Fruit Chips	1 pkg	35	0	8	7	1
FRESH						
diced	1 cup	77	tr	19	–	2
slice	1 slice	42	tr	10	–	1
Chiquita						
Bites	1 piece (2.8 oz)	40	0	9	7	tr
Cut Up	1 cup (5.8 oz)	82	0	22	16	2
FROZEN						
chunks sweetened	½ cup	104	tr	27	–	–
PINEAPPLE JUICE						
canned	1 cup	139	tr	34	–	–
frzn as prep	1 cup	129	tr	32	–	–
frzn not prep	6 oz	387	tr	96	–	–
PINK BEANS						
dried cooked	1 cup	252	1	47	–	–
PINTO BEANS						
dried cooked	1 cup	245	1	45	1	15
HamBeens						
Dried as prep	½ cup	120	1	22	1	6
Tree Of Life						
Organic	½ cup (4.6 oz)	120	0	23	2	<9
TAKE-OUT						
stewed w/ viandas	1 cup	222	8	27	2	6
PISTACHIOS						
dry roasted w/ salt	49 nuts (1 oz)	161	13	8	2	3

FOOD	PORTION	CAL	FAT	CARB	SUGAR	FIBER
dry roasted w/o salt	49 nuts (1 oz)	162	13	8	2	3
in shells	½ cup	165	13	8	2	3
Fisher						
Shelled	¼ cup (1 oz)	160	13	8	2	3
True North						
Sea Salted In Shells	½ cup	170	14	7	2	4
Wonderful						
Roasted & Salted In Shells	½ cup	170	14	8	2	3

PITANGA

FOOD	PORTION	CAL	FAT	CARB	SUGAR	FIBER
fresh	1	2	tr	1	–	–
fresh	1 cup	57	1	13	–	–

PIZZA (see also PIZZA CRUST)

FOOD	PORTION	CAL	FAT	CARB	SUGAR	FIBER
4Real						
Cheese	1 (4.2 oz)	220	4	38	2	5
Cheesy Pizza Quesadilla	1 (2.5 oz)	160	5	15	1	1
Turkey Pepperoni	1 (4.2 oz)	220	4	38	2	5
Amy's						
Cheese & Pesto Whole Wheat Crust	⅓ pie (4.6 oz)	360	18	37	4	4
Margherita	1 pie (6.2 oz)	360	17	47	4	3
Non Dairy Cheese Rice Crust	1 pie (6 oz)	460	28	46	7	4
Pocket Sandwich Spinach Feta	1 (4.5 oz)	260	9	34	4	3
Roasted Vegetable No Cheese	⅓ pie (4 oz)	270	9	42	5	2
Single Serve Spinach Light In Sodium	1 (7.2 oz)	440	18	54	5	3
Soy Cheese	⅓ pie (4.3 oz)	290	11	37	3	2

FOOD	PORTION	CAL	FAT	CARB	SUGAR	FIBER
Toaster Pops Cheese Pizza	5–6 pieces (1.9 oz)	160	6	21	2	1
Cedarlane						
Zone Cheese	1 (6.5 oz)	380	14	39	4	6
Dayeinu						
Passover Pizza	1 slice (4 oz)	325	8	49	16	5
DiGiorno						
Crispy Flatbread Tuscan Chicken	⅓ pie (4.6 oz)	280	14	25	2	2
For One Thin Crust Grilled Chicken & Vegetable	1 (8.4 oz)	520	17	64	7	4
For One Traditional Crust Supreme	1 (9.9 oz)	790	36	85	11	6
Four Cheese	⅙ pie (4.7 oz)	310	11	40	6	2
Garlic Bread Pepperoni	⅙ pie (5 oz)	380	17	40	7	3
Rising Crust Four Cheese	⅓ pie (4 oz)	270	9	34	6	2
Rising Crust Italian Sausage	⅙ pie (5 oz)	350	14	40	6	2
Rising Crust Spinach Mushroom Garlic	⅙ pie (5 oz)	290	9	42	6	2
Rising Crust Three Meat	⅙ pie (5 oz)	350	15	41	6	2
Stuffed Crust Pepperoni	⅕ pie (5.3 oz)	380	16	40	7	3
Thin Crispy Crust Pepperoni	⅕ pie (4.4 oz)	320	15	31	5	2
Thin Crispy Crust Spinach Mushroom Garlic	⅕ pie (4.6 oz)	250	9	32	4	3
Ultimate Topping Four Meat	⅕ pie (5 oz)	380	19	34	5	2
Ultimate Topping Supreme	⅕ pie (5.3 oz)	360	18	35	5	2

FOOD	PORTION	CAL	FAT	CARB	SUGAR	FIBER
Dr. Praeger's						
Bagel Pizza	1 (2 oz)	120	3	17	2	2
Health Is Wealth						
Vegetarian Mini Pizza Bagels	4 (3.1 oz)	150	0	28	4	3
Hot Pockets						
Croissant Five Cheese	1 (4.5 oz)	350	17	35	10	2
Croissant Pepperoni	1 (4.5 oz)	380	22	32	7	2
Sausage	1 (4.5 oz)	330	16	36	6	2
Jeno's						
Crisp 'N Tasty Cheese	1 pie (6.8 oz)	440	21	47	5	2
Crisp 'N Tasty Pepperoni	1 (6.7 oz)	490	26	50	5	2
Crisp 'N Tasty Supreme	1 (7.2 oz)	490	25	49	5	2
Kraft						
Rising Crust Three Meat	⅓ pie (4.4 oz)	320	14	25	7	2
Lean Pockets						
Pepperoni	1 (4.5 oz)	260	7	35	9	3
Sausage & Pepperoni	1 (4.5 oz)	280	7	39	10	2
Lunchables						
Pizza Deep Dish Cheese	1 pkg	370	11	60	37	5
Totino's						
Crisp Crust Canadian Bacon	½ pie (5.1 oz)	320	15	34	4	1
Crisp Crust Combination	½ pie (5.3 oz)	380	21	34	3	1
Crisp Crust Pepperoni Trio	½ pie (5 oz)	370	21	33	4	1
Crisp Crust Three Meat	½ pie (5.2 oz)	350	18	34	3	1
Pizza Rolls Combination	6 (3 oz)	220	11	24	2	1
Pizza Rolls Supreme	6 (3 oz)	210	9	25	3	2
Pizza Rolls Mega Ultimate Combination	3 (3.3 oz)	200	8	25	3	1
TAKE-OUT						
cheese	16 in pie	3384	144	372	44	23

FOOD	PORTION	CAL	FAT	CARB	SUGAR	FIBER
cheese pie	1/8 of 16 in	423	18	46	5	3
cheese deep dish individual	1 (5.5 oz)	460	24	47	4	2
cheese & vegetables	1/8 of 16 in pie	428	16	55	5	3
ground beef	16 in pie	3753	172	392	25	20
ham & pineapple	1/8 of 16 in pie	439	16	55	7	3
no cheese	1/8 of 16 in pie	262	7	43	3	2
pepperoni	1/8 of 16 in pie	469	22	49	3	3
white pizza	1/8 of 16 in pie	484	17	61	1	2

PIZZA CRUST

FOOD	PORTION	CAL	FAT	CARB	SUGAR	FIBER
crust	1 slice (1.7 oz)	130	2	25	1	1
whole wheat	1/8 crust (2 oz)	120	2	24	0	4
Boboli						
100% Whole Wheat	1/5 crust (2 oz)	150	3	27	2	5
Original	1/8 crust (1.8 oz)	140	3	24	1	1
Original Mini	1/2 crust (2.5 oz)	190	3	35	1	1
Thin Crust	1/5 crust (2 oz)	170	4	28	1	1
French Meadow Bakery						
Gluten Free	1/4 pie (1.9 oz)	160	4	29	2	1
Martha White						
mix not prep	1/4 pkg	160	1	32	2	1
Pillsbury						
Classic	1/6 crust (2.3 oz)	160	2	31	4	tr

PLANTAINS

FOOD	PORTION	CAL	FAT	CARB	SUGAR	FIBER
cooked mashed	1 cup	232	tr	62	28	5
sliced cooked	1 cup	179	tr	48	22	4
TAKE-OUT						
mofongo	1 serv	320	3	71	31	5
ripe fried	1 serv (2.8 oz)	214	7	38	–	4

FOOD	PORTION	CAL	FAT	CARB	SUGAR	FIBER
sweet baked w/ ice cream	1 serv	285	8	57	35	3

PLUM JUICE
Nantucket Nectars
Red Plum	8 oz	120	0	30	30	0

Sunsweet
PlumSmart Light	8 oz	60	0	15	11	3

PLUMS
canned in heavy syrup	1 cup	163	tr	42	39	3
canned purple juice pack	1 cup	146	tr	38	35	2
canned purple water pack	1 cup	102	tr	27	25	2
dried japanese	1	9	tr	2	1	tr
fresh	1	30	tr	8	7	1
pickled	1	34	tr	9	9	tr

Chiquita
fresh	1 (2.3 oz)	30	0	8	7	1

Oregon
Whole In Heavy Syrup	½ cup (4.6 oz)	100	0	25	19	2

POI
poi	1 cup	240	0	65	–	1

POKEBERRY SHOOTS
cooked	½ cup	16	tr	3	–	–
fresh	½ cup	18	tr	3	–	–

POLLACK
atlantic fillet baked	5.3 oz	178	2	0	0	0
atlantic baked	3 oz	100	1	0	0	0

FOOD	PORTION	CAL	FAT	CARB	SUGAR	FIBER
POMEGRANATE						
fresh	1 (5.4 oz)	105	tr	26	26	1
Navitas Naturals						
Pomegranate Powder	1 tbsp (0.5 oz)	50	0	13	3	0
POMEGRANATE JUICE						
Arthur's						
Pom Plus	1 bottle (11 oz)	220	0	54	33	1
Smart Juice						
Organic 100% Juice	8 oz	149	0	37	33	1
Tart Is Smart						
Concentrate	0.5 oz	37	0	9	9	0
POMPANO						
smoked	2 oz	109	6	0	0	0
steamed or poached	4 oz	156	9	0	0	0
TAKE-OUT						
battered & fried	4 oz	304	21	8	tr	tr
breaded & fried	4 oz	242	15	10	1	1
POPCORN						
air popped	1 cup (0.3 oz)	31	tr	6	–	2
caramel coated	1 cup (1.2 oz)	152	5	28	14	2
caramel coated w/ peanuts	2/3 cup (1 oz)	114	2	23	11	1
cheese	1 cup (0.4 oz)	58	4	6	–	1
oil popped	1 cup (0.4 oz)	55	3	6	tr	1
Deep River Snacks						
Sharp White Cheddar	1 oz	150	10	13	3	2
Divvies						
Caramel Corn Vegan	½ cup	80	3	14	10	tr
I.M. Healthy						
Roasted Sweet Corn Original Lighly Salted	1 oz	120	5	20	1	2

FOOD	PORTION	CAL	FAT	CARB	SUGAR	FIBER
Lance						
White Cheddar	1 pkg (0.7 oz)	100	11	8	1	2
Mrs. Fields						
Clusters Butter Toffee Crunch	⅔ cup	170	5	31	20	3
Poppycock						
Cashew Lovers	½ cup (1.1 oz)	148	6	21	12	tr
Original	½ cup (1.1 oz)	160	8	20	13	1
Pecan Delight	½ cup (1.1 oz)	150	8	20	13	0
Smart Balance						
Low Fat Smart 'N Healthy as prep	5 cups	120	2	24	0	5
Tree Of Life						
Organic Lightly Salted	4 cups	100	2	21	0	5
Utz						
Butter	2 cups	170	12	13	tr	2
Cheese	2 cups	160	11	14	1	3
Puff'n Corn Original Hulless	2 cups	150	17	11	0	0
POPOVER						
home recipe as prep w/ 2% milk	1 (1.4 oz)	87	3	11	–	–
home recipe as prep w/ whole milk	1 (1.4 oz)	90	3	11	–	–
mix as prep	1 (1.2 oz)	67	2	10	–	–
POPPY SEEDS						
poppy seeds	1 tbsp	47	4	2	1	1
PORGY						
fresh	3 oz	77	tr	0	0	0

FOOD	PORTION	CAL	FAT	CARB	SUGAR	FIBER
PORK (*see also* HAM, JERKY, PORK DISHES)						
FRESH						
boneless loin lean & fat roasted	3.5 oz	195	9	0	0	0
center loin chop bone in broiled	1 (3 oz)	178	9	0	0	0
center rib chop lean & fat bone in broiled	1 (3 oz)	189	11	0	0	0
country style ribs bone in lean & fat braised	3.5 oz	288	19	0	0	0
dehydrated oriental style	1 cup (0.8 oz)	135	14	tr	0	0
fresh ham rump half lean & fat roasted	4 oz	278	16	0	0	0
fresh ham shank half lean & fat roasted	4 oz	319	22	0	0	0
fresh ham whole lean & fat roasted	4 oz	302	19	0	0	0
ground cooked	4 oz	328	23	0	0	0
ham hock cooked	1	167	12	0	0	0
shoulder chop bone in braised	1 (3 oz)	229	15	0	0	0
sirloin roast lean & fat bone in roasted	4 oz	231	13	0	0	0
spareribs bone in roasted	3 oz	304	26	0	0	0
tail simmered	3 oz	336	30	0	0	0
tenderloin roast boneless lean & fat roasted	4 oz	145	4	0	0	0
top loin chop boneless lean & fat broiled	1 (3.5 oz)	195	9	0	0	0

FOOD	PORTION	CAL	FAT	CARB	SUGAR	FIBER
Smithfield						
Boneless Smoked Pork Chop	3 oz	110	4	4	3	0
TAKE-OUT						
chicharrones pork cracklings fried	1 cup	492	38	1	0	0
chop breaded & fried	1 med (3.4 oz)	304	18	13	1	1
chop breaded & fried	1 lg (5 oz)	441	26	19	2	1
chop stewed	1 lg (4.6 oz)	315	18	0	0	0

PORK DISHES
Hormel

FOOD	PORTION	CAL	FAT	CARB	SUGAR	FIBER
Always Tender Loin Filet Honey Mustard	1 serv (4 oz)	140	5	4	4	0
Always Tender Tenderloin Apple Burbon	1 serv (4 oz)	140	4	5	4	0
Pork Roast Au Jus	1 serv (2 oz)	90	3	10	10	0
Ventera						
Pork Carnitas	1 serv (5 oz)	190	8	6	1	1
TAKE-OUT						
kalua pork	1 cup (7 oz)	497	34	1	–	0
pork satay w/ peanut sauce	5 sticks (3.5 oz)	214	13	14	–	3
pulled pork w/ barbecue sauce	1 serv (5 oz)	240	14	15	12	1
spareribs barbecued w/ sauce	2 med (2.8 oz)	248	18	3	1	tr
tourtiere	1 piece (4.9 oz)	451	34	21	–	–

PORK RINDS (see SNACKS)

FOOD	PORTION	CAL	FAT	CARB	SUGAR	FIBER
POT PIE						
Amy's						
Broccoli	1 (7.5 oz)	430	22	46	3	4
Shepherd's	1 (8 oz)	160	4	27	5	5
Shepherd's Pie Light In Sodium	1 (8 oz)	160	4	27	5	5
Vegetable	1 (7.5 oz)	360	13	50	3	4
Banquet						
Beef	1	450	27	36	7	2
Chicken	1	370	21	34	5	2
Chicken w/ Broccoli	1	350	20	32	4	2
Turkey	1	390	21	36	3	2
Hot Pockets						
Pot Pie Express Chicken	1 (4.5 oz)	330	18	34	8	2
Marie Callender's						
Beef	½ pie	540	32	46	4	3
Cheeesy Chicken	½ pie	600	37	46	5	3
Chicken	1	670	41	55	4	3
Creamy Mushroom & Chicken	½ pie	560	35	45	4	3
Turkey	1	670	41	56	6	4
Mon Cuisine						
Vegan	1 pkg (9 oz)	650	39	60	6	8
TAKE-OUT						
beef	1 (14.6 oz)	938	57	72	4	5
chicken	1 (14.6 oz)	897	52	69	5	6
ham	1 serv (11 oz)	752	45	58	3	4
oyster	1 serv (11.5 oz)	817	53	67	6	3
puerto rican pastelon de carne	1 piece (5 oz)	666	48	35	1	2
st. stephen's day pie	1 serv (16.7 oz)	549	29	38	5	6

FOOD	PORTION	CAL	FAT	CARB	SUGAR	FIBER
tuna	1 (27 oz)	1715	102	126	10	10
vegetarian w/ meat substitute	1 (8 oz)	511	32	39	3	5

POTATO (see also CHIPS, KNISH, PANCAKES)
CANNED

FOOD	PORTION	CAL	FAT	CARB	SUGAR	FIBER
potatoes	½ cup	54	tr	12	–	–
Butterfield						
Whole White	3.5 pieces (5.8 oz)	90	0	20	0	2
S&W						
New Whole	2 (5.5 oz)	60	0	13	0	2
Sunshine						
Whole White	3 pieces (5.9 oz)	90	0	20	0	2
FRESH						
baked skin only	1 skin (2 oz)	115	tr	27	–	2
baked w/ skin	1 (6.5 oz)	220	tr	51	–	–
baked w/o skin	½ cup	57	tr	13	–	1
baked w/o skin	1 (5 oz)	145	tr	34	–	2
boiled	½ cup	68	tr	16	–	1
microwaved	1 (7 oz)	212	tr	49	–	–
microwaved w/o skin	½ cup	78	tr	18	–	–
raw w/o skin	1 (3.9 oz)	88	tr	20	–	–
red new boiled	5 sm (5 oz)	120	0	27	3	2
FROZEN						
french fries	10 strips	111	4	17	–	2
french fries thick cut	10 strips	109	4	17	–	–
hash browns	½ cup	170	9	22	–	–
potato puffs	1	16	1	2	–	–
potato puffs	½ cup	138	7	19	–	–
Cascadian Farm						
Organic Country Style	¾ cup	50	0	12	0	1
Organic Hash Browns	1 cup	60	0	14	0	1

FOOD	PORTION	CAL	FAT	CARB	SUGAR	FIBER
Green Giant						
Roasted Potatoes w/ Garlic & Herb Sauce as prep	½ cup	90	2	15	1	1
Health Is Wealth						
Twice Baked Cheddar Cheese	1 (5 oz)	200	10	25	2	2
Vegetarian Potato Skins	2 (2.7 oz)	110	7	8	0	1
Joy Of Cooking						
Elegant Scalloped	1 cup (8 oz)	300	17	21	2	2
Red Skin Mashed	1 cup (4.2 oz)	160	9	17	2	2
MIX						
au gratin as prep	½ cup	160	9	14	–	–
instant mashed flakes as prep w/ whole milk & butter	½ cup	118	6	16	–	–
instant mashed flakes not prep	½ cup	78	tr	18	–	–
instant mashed granules as prep w/ whole milk & butter	½ cup	114	5	15	–	–
instant mashed granules not prep	½ cup	372	1	86	–	–
scalloped	½ cup	105	5	13	–	–
Betty Crocker						
Au Gratin as prep	⅔ cup	150	5	24	0	1
Cheddar & Bacon as prep	⅔ cup	120	3	21	1	1
Cheesy Scalloped as prep	½ cup	120	3	21	1	1
Julienne as prep	⅔ cup	140	5	20	1	1
Mashed Four Cheese as prep	½ cup	170	7	21	1	1

FOOD	PORTION	CAL	FAT	CARB	SUGAR	FIBER
Mashed Sour Cream & Chives as prep	½ cup	170	7	21	1	1
Scalloped as prep	½ cup	130	4	20	1	1
Seasoned Skillets Hash Browns as prep	½ cup	120	4	19	0	2
REFRIGERATED						
Bob Evans						
Mashed Potatoes Original	½ cup (4.4 oz)	150	7	20	1	2
Country Crock						
Garlic Mashed	⅔ cup (5 oz)	160	7	22	1	2
Homestyle Mashed	⅔ cup (5 oz)	180	9	23	1	2
Loaded Mashed	⅔ cup (5 oz)	200	11	22	2	2
Reser's						
Potato Express Red Skinned Mashed	½ cup	140	5	22	1	2
Simply Potatoes						
Traditional Mashed	½ cup (4.4 oz)	120	6	15	1	2
TAKE-OUT						
au gratin w/ cheese	½ cup	178	10	17	–	–
baked topped w/ cheese sauce	1	475	29	47	–	–
baked topped w/ cheese sauce & bacon	1	451	26	44	–	–
baked topped w/ cheese sauce & broccoli	1	402	14	47	–	–
baked topped w/ cheese sauce & chili	1	481	22	56	–	–
baked topped w/ sour cream & chives	1	394	22	50	–	–
french fries	1 reg	235	12	29	–	–

FOOD	PORTION	CAL	FAT	CARB	SUGAR	FIBER
hash browns	½ cup (2.5 oz)	151	9	16	–	–
indian yogurt potatoes	1 serv	315	9	52	–	0
mashed	½ cup	111	4	18	–	–
o'brien	1 cup	157	3	30	–	–
potato pancakes	1 (1.3 oz)	101	7	11	–	–
potato salad	½ cup	179	10	14	–	2
scalloped	½ cup	127	5	18	–	–
twice baked w/ cheese	1 half (10 oz)	392	18	48	–	4

POTATO STARCH

FOOD	PORTION	CAL	FAT	CARB	SUGAR	FIBER
potato starch	1 oz	96	tr	24	–	–

POUT

FOOD	PORTION	CAL	FAT	CARB	SUGAR	FIBER
ocean baked	3 oz	86	1	0	0	0
ocean fillet baked	4.8 oz	139	2	0	0	0

PRETZELS

FOOD	PORTION	CAL	FAT	CARB	SUGAR	FIBER
chocolate covered	1 (0.4 oz)	47	1	8	2	tr
soft	1 lg (5 oz)	483	4	99	tr	2
twists salted	10 (2.1 oz)	229	2	48	–	2
twists w/o salt	10 (2.1 oz)	229	2	48	1	2
whole wheat	2 sm (1 oz)	103	1	23	–	2
yogurt covered	1 (4 g)	19	1	3	1	tr
yogurt covered	1 cup (3 oz)	391	13	61	30	1
Braids						
Honey Wheat	7 (1 oz)	110	2	23	4	1
Mini Knots	17 (1 oz)	110	1	23	tr	tr
Rold Gold						
Braided Twists	1 oz	110	1	22	tr	1
Braided Twists Honey Wheat	1 oz	110	1	23	3	1
Dipped Twists Fudge Coated	1 oz	140	6	18	11	2
Mini Sticks Honey Mustard & Onion	1 oz	140	6	19	2	1

FOOD	PORTION	CAL	FAT	CARB	SUGAR	FIBER
Pretzel Waves Cheddar	1 oz	130	5	20	tr	1
Pretzel Waves Dark Chocolate Drizzle	1 oz	130	4	20	6	2
Pretzel Waves Vanilla Yogurt Drizzle	1 oz	130	5	21	8	tr
Sourdough Hard	1	100	1	21	tr	1
Sticks Classic	1 oz	100	0	23	1	1
Tiny Twists :Salba Smart	1 oz	100	0	23	tr	1
Omega-3 Enriched	1 oz	110	2	21	1	1
Tom Sturgis						
Little Cheesers	17 (1 oz)	120	2	22	tr	2
Little Ones	17 (1 oz)	110	2	22	tr	tr
Utz						
Braided Twists Baked Honey Wheat	1 oz	110	2	23	4	1
Chocolate Covered	6 (1.1 oz)	140	5	22	11	tr
Hard	1	90	0	18	tr	tr
Special	1 oz	110	1	21	tr	1
Special Multigrain	1 oz	110	1	21	1	2
Sticks Organic Whole Grain	1 oz	120	2	22	1	3

PRUNE JUICE

FOOD	PORTION	CAL	FAT	CARB	SUGAR	FIBER
jarred	1 cup	182	tr	45	42	3
Tree Of Life						
Organic 100% Juice	8 oz	180	0	43	23	2

PRUNES

FOOD	PORTION	CAL	FAT	CARB	SUGAR	FIBER
cooked w/o sugar	½ cup	133	tr	35	31	4
dried	1	20	tr	5	3	1
Sunsweet						
Pitted	5 (1.5 oz)	100	0	24	12	3

FOOD	PORTION	CAL	FAT	CARB	SUGAR	FIBER
PUDDING						
READY-TO-EAT						
Jell-O						
Vanilla	1 serv (4 oz)	110	2	23	18	0
SoYummi						
GoLite Bavarian Cream	1 pkg (3.5 oz)	86	3	12	–	–
Mousse All Flavors	1 pkg (4.4 oz)	137	4	21	15	2
Swiss Miss						
Chocolate	1 pkg	150	4	27	22	0
Low Fat Chocolate	1 pkg	130	2	26	19	0
Pie Lover's Banana Cream	1 pkg	130	4	23	17	0
Pie Lover's Lemon Meringue	1 pkg	140	3	28	21	0
Swirl Chocolate Vanilla	1 pkg	140	4	27	20	0
ZenSoy						
Banana	1 pkg (4 oz)	100	1	21	15	1
Chocolate	1 pkg (4 oz)	130	1	29	21	2
Vanilla	1 pkg (4 oz)	110	1	23	15	1
TAKE-OUT						
blancmange	1 serv (4.7 oz)	154	5	25	–	tr
bread w/ raisins	1 cup	306	9	47	29	2
coconut	1 cup	291	9	45	38	2
corn	1 cup	328	13	43	17	4
indian pudding	½ cup	156	4	25	16	1
noodle pudding kugel	1 cup	297	10	44	15	2
plum pudding	1 slice (1.5 oz)	125	5	20	12	1
queen of puddings	1 serv (4.4 oz)	266	10	41	–	tr
rice pudding	1 cup	302	4	60	37	1
sweet potato	½ cup	107	3	19	7	3
tapioca	1 cup	236	7	35	31	0
yorkshire	1 serv (3 oz)	177	8	22	–	tr

FOOD	PORTION	CAL	FAT	CARB	SUGAR	FIBER
PUFFERFISH						
raw	3 oz	72	0	0	0	0
PUMMELO						
fresh	1	228	tr	59	–	–
sections	1 cup	71	tr	18	–	–
PUMPKIN						
butter	1 tbsp	32	0	8	8	–
canned	½ cup	41	tr	10	–	–
cooked mashed	½ cup	24	tr	6	–	–
flowers cooked	½ cup	10	tr	2	–	–
flowers raw	1	0	0	tr	–	–
leaves cooked	½ cup	7	tr	1	–	–
leaves raw	½ cup	4	tr	tr	–	–
raw cubed	½ cup	15	tr	4	–	–
Jake & Amos						
Pumpkin Butter	1 tbsp (0.5 oz)	5	0	1	1	0
Tree Of Life						
Organic Puree	½ cup (4.3 oz)	50	0	10	4	4
TAKE-OUT						
indian sago	1 serv (2.3 oz)	75	5	6	3	3
PUMPKIN SEEDS						
dried	1 oz	154	13	5	–	–
roasted	¼ cup	296	24	8	–	–
salted & roasted	¼ cup	296	24	8	–	–
whole roasted	¼ cup	71	3	9	–	–
whole roasted	1 oz	127	6	15	–	–
whole salted roasted	¼ cup	71	3	9	–	–
Mrs. May's						
Pumpkin Crunch	1 oz	164	11	8	4	1
Tree Of Life						
Seeds Roasted & Salted	¼ cup (2 oz)	300	24	8	1	4

FOOD	PORTION	CAL	FAT	CARB	SUGAR	FIBER
PURSLANE						
cooked	1 cup	21	tr	4	–	–
fresh	1 cup	7	tr	1	–	–
QUAIL						
cooked bone removed	1 (2.7 oz)	177	11	0	0	0
QUICHE						
TAKE-OUT						
cheese	⅛ (9 in) pie	566	44	27	1	1
lorraine	⅛ (9 in) pie	568	44	27	1	1
mushroom	1 slice (3 oz)	256	18	17	–	1
spinach	⅛ (9 in) pie	342	26	17	1	1
QUINCE						
fresh	1	53	tr	14	–	–
QUINOA						
cooked	1 cup (6.5 oz)	222	4	39	–	5
quinoa not prep	¼ cup (1.5 oz)	156	3	27	–	3
Ancient Harvest Quinoa						
Flakes not prep	¼ cup	159	2	28	1	3
Organic Inca Red not prep	¼ cup	163	3	29	5	4
Organic Traditional not prep	¼ cup	172	3	31	3	3
TruRoots						
Organic not prep	¼ cup (1.6 oz)	172	3	31	3	3
RABBIT						
domestic w/o bone roasted	3 oz	167	7	0	0	0
wild w/o bone stewed	3 oz	147	3	0	0	0
RACCOON						
roasted	3 oz	217	12	0	0	0

FOOD	PORTION	CAL	FAT	CARB	SUGAR	FIBER
RADICCHIO						
raw shredded	½ cup	5	tr	1	–	–
RADISHES						
chinese dried	½ cup	157	tr	37	–	–
chinese raw	1 (12 oz)	62	tr	14	–	–
chinese raw sliced	½ cup	8	tr	2	–	–
chinese sliced cooked	½ cup	13	tr	3	–	–
daikon dried	½ cup	157	tr	37	–	–
daikon raw	1 (12 oz)	62	tr	14	–	–
daikon raw sliced	½ cup	8	tr	2	–	–
daikon sliced cooked	½ cup	13	tr	3	–	–
red raw	10	7	tr	2	–	–
red sliced	½ cup	10	tr	2	–	–
white icicle raw	1 (0.5 oz)	2	tr	tr	–	–
white icicle raw sliced	½ cup	7	tr	1	–	–
Cadis						
Fresh	6 (2.6 oz)	12	tr	2	–	–
TAKE-OUT						
korean kimchee	½ cup	31	1	6	–	–
moo namul saengche korean salad	1 serv (3.7 oz)	34	tr	8	6	2
RAISINS						
cinnamon coated	¼ cup	108	tr	29	21	1
cooked	¼ cup	162	tr	42	35	1
golden seedless	¼ cup	109	tr	29	21	1
jumbo golden	¼ cup	130	0	31	29	2
milk chocolate coated	¼ cup	176	7	31	28	2
milk chocolate coated	28 (1 oz)	109	4	19	17	1
seedless	55 (1 oz)	86	tr	23	17	1
sultanas	1 oz	88	0	23	–	2
Amazin' Raisin						
All Flavors	1 pkg (1 oz)	84	0	22	20	2

FOOD	PORTION	CAL	FAT	CARB	SUGAR	FIBER
Emily's						
Milk Chocolate Covered	29 (1.4 oz)	180	8	26	24	2
Godiva						
Milk Chocolate Covered	1 pkg (1.2 oz)	150	7	21	20	1
Revolution Foods						
Organic	1 pkg (1.2 oz)	100	0	28	21	1
Sun-Maid						
Chocolate Covered	30 (1.4 oz)	170	6	26	25	1
Golden	¼ cup (1.4 oz)	130	0	31	29	2
Jumbo	¼ cup (1.4 oz)	130	0	31	29	2
Seedless	¼ cup (1.4 oz)	130	0	31	29	2
Snack Box	1 (1 oz)	90	0	22	20	2
RAMBUTAN						
canned in syrup	1 (0.3 oz)	7	tr	2	–	tr
canned in syrup	1 cup (4.3 oz)	123	tr	31	–	1
puerto rican fresh	5 (1.6 oz)	34	tr	8	8	tr
Polar						
In Syrup	½ cup	68	0	17	14	tr
RASPBERRIES						
black fresh	1 cup	70	1	16	6	9
canned in heavy syrup	½ cup	116	tr	30	26	4
canned water pack	1 cup	43	1	10	4	5
fresh	1 pt	162	2	37	14	20
fresh	1 cup	64	1	15	5	8
frzn sweetened	1 cup	129	tr	33	27	6
frzn unsweetened	1 cup	65	1	15	6	8
Cascadian Farm						
Organic frzn	1¼ cup	60	0	17	6	6
Stoneridge Orchards						
Dried Whole	⅓ cup (1.4 oz)	130	1	32	29	3

FOOD	PORTION	CAL	FAT	CARB	SUGAR	FIBER
RED BEANS						
Allens						
Red Beans	½ cup	100	1	19	1	9
RELISH						
hamburger	½ cup	158	1	42	–	–
hamburger	1 tbsp	19	tr	5	–	–
hot dog	½ cup	111	1	28	–	–
hot dog	1 tbsp	14	tr	4	–	–
piccalilli	1.4 oz	13	tr	2	–	1
sweet	½ cup	159	1	43	–	–
sweet	1 tbsp	19	tr	5	–	–
tomato	¼ cup (2.8 oz)	119	tr	28	26	1
Cascadian Farm						
Organic Sweet Relish	1 tbsp (0.5 oz)	15	0	4	4	0
Claussen						
Sweet Pickle	1 tbsp (0.5 oz)	15	0	3	2	0
Gedney						
Hot Dog	1 tbsp	18	0	4	3	0
Organic Sweet	1 tbsp	15	0	4	3	0
Texas Sassy						
Pickle Relish	1 tbsp (0.5 oz)	30	0	7	7	–
Tree Of Life						
Organic Sweet Pickle	1 tbsp (0.5)	15	0	4	3	0
RENNIN						
tablet	1 (0.9 g)	1	0	tr	–	–
RHUBARB						
fresh	½ cup	13	tr	3	–	–
frozen	½ cup	60	tr	3	–	–
frzn as prep w/ sugar	½ cup	139	tr	37	–	–
RICE (see also RICE CAKES, WILD RICE)						
arborio	½ cup	100	0	22	–	–

FOOD	PORTION	CAL	FAT	CARB	SUGAR	FIBER
brown long grain cooked	1 cup (6.8 oz)	216	2	45	–	4
brown medium grain cooked	1 cup (6.8 oz)	218	2	46	–	4
glutinous cooked	1 cup (6.1 oz)	169	tr	37	–	2
starch	1 oz	98	0	24	–	–
white long grain cooked	1 cup (5.5 oz)	205	tr	45	–	1
white long grain instant cooked	1 cup (5.8 oz)	162	tr	35	–	1
white medium grain cooked	1 cup (6.5 oz)	242	tr	53	–	1
white short grain cooked	1 cup (6.5 oz)	242	tr	53	–	–
Amy's						
Bowls Brown Rice Black-Eyed Peas & Veggies	1 pkg (8.9 oz)	290	11	38	5	8
Bowls Brown Rice & Vegetables	1 pkg (9.9 oz)	260	9	36	7	5
Betty Crocker						
Bowl Appetit! Teriyaki Rice	1 bowl (2.5 oz)	260	3	54	6	2
Carolina						
Saffron Yellow Mix not prep	1 serv	190	0	43	1	1
Country Crock						
Cheddar Broccoli Rice	1 cup (7 oz)	270	11	35	3	1
Green Giant						
Rice Pilaf	1 pkg (9.9 oz)	200	3	40	3	3
White & Wild & Green Beans	1 pkg (9.9 oz)	260	5	48	3	3
Minute						
Boil-In-Bag White as prep	1 cup	180	0	41	0	1

FOOD	PORTION	CAL	FAT	CARB	SUGAR	FIBER
Brown as prep	1 cup	150	2	34	0	2
Ready To Serve Brown	1 pkg (4.4 oz)	170	5	28	0	2
Ready To Serve White	1 pkg (4.4 oz)	190	4	34	0	0
Ready To Serve Yellow	1 pkg (4.4 oz)	190	4	35	0	1
White as prep	1 cup	200	0	45	0	0
Near East						
Long Grain & Wild Original as prep	1 cup	220	4	43	0	2
Pilaf Curry as prep	1 cup	220	4	44	0	2
Pilaf Original as prep	1 cup	220	4	43	0	1
Pilaf Sesame Ginger as prep	1 cup	270	4	55	6	1
Pilaf Spanish Rice as prep	1 cup	310	7	54	2	2
Whole Grains Brown Rice as prep	1 cup	210	4	41	1	3
Thai Kitchen						
Jasmine not prep	2 tbsp (1.5 oz)	160	0	36	0	tr
Uncle Ben's						
Long Grain & Wild Herb Roasted Chicken as prep	1 cup	190	1	39	1	3
Long Grain & Wild Sun-Dried Tomato Florentine as prep	1 cup	180	1	39	1	3
Zatarain's						
Black Beans & Rice as prep	1 cup	230	1	47	0	6
Caribbean Rice Mix as prep	1 cup	160	2	34	0	1
Yellow as prep	½ cup	110	0	23	0	0
TAKE-OUT						
coconut rice	1 serv	500	42	30	–	2
congee	½ cup (4.1 oz)	44	–	10	–	–

FOOD	PORTION	CAL	FAT	CARB	SUGAR	FIBER
dirty rice w/ chicken giblets	1 cup (6.9 oz)	291	10	38	tr	1
nasi goreng indonesian rice & vegetables	1 cup (4.9 oz)	130	0	28	1	1
pea palau rice & peas fried in ghee	1 serv	144	5	21	1	2
pilaf	½ cup	84	3	11	–	3
risotto	1 serv (6.6 oz)	426	18	65	–	3
spanish	¾ cup	363	27	19	–	–

RICE CAKES
Hain

FOOD	PORTION	CAL	FAT	CARB	SUGAR	FIBER
Mini Munchies Apple Cinnamon	9 (0.5 oz)	60	1	14	2	tr

ROCKFISH

FOOD	PORTION	CAL	FAT	CARB	SUGAR	FIBER
pacific cooked	3 oz	103	2	0	0	0
pacific cooked	1 fillet (5.2 oz)	180	3	0	0	0
pacific raw	3 oz	80	1	0	0	0

ROE (see also individual fish names)

FOOD	PORTION	CAL	FAT	CARB	SUGAR	FIBER
fresh baked	1 oz	58	2	1	–	0

ROLL
FROZEN
Joy Of Cooking

FOOD	PORTION	CAL	FAT	CARB	SUGAR	FIBER
Ciabatta Olive Oil Rosemary	1 (1.7 oz)	120	2	21	0	1
French Baguettes Mini	1 (1.6 oz)	100	0	20	0	1

Pillsbury

FOOD	PORTION	CAL	FAT	CARB	SUGAR	FIBER
Dinner Rolls Crusty Sourdough	1 (1.2 oz)	90	1	17	0	tr
Dinner Rolls Crusty French	1 (1.2 oz)	90	1	15	1	tr

FOOD	PORTION	CAL	FAT	CARB	SUGAR	FIBER
Dinner Rolls Whole Wheat	1 (1.2 oz)	90	1	17	2	3
READY-TO-EAT						
bialy	1 (2.2 oz)	138	0	32	–	1
brioche sweet roll	1 (3.5 oz)	410	23	41	5	3
cheese	1 (2.3 oz)	238	12	29	–	1
cinnamon raisin	1 (2.1 oz)	223	10	31	19	1
dinner	1 (1 oz)	78	1	14	2	1
egg	1 (1.2 oz)	107	2	18	2	1
french	1 (1.3 oz)	105	2	19	tr	1
garlic	1 (1.5 oz)	133	3	22	2	1
hamburger or hot dog	1 (1.5 oz)	120	2	21	3	1
hamburger or hot dog multi grain	1 (1.5 oz)	113	3	19	3	2
hamburger or hot dog reduced calorie	1 (1.5 oz)	84	1	18	2	3
hamburger or hot dog whole wheat	1 (1.5 oz)	114	2	22	4	3
hard	1 (2 oz)	167	2	30	1	1
hoagie or submarine roll whole wheat roll whole wheat	1 (4.7 oz)	359	6	69	11	10
hot cross bun	1	202	4	38	–	1
mexican bolillo	1 (4.1 oz)	305	2	60	tr	2
oat bran	1 (1.2 oz)	78	2	13	2	1
oatmeal	1 (1.3 oz)	103	2	17	2	1
pumpernickel	1 (1.3 oz)	100	1	19	tr	2
rye	1 med (1.3 oz)	103	1	19	tr	2
sourdough	1 (1.6 oz)	130	1	25	1	1
wheat	1 (1 oz)	76	2	13	tr	1
whole wheat	1 med (1.3 oz)	96	2	18	3	3

FOOD	PORTION	CAL	FAT	CARB	SUGAR	FIBER
Arnold						
Whole Grains Sandwich 100% Whole Wheat	1 (2.2 oz)	160	2	26	4	4
Calise						
Kaiser 100% Whole Wheat	1 (2.5 oz)	190	3	33	5	3
Ecce Panis						
Focaccia	1 (3.2 oz)	260	5	49	tr	2
French Meadow Bakery						
Gluten Free Italian	1 (4.4 oz)	340	9	63	7	8
J.J. Cassone						
Sandwich	1 (2.5 oz)	190	2	38	2	2
Mrs Baird's						
Home Bake	1 (1 oz)	80	2	13	2	tr
Natural Ovens						
Better Wheat Buns	1 (2.2 oz)	170	3	30	5	4
Pepperidge Farm						
Sandwich Buns Sesame Seeds	1 (1.6 oz)	130	3	22	3	1
S. Rosen's						
Brat & Sausage Rolls	1 (2.1 oz)	160	3	28	2	1
Klassic Kaiser	1 (2.6 oz)	230	3	46	7	1
Weight Watchers						
Sandwich Wheat	1 (2 oz)	140	2	28	2	5
REFRIGERATED						
crescent	1 (1 oz)	78	1	14	2	1
Pillsbury						
Crescent Big & Buttery	1 (1.7 oz)	170	10	20	4	tr
Crescent Butter Flake	1 (1 oz)	110	6	11	2	0
Crescent Original	1 (1 oz)	110	6	11	2	0
Crescent Reduced Fat	1 (1 oz)	90	5	12	2	0

FOOD	PORTION	CAL	FAT	CARB	SUGAR	FIBER
ROSE APPLE						
fresh	3.5 oz	32	tr	7	–	–
ROSE HIP						
fresh	1 oz	26	0	5	–	–
ROSELLE						
fresh	1 cup	28	tr	6	–	–
ROSEMARY						
dried	1 tsp	4	tr	1	–	1
fresh	1 tbsp	1	tr	tr	–	tr
ROUGHY						
orange baked	3 oz	75	1	0	0	0
RUBS (see HERBS/SPICES)						
RUTABAGA						
cooked mashed	1 cup	94	1	21	14	4
cubed cooked	1 cup	66	tr	14	10	3
Sunshine						
Diced	½ cup	30	0	7	2	1
SABLEFISH						
baked	3 oz	213	17	0	0	0
fillet baked	5.3 oz	378	30	0	0	0
smoked	3 oz	218	17	0	0	0
smoked	1 oz	72	6	0	0	0
SAFFLOWER						
seeds dried	1 oz	147	11	10	–	–
SAFFRON						
dried	1 tsp	2	tr	tr	–	tr
SAGE						
ground	1 tsp	2	tr	tr	tr	tr

FOOD	PORTION	CAL	FAT	CARB	SUGAR	FIBER
SALAD (*see also* SALAD TOPPINGS)						
Dole						
Field Greens	1½ cups (3 oz)	20	0	4	2	2
Fresh Express						
50/50 Mix	3 cups	10	0	5	2	4
Asian Supreme w/ Dressing as prep	2½ cups	170	10	17	8	2
Caesar Lite w/ Dressing as prep	2½ cups	100	7	8	2	2
Caesar w/ Dressing as prep	2½ cups	150	13	8	2	2
Fancy Field Greens	3 cups	20	0	3	1	2
Gourmet Cafe Caribbean Chicken as prep	1 pkg (3.5 oz)	120	6	14	8	1
Gourmet Cafe Chicken Caesar w/ Crostini as prep	1 pkg (3.5 oz)	150	11	5	1	1
Gourmet Cafe Chopped Turkey Chef as prep	1 pkg (3.5 oz)	120	9	7	4	tr
Gourmet Cafe Orchard Harvest as prep	1 pkg (3.5 oz)	230	18	13	9	2
Gourmet Cafe Tuscan Pesto Chicken as prep	1 pkg (3.5 oz)	130	8	6	3	1
Gourmet Cafe Waldorf Chicken as prep	1 pkg (3.5 oz)	190	10	19	14	2
More Carrots American	1½ cups	15	0	3	2	1
Organic Italian	2½ cups	15	0	3	2	1
Original Iceberg Garden With Zip	1½ cups	15	0	3	2	4
Pacifica! Veggie Supreme w/ Dressing as prep	3 cups	220	15	18	14	2

FOOD	PORTION	CAL	FAT	CARB	SUGAR	FIBER
Spring Mix	3 cups	15	0	3	1	2
Sweet Baby Greens	3 cups	10	0	2	1	1
Veggie Lover's	2 cups	20	0	4	2	1
Lifestyle Foods						
Asian w/ Chicken	1 pkg (8.9 oz)	340	16	36	21	3
Casear	1 pkg (5 oz)	210	11	22	6	2
Garden	1 pkg (6.6 oz)	180	12	14	4	2
Greek	1 pkg (6 oz)	130	11	6	2	2
Mann's						
Rainbow	3 oz	25	0	5	2	2
TAKE-OUT						
7-layer salad	2 cups	557	51	15	8	3
caesar	4 cups	734	61	28	6	7
chef salad w/o dressing	3 cups	535	32	9	–	–
cobb w/ dressing	4 cups	645	49	23	9	11
greek w/ dressing	4 cups	424	29	14	8	4
mixed salad greens shredded	1 cup	9	tr	2	tr	1
somen w/ lettuce egg fish pork	2 cups	550	17	57	4	4
spinach w/o dressing	4 cups	429	19	45	5	6
tossed w/ avocado w/o dressing	2 cups	90	6	9	4	5
tossed w/ chicken w/o dressing	3 cups	194	4	5	3	2
tossed w/ egg w/o dressing	2 cups	93	5	6	4	2
tossed w/ seafood w/o dressing	3 cups	120	1	8	5	3
tossed w/ shrimp & egg w/o dressing	3 cups	185	5	5	3	2
tossed w/o dressing	2 cups	22	tr	5	3	2
waldorf	1 cup	242	21	15	10	3

FOOD	PORTION	CAL	FAT	CARB	SUGAR	FIBER
wilted lettuce w/ bacon dressing	1 cup	99	8	3	1	1

SALAD DRESSING (see also SALAD TOPPINGS)
MIX
Good Seasons
Italian as prep	2 tbsp	130	13	3	tr	–
Italian not prep	⅛ pkg (3 g)	5	0	1	tr	–

READY-TO-EAT
blue cheese	1 tbsp	77	8	1	–	–
french	1 tbsp	67	6	3	–	–
french reduced calorie	1 tbsp	22	1	4	–	–
italian	1 tbsp	69	7	2	–	–
italian reduced calorie	1 tbsp	16	2	1	–	–
russian	1 tbsp	76	8	2	–	–
russian reduced calorie	1 tbsp	23	1	5	–	–
sesame seed	1 tbsp	68	7	1	–	–
thousand island	1 tbsp	59	6	2	–	–
thousand island reduced calorie	1 tbsp	24	2	3	–	–

Bragg
Ginger & Sesame	2 tbsp	150	12	2	2	0
Organic Vinaigrette	2 tbsp	150	15	3	2	0

Follow Your Heart
Lemon Herb	2 tbsp (1 oz)	100	11	1	0	0
Sesame Miso	2 tbsp (1 oz)	64	6	3	2	0
Thousand Island	2 tbsp (1 oz)	80	8	3	0	tr

Gotta Luv It
Chipotle Lime	2 tbsp	110	11	3	2	0
Raspberry Balsamic Vinaigrette	2 tbsp	150	14	6	5	0
Sweet & Tangy Italian	2 tbsp	140	15	2	2	0

Kraft
Honey Dijon	2 tbsp	100	9	6	5	0

FOOD	PORTION	CAL	FAT	CARB	SUGAR	FIBER
Italian Creamy	2 tbsp	100	11	2	2	0
Light Done Right Caesar	2 tbsp	60	5	3	1	0
Light Done Right Red Wine Vinaigrette	2 tbsp	45	4	3	2	0
Ranch Garlic	2 tbsp	120	12	3	2	0
Special Collection Classic Italian Vinaigrette	2 tbsp	60	4	5	2	0
Special Collection Parmesan Romano	2 tbsp	140	14	2	1	0
Special Collection Tangy Tomato Bacon	2 tbsp	100	6	10	9	0
Thousand Island w/ Bacon	2 tbsp	100	8	7	6	0
LiteHouse						
Bleu Cheese Bacon	2 tbsp	150	16	1	1	0
Organic Vinaigrette Raspberry Lime	2 tbsp	40	2	5	5	0
Ranch Homestyle	2 tbsp	120	12	2	1	0
Ranch Lite	2 tbsp	70	6	2	2	0
Sesame Ginger	2 tbsp	35	0	8	7	0
Spinach Salad	2 tbsp	50	0	11	7	0
Vinaigrette Huckleberry	2 tbsp	20	0	4	4	0
Vinaigrette Lite Honey Dijon	2 tbsp	130	13	3	2	0
Lucini						
Delicate Cucumber & Shallots	2 tbsp (1 oz)	120	12	2	1	–
Fig & Walnut Savory Balsamic	2 tbsp (1 oz)	110	10	4	3	–
Roasted Hazelnut & Extra Virgin Olive Oil	2 tbsp (1 oz)	120	11	3	2	–
Naturally Fresh						
Balsamic Vinaigrette	2 tbsp	10	0	2	1	0

FOOD	PORTION	CAL	FAT	CARB	SUGAR	FIBER
Bleu Cheese	2 tbsp	170	18	1	0	0
Bleu Cheese Bacon	2 tbsp	170	18	1	0	0
Bleu Cheese Lite	2 tbsp	100	10	1	1	0
Buffalo Ranch	2 tbsp	110	10	4	3	0
Classic Oriental	2 tbsp	100	11	9	8	0
Ginger	2 tbsp	70	7	1	0	0
Greek Feta	2 tbsp	100	12	1	0	0
Honey French	2 tbsp	100	11	5	5	0
Honey Mustard	2 tbsp	140	13	5	4	0
Orange Miso	2 tbsp	100	9	4	3	0
Ranch Classic	2 tbsp	150	16	1	1	0
Ranch Lite	2 tbsp	80	8	2	1	0
Slaw	2 tbsp	90	10	6	6	0
Newman's Own						
Lighten Up Light Balsamic Vinaigrette	2 tbsp (1 oz)	45	4	2	1	0
OrganicVille						
Herbs De Provence	2 tbsp (1 oz)	100	11	tr	0	0
Miso Ginger	2 tbsp (1 oz)	100	10	1	tr	0
Orange Cranberry	2 tbsp (1 oz)	100	10	3	3	0
Pomegranate	2 tbsp (1 oz)	100	10	2	2	0
Ranch Non Dairy	2 tbsp (1 oz)	90	9	1	1	0
Sesame Goddess	2 tbsp (1 oz)	130	13	2	tr	0
Petrini's						
Italian Original	2 tbsp (1 oz)	106	12	tr	0	tr
Italian Ranch	2 tbsp (1 oz)	140	14	1	–	–
Soy Vay						
Cha-Cha Chinese Chicken	3 tbsp	190	15	11	9	0
Texas Sassy						
Vinaigrette	2 tbsp (1 oz)	80	8	4	4	–
Three Acre Kitchen						
Balsamic Vinaigrette	2 tbsp (1.1 oz)	130	14	3	2	–

FOOD	PORTION	CAL	FAT	CARB	SUGAR	FIBER
Wild Thymes Farm						
Salad Refreshers Black Currant	1 tbsp	36	3	3	3	tr
Salad Refreshers Meyer Lemon	1 tbsp	35	3	3	3	tr
Salad Refreshers Morello Cherry	1 tbsp	34	3	3	2	tr
Salad Refreshers Pomegrante	1 tbsp	33	3	3	2	0
Vinaigrette Mandarin Orange Basil	1 tbsp	43	4	2	1	tr
Vinaigrette Raspberry Pear	1 tbsp	43	4	1	1	tr
Vinaigrette Roasted Apple Shallot	1 tbsp	42	4	2	1	tr
Vinaigrette Toasted Sesame Wasabi	1 tbsp	42	4	1	1	tr
Wishbone						
Bountifuls Berry Delight	2 tbsp	35	0	8	6	–
Bountifuls Tuscan Romano Basil	2 tbsp	25	1	4	3	–
Western	2 tbsp (1 oz)	160	12	11	11	0
Western Fat Free	2 tbsp (1 oz)	50	0	12	11	0
Western Light Just 2 Good	2 tbsp (1 oz)	70	2	13	12	0
TAKE-OUT						
vinegar & oil	1 tbsp	72	8	tr	–	–
SALAD TOPPINGS						
Naturally Fresh						
Fruit & Nut Mix	½ tbsp	45	4	2	1	1
Glazed Almond & Pecan Pieces	½ tbsp	40	3	3	2	1

FOOD	PORTION	CAL	FAT	CARB	SUGAR	FIBER
SALBA						
Salba Smart						
Ground	2 tbsp	65	4	5	–	4
Whole Grain	1 tbsp	65	4	5	–	4
SALMON						
CANNED						
w/ bone	½ cup	106	5	0	0	0
Polar						
Pink	¼ cup	90	5	0	0	0
Sockeye Red	¼ cup	110	7	0	0	0
FRESH						
atlantic farmed baked	4 oz	233	14	0	0	0
coho wild poached	4 oz	209	9	0	0	0
pink baked	4 oz	169	5	0	0	0
roe raw	1 oz	59	3	tr	–	–
sockeye baked	4 oz	245	12	0	0	0
FROZEN						
Dr. Praeger's						
Salmon Cakes	1 (2.9 oz)	190	10	15	0	3
Gorton's						
Fillets Classic Grilled	1 (3 oz)	100	3	2	1	–
SMOKED						
lox	1 oz	33	1	0	0	0
TAKE-OUT						
guisado salmon stew	1 serv (7.4 oz)	320	16	18	3	3
roulette w/ spinach stuffing	1 serv (4 oz)	160	6	10	0	tr
salmon cake	1 (4.2 oz)	264	16	14	1	1
salmon loaf	1 slice (3.7 oz)	206	11	9	2	tr
SALSA						
black bean & corn	2 tbsp	15	0	3	1	tr

FOOD	PORTION	CAL	FAT	CARB	SUGAR	FIBER
citrus	2 tbsp (1 oz)	10	0	2	2	0
peach	2 tbsp	15	0	4	4	0
tomatoless corn & chile	2 tbsp	45	0	10	6	tr
Amy's						
Organic Black Bean & Corn	2 tbsp (1 oz)	15	0	3	1	tr
Organic Medium	2 tbsp (1 oz)	10	0	2	1	0
Chukar Cherries						
Peach Cherry	1 tbsp	13	0	3	2	tr
Clint's						
Texas Medium	2 tbsp (1 oz)	5	0	1	1	–
Dave's Gourmet						
Insanity	2 tbsp (1 oz)	15	0	2	2	–
Dei Fratelli						
Casera Mild	2 tbsp (1.1 oz)	5	0	2	1	0
DelGrosso						
Chunky Hot	2 tbsp (1.1 oz)	10	0	3	2	tr
Chunky Mild	2 tbsp (1.1 oz)	10	0	3	2	tr
Emerald Valley						
Organic Fiesta	1 tbsp (1 oz)	20	0	4	tr	tr
Organic Green	2 tbsp (1 oz)	10	0	2	tr	tr
Jala-Fresca						
Green Stuff Medium	2 tbsp	10	0	2	1	0
Muir Glen						
Organic Medium	2 tbsp	10	0	3	1	0
Number 9						
Black Bean & Corn	2 tbsp (1.1 oz)	20	0	4	1	1
Hot	2 tbsp (1.1 oz)	15	0	2	1	1
Mild	2 tbsp (1.1 oz)	15	0	2	1	1
OrganicVille						
Mild	2 tbsp (1 oz)	15	0	3	1	0
Pineapple	2 tbsp (1 oz)	15	0	4	3	0

FOOD	PORTION	CAL	FAT	CARB	SUGAR	FIBER
Salba Smart						
Organic Omega-3 Enriched	2 tbsp	12	0	2	0	1
Utz						
Sweet	2 tbsp	10	0	2	1	tr
SALSIFY						
fresh sliced cooked	½ cup	46	tr	10	–	–
SALT SUBSTITUTES						
gomasio sesame salt	2 tsp	34	3	2	–	1
AlsoSalt						
Butter Flavored	¼ tsp	1	0	0	0	0
Garlic Flavored	¼ tsp	1	0	0	0	0
Original	¼ tsp	1	0	0	0	0
Nu-Salt						
Salt Substitute	1 pkg (1 g)	0	0	0	0	0
SALT/SEASONED SALT						
kosher	¼ tsp	0	0	0	0	0
salt	1 tsp (6 g)	0	0	0	0	0
salt	1 dash (0.4 g)	0	0	0	0	0
salt	1 tbsp (0.6 oz)	0	0	0	0	0
sea salt coarse	1 tsp	0	0	0	0	0
sea salt fine	¼ tsp	0	0	0	0	0
Maine Coast						
Sea Salt w/ Sea Veg	¼ tsp	0	0	0	0	0
Ocean's Flavor						
Natural Sea Salt	¼ tsp	0	0	0	0	0
SANDWICHES						
Alexia						
Panini Tuscan Four Cheese w/ Roasted Tomato & Basil	1 pkg (6 oz)	380	15	42	5	6

FOOD	PORTION	CAL	FAT	CARB	SUGAR	FIBER
Panini Tuscan Grilled Chicken w/ Mozzarella	1 pkg (6 oz)	400	18	37	2	5
Panini Tuscan Grilled Steak w/ Mushrooms & Onions	1 pkg (6 oz)	370	12	43	9	5
Panini Tuscan Smoked Chicken w/ Fire Roasted Vegetables & Parmesan	1 pkg (6 oz)	410	19	37	3	5
Amy's						
Pocket Sandwich Tofu Scramble	1 (4 oz)	180	6	23	2	tr
Pocket Sandwich Vegetable Pie	1 (5 oz)	300	9	45	5	3
Wrap Indian Somosa	1 (5 oz)	250	9	35	2	4
Aunt Trudy's						
Fillo Pocket Cheese & Tomato	1 (5 oz)	320	15	36	1	2
Fillo Pocket Classic Samosa	1 (5 oz)	280	10	43	1	3
Fillo Pocket Mediterranean Olive & Veggies	1 (5 oz)	270	10	41	1	2
Organic Fillo Pocket Roasted Sweet Potato	1 (5 oz)	310	12	45	0	4
Cedarlane						
Wrap Low Fat Couscous & Vegetable Veggie	1 (6 oz)	220	3	36	2	3
DiGiorno						
Flatbread Melts Chicken Parmesan	1 (6 oz)	380	14	45	4	2
Fillo Factory						
Organic Fillo Pocket Asian Vegetable	1 (5 oz)	240	10	34	2	3

FOOD	PORTION	CAL	FAT	CARB	SUGAR	FIBER
Guiltless Gourmet						
Wrap Black Bean Chipotle	1 (5.7 oz)	270	3	51	6	7
Wrap California Veggie	1 (5.7 oz)	300	5	53	2	6
Wrap Mediterranean Spinach	1 (5.7 oz)	270	5	45	4	4
Hot Pockets						
Bacon Egg & Cheese	1 (2.2 oz)	160	8	17	4	1
Barbecue Beef	1 (4.5 oz)	310	10	42	11	1
Biscuit Sausage Egg & Cheese	1 (4.5 oz)	270	11	32	7	2
Calzone Four Meat & Four Cheese	½ (4.2 oz)	300	13	35	13	2
Calzone Pepperoni & Three Cheese	½ (4.2 oz)	330	15	39	14	2
Chicken Melt	1 (4.5 oz)	300	11	36	8	1
Croissant Chicken Parmesan	1 (4.5 oz)	340	15	41	10	3
Croissant Turkey Bacon Club	1 (4.5 oz)	320	15	34	10	1
Ham & Cheese	1 (4.5 oz)	290	11	36	9	1
Meatballs & Mozzarella	1 (4.5 oz)	300	12	36	7	2
Philly Steak & Cheese	1 (4.5 oz)	270	9	34	6	2
Steak Fajita	1 (4.5 oz)	280	12	33	8	2
Turkey & Ham w/ Cheese	1 (4 .5 oz)	280	10	35	8	1
Jimmy Dean						
Bagel Sausage Egg & Cheese	1 (4.8 oz)	380	21	34	3	1
Biscuit Sausage Egg & Cheese	1 (4.5 oz)	440	31	27	5	1
Croissant Sausage Egg & Cheese	1 (4.5 oz)	430	29	30	6	1

FOOD	PORTION	CAL	FAT	CARB	SUGAR	FIBER
D-Lights Croissants Turkey Sausage Egg White & Cheese	1 (4.8 oz)	300	12	31	4	4
D-Lights Honey Wheat Muffin Canadian Bacon Egg White & Cheese	1 (4.5 oz)	230	6	30	3	2
Muffin Sausage Egg & Cheese	1 (4.6 oz)	350	21	28	3	1
Lean Pockets						
Bacon Egg & Cheese	1 (2.2 oz)	150	5	18	3	1
Barbecue Beef	1 (4.5 oz)	290	7	46	11	2
Chicken Cheddar & Broccoli	1 (4.5 oz)	260	7	40	11	2
Chicken Fajita	1 (4.5 oz)	240	7	35	6	3
Chicken Parmesan	1 (4.5 oz)	290	7	45	5	3
Ham & Cheese	1 (4.5 oz)	270	7	39	11	2
Meatballs & Mozzarella	1 (4.5 oz)	260	7	35	9	4
Philly Steak & Cheese	1 (4.5 oz)	270	7	38	8	1
Sausage Egg & Cheese	1 (2.2 oz)	140	5	18	6	1
Steak Fajita	1 (4.5 oz)	250	7	36	8	4
Three Cheese & Chicken Quesadilla	1 (4.5 oz)	260	7	34	6	3
Turkey & Ham w/ Cheddar	1 (4.5 oz)	280	7	40	9	2
Turkey Broccoli & Cheese	1 (4.5 oz)	270	7	39	12	2
Lunchables						
Cracker Stackers Bologna & American	1 pkg (4.1 oz)	390	22	34	12	1
Cracker Stackers Ham & Swiss	1 pkg (4.5 oz)	340	18	23	6	1
Sub Ham + American	1 pkg	350	11	49	21	2
Sub Turkey + Cheddar	1 pkg	360	8	62	22	4

FOOD	PORTION	CAL	FAT	CARB	SUGAR	FIBER
Oscar Mayer						
Deli Creations Honey Ham & Swiss	1 pkg (6.8 oz)	440	14	51	15	4
Deli Creations Steakhouse Cheddar	1 pkg (7.1 oz)	450	15	50	14	3
Deli Creations Turkey & Cheddar Dijon	1 pkg (6.7 oz)	430	15	48	12	5
PBJammerz						
Peanut Butter & Jelly All Flavors	1 (2 oz)	220	13	22	10	3
Pillsbury						
Toaster Scrambles Cheese Egg & Bacon	1 (1.6 oz)	180	12	15	1	0
Toaster Scrambles Cheese Egg & Sausage	1 (1.6 oz)	180	12	15	1	0
Van's						
Breakfast In A Pocket Sandwich Ham Egg & Cheese	1 (4.5 oz)	370	22	30	3	tr
Breakfast In A Pocket Sandwich Veggie Egg & Cheese	1 (4.5 oz)	340	19	31	3	1
Breakfast Panini Huevos Rancheros	1 (4.5 oz)	270	11	33	2	5
Breakfast Panini Sausage Egg & Cheese	1 (4.5 oz)	290	13	28	1	3
TAKE-OUT						
bacon & egg	1 (6.2 oz)	388	21	28	4	1
bacon lettuce & tomato w/ mayo	1 (5.8 oz)	344	17	35	5	3
beef barbecue w/ bun	1 (6.7 oz)	417	12	42	6	2
calzone beef & cheese	1 (14 oz)	1476	76	131	1	6
calzone cheese	1 (15 oz)	1632	93	117	2	5

FOOD	PORTION	CAL	FAT	CARB	SUGAR	FIBER
chicken fillet	1 (6.4 oz)	515	29	39	–	–
chicken fillet w/ cheese	1 (8 oz)	632	39	42	–	–
chicken salad	1 (5 oz)	333	16	28	3	2
crab cake w/ bun	1	308	8	36	4	2
crispy chicken fillet w/ lettuce tomato & mayo	1 (7.7 oz)	537	26	49	tr	3
croque monsieur	1 (12.4 oz)	765	46	43	9	2
egg salad	1 (5.6 oz)	485	35	28	3	1
french dip w/ roll	1 (6.8 oz)	357	13	34	4	1
fried egg	1 (3.4 oz)	226	9	26	3	1
grilled cheese	1 (2.9 oz)	290	16	28	4	1
gyro	1 (13.7 oz)	593	12	74	8	4
ham & egg	1 (4.4 oz)	272	11	27	3	2
ham w/ cheese lettuce & mayo	1 (5.4 oz)	369	18	32	4	2
hot turkey w/ gravy	1	389	10	32	2	2
peanut butter & banana	1	617	14	43	11	4
peanut butter & jelly	1 (3.3 oz)	327	14	42	12	3
reuben w/ sauerkraut & cheese	1 (6.4 oz)	463	29	30	7	4
roast beef w/ gravy	1 (7.8 oz)	386	16	30	2	2
sloppy joe pork on bun	1 (6.5 oz)	318	9	34	6	2
tuna melt	1 (5.3 oz)	350	16	30	6	1
tuna salad w/ lettuce	1 (5.9 oz)	289	7	37	6	2
turkey w/ mayo	1 (5 oz)	329	11	26	2	1

SAPODILLA

FOOD	PORTION	CAL	FAT	CARB	SUGAR	FIBER
fresh	1	140	2	34	–	–
fresh cut up	1 cup	199	3	48	–	–

SAPOTES

FOOD	PORTION	CAL	FAT	CARB	SUGAR	FIBER
fresh	1	301	1	76	–	–

FOOD	PORTION	CAL	FAT	CARB	SUGAR	FIBER
SARDINES						
CANNED						
atlantic in oil w/ bone	1 can (3.2 oz)	192	11	0	0	0
atlantic in oil w/ bone	2	50	3	0	0	0
pacific in tomato sauce w/ bone	1 (1.3 oz)	68	5	0	0	0
pacific in tomato sauce w/ bone	1 can (13 oz)	658	44	0	0	0
King Oscar						
In Olive Oil	1 can (3.75 oz)	150	11	0	0	0
Skinless Boneless In Soya Oil	3 pieces (1.9 oz)	120	7	0	0	0
Polar						
In Mustard	1 can (4.5 oz)	170	7	10	1	0
In Tomato Sauce	1 can (4.5 oz)	120	4	5	tr	0
In Water	1 can (3 oz)	100	3	tr	tr	0
FRESH						
raw	3.5 oz	135	5	0	0	0
SAUCE (see also BARBECUE SAUCE, GRAVY, SPAGHETTI SAUCE)						
adobo fresco	2 tbsp	81	8	7	tr	1
bearnaise	1 oz	177	19	1	–	tr
cheese mix as prep w/ milk	1 cup	307	17	23	–	–
curry mix as prep	1 cup	120	6	14	–	–
curry mix as prep w/ milk	1 cup	270	15	26	–	–
enchilada sauce green	¼ cup	46	4	3	2	1
enchilada sauce red	¼ cup	79	8	2	1	1
fish sauce chinese	1 tbsp	9	0	tr	–	0
fish sauce vietnamese nuoc mam	1 tbsp	6	0	1	–	0
hoisin	1 tbsp	35	1	7	–	tr

FOOD	PORTION	CAL	FAT	CARB	SUGAR	FIBER
moroccan tagine	½ cup (4 oz)	70	3	10	10	1
mushroom mix as prep w/ milk	1 cup	228	10	24	–	–
oyster	1 tbsp	8	0	2	–	0
plum sauce	0.5 oz	42	0	10	10	0
satay peanut sauce	1 oz	77	6	3	3	1
sour cream mix as prep w/ milk	1 cup	509	30	45	–	–
stroganoff mix as prep	1 cup	271	11	34	–	–
sweet & sour mix as prep	1 cup	294	tr	73	–	–
teriyaki	1 tbsp	15	0	3	–	–
teriyaki mix as prep	1 cup	131	1	28	–	–
white sauce mix as prep w/ milk	1 cup	241	13	21	–	–
Ahh!Gourmet						
Perky Savory Coffee Sauce	4 tbsp	71	0	17	15	tr
Ritzy Kumquat Plum Sauce	4 tbsp	98	0	24	21	1
Spicy Garlicky Sweet Sauce Paste	4 tbsp	101	4	16	13	2
Spicy Ginger Soy Sauce Paste	4 tbsp	137	8	15	13	2
Bear-Man						
Sap-Happy Golden Bear	2 tbsp	60	0	20	17	0
Burbon Chicken						
Marinade Original	1 tbsp (0.6 oz)	5	0	1	0	–
Chef Hymie Grande						
New Mexico Sweet Basting Sauce	2 tbsp (1.2 oz)	35	0	8	6	–
China Pride						
Duck Sauce Sweet & Pungent	2 tbsp	80	0	19	11	1

FOOD	PORTION	CAL	FAT	CARB	SUGAR	FIBER
Dave's Gourmet						
Hot Sauce Roasted Garlic	1 tsp (5 g)	0	0	0	0	0
Insanity Sauce	1 tsp (5 g)	10	1	0	0	0
Jammin' Jerk	1 tsp (5 g)	5	0	1	–	–
Steak Sauce	1 tbsp (0.6 oz)	20	0	5	4	–
Dei Fratelli						
Sloppy Joe Sauce	¼ cup (2.2 oz)	35	0	9	5	1
DelGrosso						
Sloppy Joe Sauce	¼ cup (2.2 oz)	60	1	13	10	1
D'Oni						
Happy Together Orange Chili Garlic	2 tbsp	50	0	12	11	–
Moondance Marinade	1 tbsp	10	0	0	0	–
Ethnic Gourmet						
Punjab Saag Spinach	4 oz	60	3	6	3	1
Simmer Sauce Calcutta Masala	4 oz	90	5	10	8	1
Simmer Sauce Delhi Korma	4 oz	100	7	9	1	2
Fortun's						
Asian Style Pepper	¼ cup (2 oz)	40	1	5	2	0
Lemon Dill Caper w/ White Wine	¼ cup (2 oz)	20	1	3	1	0
Marsala & Mushroom	¼ cup (2 oz)	40	1	5	2	0
Spicy Mustard w/ Brandy	¼ cup (2 oz)	35	2	2	1	0
Stroganoff	¼ cup (2 oz)	45	3	3	1	0
La Choy						
Sweet & Sour	2 tbsp (1.2 oz)	60	0	14	11	0
Teriyaki	1 tbsp (0.6 oz)	40	0	10	8	0
Lea & Perrins						
Worcestershire	1 tsp (0.2 oz)	5	0	1	1	–

FOOD	PORTION	CAL	FAT	CARB	SUGAR	FIBER
Manwich						
Sloppy Joe Original	¼ cup (2.2 oz)	30	0	7	5	1
Mrs. Dash						
10 Minute Marinade Lemon Herb Peppercorn	1 tbsp (0.5 oz)	25	2	2	1	–
10 Minute Marinade Mesquite Grille	1 tbsp (0.5 oz)	25	2	2	1	–
10 Minute Marinade Spicy Teriyaki	1 tbsp (0.5 oz)	25	1	5	3	–
10 Minute Marinade Zesty Garlic Herb	1 tbsp (0.5 oz)	25	2	3	1	–
Naturally Fresh						
Seafood Cocktail	2 tbsp	25	0	5	5	0
Tartar Sauce	2 tbsp	130	14	2	2	0
OrganicVille						
Island Teriyaki	1 tbsp (0.5 oz)	25	1	4	3	0
Simply Boulder						
Coconut Peanut	2 tbsp (1 oz)	90	7	6	5	0
Lemon Pesto	2 tbsp (1 oz)	50	5	3	2	0
Zesty Pineapple	2 tbsp (1 oz)	45	3	7	5	0
Soy Vay						
Hoisin Garlic Asian Glaze & Marinade	1 tbsp	40	1	7	7	0
Veri Veri Teriyaki	1 tbsp	35	1	6	5	0
Texas Sassy						
Marinade Salsa	1 tbsp (0.5 oz)	15	0	3	3	–
Pickle Sauce	1 tbsp (0.5 oz)	30	0	7	7	–
Thai Kitchen						
Premium Fish Sauce	1 tbsp (0.5 oz)	10	0	0	0	0
The Gracious Gourmet						
Pesto Lemon Artichoke	2 tbsp (1 oz)	50	5	2	0	1

FOOD	PORTION	CAL	FAT	CARB	SUGAR	FIBER
Three Acre Kitchen						
Marinade Balsamic w/ Juniper & Rosemary	1 tbsp (0.5 oz)	50	5	2	1	–
Wild Thymes Farm						
Marinade Hawaiian Teryaki	1 tbsp	19	1	3	2	tr
Marinade Korean Ginger Scallion	1 tbsp	20	1	3	2	tr
Marinade New Orleans Creole	1 tbsp	11	0	3	1	tr
World Harbors						
Buccaneer Blends Pirate's Original	1 tbsp (0.6 oz)	20	0	4	10	0
Chimichurri	2 tbsp (1.2 oz)	40	0	9	8	0
Fajita	2 tbsp (1.1 oz)	45	0	10	8	0
Jerk	2 tbsp (1 oz)	70	0	18	16	0
Lemon Pepper & Garlic	2 tbsp (1 oz)	35	0	8	7	0
Thai	2 tbsp (1 oz)	40	0	8	7	0
Zatarain's						
Cocktail	¼ cup	70	0	17	13	0
Etouffee Base as prep	½ cup	35	0	7	0	1
TAKE-OUT						
cucumber yogurt sauce	1½ tbsp	20	0	3	–	0
SAUERKRAUT						
canned	½ cup	22	tr	5	–	–
Ba-Tampte						
Kosher	2 tbsp (1 oz)	5	0	1	0	1
Dei Fratelli						
Sauerkraut	2 tbsp (1 oz)	5	0	1	0	tr
Gedney						
Sauerkraut	½ cup	15	0	3	0	0
Tree Of Life						
Organic	½ cup (3.6 oz)	15	0	3	0	<3

FOOD	PORTION	CAL	FAT	CARB	SUGAR	FIBER
SAUSAGE						
beef & pork	1 link (2.3 oz)	196	17	1	0	0
beef & pork w/ cheddar cheese	1 link (2.7 oz)	228	20	2	tr	0
bierschinken	3.5 oz	174	11	tr	–	–
bierwurst	3.5 oz	258	21	0	0	0
blutwurst uncooked	3.5 oz	424	39	0	0	0
bockwurst	3.5 oz	276	25	0	0	0
bratwurst chicken cooked	1 (3 oz)	148	9	0	0	0
bratwurst pork cooked	1 link (2.5 oz)	226	19	2	2	0
brotwurst pork & beef	1 link (2.5 oz)	226	19	2	2	0
chipolata	3.5 oz	342	32	1	1	0
chorizo	1 link (2.1 oz)	273	23	1	0	0
fleischwurst	3.5 oz	305	29	0	0	0
free range chicken breakfast	2 links (2.7 oz)	110	6	1	1	0
gelbwurst uncooked	3.5 oz	363	33	0	0	0
italian pork cooked	1 (2.4 oz)	230	18	3	1	1
jagdwurst	3.5 oz	211	16	0	0	0
knockwurst pork & beef	1 (2.5 oz)	221	20	2	0	0
mettwurst uncooked	3.5 oz	483	45	0	0	0
plockwurst uncooked	3.5 oz	312	45	0	0	0
polish kielbasa	2 oz	127	10	2	0	0
pork cooked	2 links (1.7 oz)	163	14	0	0	0
regensburger uncooked	3.5 oz	354	31	0	0	0
turkey italian smoked	1 (2 oz)	88	5	3	2	1
vienna canned	1 can (4 oz)	260	22	3	0	0
vienna canned	1 link (0.5 oz)	37	3	tr	0	0
weisswurst uncooked	3.5 oz	305	27	0	0	0
zungenwurst (tongue)	3.5 oz	285	24	0	0	0

FOOD	PORTION	CAL	FAT	CARB	SUGAR	FIBER
Applegate Farms						
Organic Andouille	1 (3 oz)	120	6	3	1	1
Organic Spinach & Feta	1 (3 oz)	120	7	2	0	0
Armour						
Sizzle & Serve Turkey	3 (1.8 oz)	130	9	2	1	0
Banquet						
Brown 'N Serve Lite Original	3 (2.1 oz)	120	9	2	1	0
Butterball						
Bratwurst Turkey	1 (3.2 oz)	140	8	1	–	–
Breakfast Turkey	3 (3 oz)	130	7	0	0	0
Polska Kielbasa Turkey	2 oz	100	6	4	1	0
Sweet Italian Turkey	1 (3.2 oz)	140	8	1	–	–
Healthy Ones						
Smoked	2 oz	80	3	6	2	0
Jimmy Dean						
Fully Cooked Original Links	3 (2.4 oz)	240	22	1	1	0
Fully Cooked Original Patties	2 (2.4 oz)	240	23	1	2	0
Fully Cooked Turkey Links	3 (2.4 oz)	120	7	1	1	0
Fully Cooked Turkey Patties	2 (2.4 oz)	120	7	1	1	0
Original Links	3 (2 oz)	170	14	1	1	0
Original Patties cooked	2 (2.4 oz)	240	23	1	0	0
Pork All Natural cooked	2 oz	190	15	1	1	0
Pork Light cooked	2 oz	140	11	1	0	0
Jones						
All Natural Light	3 (2.1 oz)	130	9	3	–	–
Libby's						
Vienna Sausage BBQ	3	140	12	4	2	1

FOOD	PORTION	CAL	FAT	CARB	SUGAR	FIBER
Perdue						
Turkey Sweet Italian cooked	1 link (2.8 oz)	150	8	4	1	–
Turkey Breakfast	2 oz	80	5	0	0	0
Wampler						
Bratwurst as prep	1 (2.5 oz)	230	20	0	0	0
Breakfast Links as prep	2 (1.2 oz)	130	11	0	0	0
Breakfast Patties as prep	1 (1.1 oz)	120	11	0	0	0
Italian as prep	1 (2.5 oz)	230	20	0	0	0

SAUSAGE DISHES
TAKE-OUT

FOOD	PORTION	CAL	FAT	CARB	SUGAR	FIBER
italian sausage w/ peppers & onions	1 cup	210	11	14	–	–
sausage roll	1 (2.3 oz)	311	24	22	–	1

SAUSAGE SUBSTITUTES

FOOD	PORTION	CAL	FAT	CARB	SUGAR	FIBER
meatless	1 link (0.9 oz)	64	5	2	0	1
meatless	1 patty (1.3 oz)	98	7	4	0	1

SAVORY

FOOD	PORTION	CAL	FAT	CARB	SUGAR	FIBER
ground	1 tsp	4	tr	1	–	tr

SCALLOP

FOOD	PORTION	CAL	FAT	CARB	SUGAR	FIBER
raw	3 oz	75	1	2	–	–

TAKE-OUT

FOOD	PORTION	CAL	FAT	CARB	SUGAR	FIBER
breaded & fried	2 lg	67	3	3	–	–

SCONE
TAKE-OUT

FOOD	PORTION	CAL	FAT	CARB	SUGAR	FIBER
apricot	1	232	7	39	–	–
blueberry	1 (3 oz)	270	9	41	7	2
cheese	1 (3.5 oz)	364	18	44	–	2
orange poppy	1 (3 oz)	260	6	47	12	2
plain	1 (3.5 oz)	362	14	54	–	2
raisin	1 (3 oz)	270	8	43	12	2

FOOD	PORTION	CAL	FAT	CARB	SUGAR	FIBER
SCUP						
fresh baked	3 oz	115	3	0	0	0
SEA BASS (see BASS)						
SEA CUCUMBER						
dried	1 oz	74	1	1	–	0
fresh	1 oz	20	tr	tr	–	0
SEA URCHIN						
canned	1 oz	39	1	3	–	0
fresh	1 oz	36	1	3	–	tr
roe paste	1 tbsp	19	tr	3	–	0
SEATROUT (see TROUT)						
SEAWEED						
agar dried	1 oz	87	tr	23	–	–
agar fresh	1 oz	tr	tr	2	–	–
hijiki dried	1 tbsp	9	0	2	–	1
irishmoss fresh	1 oz	14	tr	4	–	–
kelp fresh	1 oz	12	tr	3	–	–
kombu fresh	1 oz	12	tr	3	–	–
laver fresh	1 oz	10	tr	1	–	–
nori fresh	1 oz	10	tr	1	–	–
nori sheet dried	1 (8 x 8 in)	5	0	1	–	1
seahair dried	1 tbsp	13	0	3	–	tr
spirulina dried	1 oz	83	2	7	–	–
spirulina fresh	1 oz	7	tr	1	–	–
tangle fresh	1 oz	12	tr	3	–	–
wakame fresh	1 oz	13	tr	3	–	–
Maine Coast						
Organic Alaria Whole Leaf	1/3 cup	18	tr	3	–	3
Organic Dulse Whole Leaf	1/2 cup	19	tr	3	–	2

FOOD	PORTION	CAL	FAT	CARB	SUGAR	FIBER
Organic Dulse Granules	1 tsp	6	0	2	–	–
Organic Kelp Whole Leaf	1/3 cup	17	tr	3	–	2
Organic Kelp Granules	1/2 tsp	5	0	2	–	–
Organic Laver Whole Leaf	1/3 cup	22	tr	3	–	2

SEITAN (see WHEAT)

SEMOLINA

dry	1 cup (5.9 oz)	601	2	122	–	7

SESAME

seeds	1 tsp	16	2	tr	–	–
sesame butter	1 tbsp	95	8	4	–	1
sesame crunch candy	1 oz	146	9	14	–	–
sesame crunch candy	20 pieces (1.2 oz)	181	12	18	–	–
tahini from roasted & toasted kernels	1 tbsp	89	8	3	–	–
tahini from stone ground kernels	1 tbsp	86	7	4	–	–
tahini from unroasted kernels	1 tbsp	85	8	3	–	–
Mrs. May's						
Black Sesame Crunch	1 oz	165	11	14	5	4
Tree Of Life						
Organic Sesame Tahini	2 tbsp	108	15	8	–	5
Seeds	1/4 cup (1.3 oz)	210	18	8	0	3

SESBANIA

flower	1	1	0	tr	–	–
flowers	1 cup	5	tr	1	–	–
flowers cooked	1 cup	23	tr	5	–	–

SHAD

american baked	3 oz	214	15	0	0	0

FOOD	PORTION	CAL	FAT	CARB	SUGAR	FIBER
cooked	1 oz	55	3	1	tr	0
roe baked w/ butter & lemon	1 oz	36	1	tr	–	–

SHALLOTS (see ONION)

SHARK
| raw | 3 oz | 111 | 4 | 0 | 0 | 0 |

TAKE-OUT
| batter-dipped & fried | 3 oz | 194 | 12 | 5 | – | – |

SHEEPSHEAD FISH
cooked	1 fillet (6.5 oz)	234	3	0	0	0
cooked	3 oz	107	1	0	0	0
raw	3 oz	92	2	0	0	0

SHELLFISH (see individual names, SHELLFISH SUBSTITUTES)

SHELLFISH SUBSTITUTES
crab imitation	1 cup (4.4 oz)	144	1	16	0	tr
scallop imitation	3 oz	84	tr	9	–	–
shrimp imitation	3 oz	86	1	8	–	–
surimi	1 oz	28	tr	2	–	–
surimi	3 oz	84	1	6	–	–

TAKE-OUT
| crab salad | 1 cup | 395 | 26 | 21 | 1 | 1 |

SHELLIE BEANS
| canned | ½ cup | 37 | tr | 8 | – | – |

SHERBET
orange	½ gal	2158	31	469	–	–
orange	1 bar (2.75 fl oz)	91	1	20	–	–
orange	½ cup (4 fl oz)	132	2	29	–	–

FOOD	PORTION	CAL	FAT	CARB	SUGAR	FIBER
Ciao Bella						
Lemon	1 pkg (3.5 oz)	120	0	31	29	–
Mango	1 pkg (3.5 oz)	100	0	25	24	1
Raspberry	1 pkg (3.5 oz)	110	0	28	25	2
Dippin' Dots						
Lemon Lime	½ cup	97	1	22	19	0
Hershey's						
Lemon	½ cup (3.4 oz)	100	1	23	22	tr
Orange	½ cup (3.4 oz)	100	1	23	22	0
Strawberry	½ cup (3.4 oz)	110	1	25	24	tr
Hola Fruta						
Bar Pomegranate & Blueberry	1 (2.5 oz)	100	1	22	14	0
Mango	½ cup	130	0	31	20	0
Land O Lakes						
Orange	½ cup (3.2 oz)	130	2	28	27	1
Turkey Hill						
Fruit Rainbow	½ cup	120	1	26	17	0
Orange Grove	½ cup	120	1	26	18	0
SHRIMP						
CANNED						
canned	1 can (6 oz)	136	2	1	0	0
chinese shrimp paste	1 tbsp	46	0	10	8	tr
Polar						
Tiny Peeled	¼ cup (2 oz)	44	0	1	1	0
DRIED						
dried	10	15	tr	tr	0	0
FRESH						
broiled	6 med	46	2	tr	0	0
steamed	6 med	41	1	tr	0	0

FOOD	PORTION	CAL	FAT	CARB	SUGAR	FIBER
FROZEN						
Blue Horizon Organic						
Garlic Shrimp	1 serv (3.5 oz)	160	2	21	0	1
Panko Shrimp	1 serv (3.5 oz)	160	2	22	0	1
Popcorn Shrimp	1 serv (3.5 oz)	160	2	21	0	1
Tempura Shrimp	1 serv (3.5 oz)	160	2	21	0	1
Gorton's						
Popcorn Crunchy Golden	20 (3.2 oz)	240	12	24	2	0
Temptations Breaded Butterfly	5 (3.5 oz)	250	11	27	4	4
Temptations Scampi Sauced	1 serv (4 oz)	120	6	8	–	tr
TAKE-OUT						
breaded & fried	6 med (2.3 oz)	162	8	8	tr	tr
cocktail w/ sauce	4 shrimp	87	1	7	4	2
curried	1 cup	295	14	14	8	tr
jambalaya	1 cup	309	9	28	2	1
scampi	1 cup	310	22	1	tr	0
shrimp newburg	1 serv (6.4 oz)	456	37	8	tr	tr
shrimp salad	¾ cup	212	12	4	1	1
shrimp w/ crab stuffing	5	158	8	5	tr	tr
SMELT						
rainbow cooked	3 oz	106	3	0	0	0
rainbow raw	3 oz	83	2	0	0	0
SMOOTHIES (see also FRUIT DRINKS, YOGURT DRINKS)						
Arthur's						
Carrot Energizer	1 bottle (11 oz)	200	1	47	37	3

FOOD	PORTION	CAL	FAT	CARB	SUGAR	FIBER
Green Energy	1 bottle (11 oz)	230	1	53	39	3
SNACKS						
cheese puffs	1 oz	122	3	21	2	3
oriental mix	1 oz	155	12	9	–	–
pork skins	1 oz	154	9	0	0	0
pork skins barbecue	1 oz	152	9	1	–	–
Barbara's Bakery						
Cheese Puffs Bakes Original	¾ cup	160	11	13	1	–
Cheese Puffs Original	¾ cup (1 oz)	150	10	16	0	–
Cheez It						
Right Bites Party Mix	1 pkg (0.74 oz)	100	4	15	tr	tr
Lance						
Cheese Puffs	9 (1 oz)	170	12	13	1	0
Gold-N-Chees	1 oz	150	8	17	0	tr
Lifestyle Foods						
Awake	1 pkg (5 oz)	170	0	55	38	5
Essential	1 pkg (5.6 oz)	200	10	21	13	3
Miami	1 pkg (7.5 oz)	180	0	36	29	3
Power Up	1 pkg (6.7 oz)	670	33	77	17	9
Medora Snacks						
Corners	1 oz	130	3	22	0	0
Sea Salt						
Pucci Garlic	1 oz	120	4	17	2	1
Pucci Tomato Basil	1 oz	120	4	17	2	1
Sotos Cheese Olive Oil & Lemon	1 oz	120	4	19	3	2
Michael Season's						
Cheese Puffs & Curls	1½ cups	180	13	13	3	2
Robert's American Gourmet						
Booty Barbeque	1 oz	130	5	20	1	1

FOOD	PORTION	CAL	FAT	CARB	SUGAR	FIBER
Booty Pirate's	1 oz	130	5	18	0	1
Booty Veggie	1 oz	130	6	17	1	1
Smart Puffs	1 oz	130	6	17	1	0
Tings	1 oz	160	8	17	0	0
Silhouette Solution						
Puffs BBQ	1 pkg (1.06 oz)	120	4	8	3	0
Snikiddy						
Puffs Grilled Cheese	1 pkg (0.6 oz)	80	3	10	0	1
Puffs Rockin' Ranch	1 pkg (0.6 oz)	83	0	11	0	1
Sweet Emotions						
Chocolate Passion	1 pkg (0.5 oz)	60	3	10	2	2
Cinnamon Joy	1 pkg (0.5 oz)	60	3	10	2	2
T.G.I. Friday's						
Mozzarella Sticks	20 (1 oz)	150	9	14	1	1
Utz						
Cheese Balls	50 (1 oz)	150	9	16	tr	tr
Cheese Curls	18 (1 oz)	150	9	16	tr	tr
Onion Rings	41 (1 oz)	130	5	20	2	0
Party Mix	1 oz	150	7	19	tr	1
Pork Cracklins	0.5 oz	90	7	0	0	0
Pork Rinds Original	0.5 oz	80	5	0	0	0
SNAIL						
cooked	3 oz	233	1	13	–	–
raw	3 oz	117	tr	7	–	–
TAKE-OUT						
escargot cooked	5	25	0	1	–	0
SNAKE						
fresh	3 oz	78	tr	3	–	0
SNAPPER						
cooked	1 fillet (6 oz)	217	3	0	0	0
cooked	3 oz	109	1	0	0	0
raw	3 oz	85	1	0	0	0

FOOD	PORTION	CAL	FAT	CARB	SUGAR	FIBER
SODA						
club	12 oz	0	0	0	0	0
cola	12 oz	151	tr	39	–	–
cream	12 oz	191	0	49	–	–
diet cola	12 oz	2	0	tr	–	–
ginger ale	12 oz can	124	0	32	–	–
grape	12 oz	161	0	42	–	–
lemon lime	12 oz	149	0	38	–	–
orange	12 oz	177	0	46	–	–
pepper type	12 oz	151	tr	38	–	–
quinine	12 oz	125	0	32	–	–
root beer	12 oz	152	0	39	–	–
shirley temple	1 serv	159	0	41	–	0
tonic water	12 oz	125	0	32	–	–
Ale 8 One						
Soft Drink	1 bottle (12 oz)	120	0	30	30	–
DRY						
Juniper Berry	1 bottle (12 oz)	55	0	15	15	–
Vanilla Bean	1 bottle (12 oz)	60	0	16	16	–
Goya						
Ginger Beer	1 bottle (12 oz)	190	0	43	27	0
GuS						
Dry Cola	1 bottle (12 oz)	95	0	24	24	–
Dry Crimson Grape	1 bottle (12 oz)	90	0	22	22	–
Dry Pomegranate	1 bottle (12 oz)	98	0	24	24	–
Star Ruby Grapefruit	1 bottle (12 oz)	90	0	22	22	–
Hansen's						
Blackberry	1 bottle	150	0	37	–	–
Health Cola						
Soda	1 bottle (12 oz)	140	0	35	35	–

FOOD	PORTION	CAL	FAT	CARB	SUGAR	FIBER
HotLips						
Apple	1 bottle	136	0	34	–	–
Boysenberry	1 bottle	152	0	37	–	–
Pear	1 bottle	142	1	34	–	–
Lucozade						
Soda	7 oz	136	0	36	–	0
Nutrisoda						
Calm Sparkling Wild Berry & Citron	1 can (8.7 oz)	0	0	1	0	–
Flex Sparkling Black Cherry & Apple	1 can (8.7 oz)	5	0	1	0	–
Immune Sparkling Tangerine & Lime	1 can (8.7 oz)	15	0	1	0	–
Slender Sparkling Guava & Grapefruit	1 can (8.7 oz)	10	0	1	0	–
Oogave Natural						
All Flavors	8 oz	68	0	17	17	0
Orangina						
Sparkling Citrus	8 oz	100	0	26	26	–
Pepsi						
Cola	8 oz	100	0	28	28	–
Diet	8 oz	0	0	0	0	0
Diet Vanilla	8 oz	0	0	0	0	0
One	8 oz	1	0	0	0	–
Wild Cherry	8 oz	100	0	28	28	–
Reed's						
Ginger Brew Original	1 bottle (12 oz)	145	0	37	37	0
Santa Cruz						
Organic Cherry	1 can (12 oz)	140	0	34	32	0
Organic Ginger Ale	1 can (12 oz)	150	0	37	35	0
Organic Root Beer	1 can (12 oz)	150	0	36	36	0
Organic Vanilla Creme	1 can 12 oz)	160	0	38	38	0

FOOD	PORTION	CAL	FAT	CARB	SUGAR	FIBER
Sprite						
Diet Zero	8 oz	0	0	0	0	0
Stirrings						
Ginger Ale	8 oz	120	0	31	30	0
Tava						
Sparkling Brazilian Samba	8 oz	0	0	0	0	0
Sparkling Mediterranean Fiesta	8 oz	0	0	0	0	0
Thomas Kemper						
Black Cherry	1 bottle (12 oz)	170	0	40	40	–
Ginger Ale	1 bottle (12 oz)	150	0	36	35	–
Orange Cream	1 bottle (12 oz)	170	0	42	40	–
Root Beer	1 bottle (12 oz)	160	0	41	40	–
Root Beer Low Calorie	1 bottle (12 oz)	20	0	5	1	–
Vanilla Cream	1 bottle (12 oz)	150	0	38	34	–
Tropicana						
Twister Orange	1 can (12 oz)	180	0	52	52	–
Vignette						
Wine Country Soda Chardonnay	1 bottle (12 oz)	130	0	33	31	–
Wine Country Soda Pinot Noir	1 bottle (12 oz)	130	0	31	31	–
Virgil's						
Micro Brewed Root Beer	1 bottle (12 oz)	160	0	42	42	–

SOUP 417

FOOD	PORTION	CAL	FAT	CARB	SUGAR	FIBER
SOLE						
cooked	3 oz	99	1	0	0	0
cooked	1 fillet (4.5 oz)	148	2	0	0	0
lemon raw	3.5 oz	85	1	0	0	0
TAKE-OUT						
breaded & fried	3.2 oz	211	11	15	–	–
SORGHUM						
sorghum	1 cup (6.7 oz)	651	6	143	–	–
SOUFFLE						
Heavenly Souffle						
Chocolate	1 (2.6 oz)	262	16	29	26	0
TAKE-OUT						
cheese	1 cup	194	15	6	3	tr
chicken	1 cup (5.6 oz)	278	18	9	4	tr
corn	1 cup	257	11	34	11	3
lime chilled	1 cup	388	18	48	45	2
seafood	1 cup	245	15	9	4	tr
spinach	1 cup	124	8	7	3	1
SOUP						
CANNED						
Allens						
Chicken Broth	1 cup	10	0	1	1	0
Amy's						
Organic Butternut Squash Light In Sodium	1 cup (8.6 oz)	100	3	20	4	2
Organic Chunky Tomato Bisque	1 cup (8.4 oz)	120	4	21	14	2
Organic Chunky Tomato Bisque Light In Sodium	1 cup (8.6 oz)	120	4	21	14	2
Organic Cream Of Mushroom	¾ cup (6.5 oz)	150	9	13	3	2

FOOD	PORTION	CAL	FAT	CARB	SUGAR	FIBER
Organic Lentil Light In Sodium	1 cup (8.6 oz)	180	5	25	3	6
Organic No Chicken Noodle Soup	1 cup (8.6 oz)	100	3	13	3	2
Organic Pasta & 3 Bean	1 cup (8.6 oz)	150	4	22	5	4
Organic Southwestern Vegetable	1 cup (8.7 oz)	140	4	21	4	4
Organic Split Pea	1 cup (8.6 oz)	100	0	19	4	3
Split Pea Light In Sodium	1 cup (8.6 oz)	100	0	19	4	4
Tom Kha Phak Thai Coconut	1 cup (7 oz)	140	10	9	4	2
Campbell's						
25% Less Sodium Chicken Noodle as prep	1 cup	60	2	8	1	1
Chicken & Stars as prep	1 cup	70	2	11	1	1
Chicken Alphabet as prep	1 cup	70	2	12	1	1
Chicken Noodle O's as prep	1 cup	90	3	15	2	1
Curly Noodle as prep	1 cup	80	2	11	1	1
Double Noodle Chicken as prep	1 cup	110	2	20	1	1
Goldfish Pasta Meatball as prep	1 cup	90	3	11	1	1
Mega Noodle as prep	1 cup	90	2	15	1	1
Select Vegetable Beef	1 cup	110	2	16	2	3
Select Harvest Caramelized French Onion	1 cup (8.4 oz)	80	3	12	4	1
Select Harvest Chicken Tuscany	1 cup	90	2	12	4	4
Select Harvest Chicken w/ Egg Noodles	1 cup	100	3	11	2	1

FOOD	PORTION	CAL	FAT	CARB	SUGAR	FIBER
Select Harvest Chicken w/ Whole Grain Pasta	1 cup (8.4 oz)	100	2	14	1	1
Select Harvest Italian Style Wedding	1 cup (8.4 oz)	130	5	13	3	1
Select Harvest Light Minestrone w/ Whole Grain Pasta	1 cup	80	1	14	4	4
Select Harvest Light Savory Chicken w/ Vegetables	1 cup	80	1	15	3	4
Select Harvest Light Southwestern Style Vegetable	1 cup	50	0	13	4	3
Select Harvest Light Vegetable & Pasta	1 cup	60	0	13	3	4
V8 Garden Broccoli	1 cup	80	2	15	6	3
V8 Golden Butternut Squash	1 cup	140	2	28	6	3
V8 Sweet Red Pepper	1 cup	120	2	22	10	4
V8 Tomato Herb	1 cup	90	0	19	14	3
Comfort Care						
Hearty Beef Barley	1 cup (8 oz)	190	7	23	9	4
Savory Chicken	1 cup (8 oz)	200	7	25	9	5
Tomato Cheddar Jack	1 cup (8 oz)	90	2	13	7	5
Dr. McDougall's						
Chunky Tomato Gluten Free Vegan	1 cup (8.6 oz)	90	0	20	8	3
Vegetable Gluten Free Vegan	1 cup (3.3 oz)	230	13	25	24	0
Go Appetit						
Carrot Bisque	8 oz	110	5	13	7	3
Gazpacho	8 oz	100	7	9	3	1
Mango Melange	8 oz	150	5	27	24	1

FOOD	PORTION	CAL	FAT	CARB	SUGAR	FIBER
Health Valley						
Beef Broth Fat Free	1 cup	10	0	0	0	0
Chicken Broth Fat Free	1 cup	20	0	0	0	0
Chicken Broth Fat Free No Salt Added	1 cup	35	2	0	0	0
Chicken Broth Low Fat	1 cup	35	2	0	0	0
Clam Chowder Manhattan	1 cup	90	3	13	5	1
Clam Chowder New England	1 cup	110	4	15	5	0
Corn & Vegetable Fat Free	1 cup	70	0	17	8	7
Garden Vegetable Fat Free	1 cup	80	0	18	6	4
Lentil & Carrot Fat Free	1 cup	100	0	25	7	7
Organic Black Bean	1 cup	130	1	25	7	5
Organic Cream Of Mushroom	1 cup	90	5	11	0	0
Organic Minestrone	1 cup	100	2	20	3	5
Organic Minestrone No Salt Added	1 cup	70	0	17	5	3
Organic Mushroom Barley	1 cup	70	0	17	4	3
Organic Mushroom Barley No Salt Added	1 cup	70	0	17	4	3
Organic Tomato	1 cup	80	0	18	14	1
Organic Tomato No Salt Added	1 cup	80	0	18	14	1
Tomato Vegetable Fat Free	1 cup	80	0	17	9	5
Vegetable Broth Fat Free	1 cup	20	0	5	1	0
Healthy Choice						
Bean & Ham	1 cup	180	2	29	4	10

FOOD	PORTION	CAL	FAT	CARB	SUGAR	FIBER
Chicken & Dumplings	1 cup	140	3	21	2	3
Country Vegetable	1 cup (8.6 oz)	110	1	19	4	4
Hormel						
Bean & Ham	1 pkg (7.5 oz)	190	4	29	2	7
Beef Vegetable	1 pkg (7.5 oz)	100	1	16	3	1
Chicken Noodle	1 pkg (7.5 oz)	100	3	12	0	0
Chicken w/ Rice	1 pkg (7.5 oz)	110	3	18	3	1
New England Clam Chowder	1 pkg (7.5 oz)	140	5	18	0	1
Lucini						
Roman Tomato Cream	1 cup (8.6 oz)	170	9	18	10	4
Umbrian Lentil	1 cup (8.6 oz)	160	5	23	6	9
Manischewitz						
Beef Broth	1 cup (8.4 oz)	150	1	1	1	0
Chicken Broth	1 cup (8.4 oz)	15	1	1	1	0
Chicken Broth Low Sodium	1 cup (8.4 oz)	15	1	1	1	0
Muir Glen						
Organic Garden Vegetable	1 cup	80	1	16	5	3
Organic Southwest Black Bean	1 cup	140	1	27	4	8
Original SoupMan						
Italian Wedding	1 cup	120	6	18	4	4
New England Clam Chowder	1 cup	290	19	16	1	1
Organic Butternut Squash	1 cup	250	13	33	12	3
Tomato Basil	1 cup	140	7	18	11	4
Turkey Chili	1 cup	210	7	18	4	5
Progresso						
40% Less Sodium Italian Style Wedding	1 cup (8.7 oz)	90	2	11	2	1

FOOD	PORTION	CAL	FAT	CARB	SUGAR	FIBER
50% Less Sodium Garden Vegetable	1 cup (8.8 oz)	100	0	22	4	3
50% Less Sodium Zesty Chicken Gumbo	1 cup (8.7 oz)	110	2	18	2	2
High Fiber Creamy Tomato Basil	1 cup (8.8 oz)	130	4	26	13	7
Light Beef Pot Roast	1 cup (8.4 oz)	80	1	12	4	2
Light Chicken Vegetable Rotini	1 cup (8.3 oz)	70	2	10	2	2
Light Italian Style Vegetable	1 cup (8.6 oz)	60	0	12	3	4
Light Savory Vegetable Barley	1 cup (8.5 oz)	60	0	14	3	4
Light Vegetable	1 cup (8.4 oz)	60	0	14	4	4
Light Vegetable & Noodle	1 cup (8.7 oz)	60	1	12	2	4
Reduced Sodium Chicken Broth	1 cup (8.4 oz)	20	0	2	1	–
Rich & Hearty Beef Pot Roast	1 cup (8.7 oz)	120	2	20	4	2
Rich & Hearty Chicken & Homestyle Noodles	1 cup (8.6 oz)	100	2	14	1	1
Rich & Hearty Chicken Pot Pie	1 cup (8.6 oz)	170	6	21	3	2
Rich & Hearty Savory Beef Barley Vegetable	1 cup (8.6 oz)	130	1	22	4	3
Rich & Hearty Sirloin Steak & Vegetables	1 cup	130	2	21	5	2
Rich & Hearty Slow Cooked Vegetable Beef	1 cup (8.6 oz)	120	1	20	6	3
Rich & Hearty Steak & Roasted Russet Potatoes	1 cup (8.6 oz)	140	2	23	3	2

FOOD	PORTION	CAL	FAT	CARB	SUGAR	FIBER
Traditional Beef & Vegetable	1 cup (8.7 oz)	120	2	18	4	2
Traditional Beef Barley	1 cup (8.5 oz)	120	2	20	3	4
Traditional Chickarina	1 cup (8.3 oz)	120	5	12	1	2
Traditional Chicken & Sausage Gumbo	1 cup (8.7 oz)	130	4	18	2	1
Traditional Chicken & Wild Rice	1 cup (8.4 oz)	100	2	15	1	1
Traditional Chicken Noodle	1 cup (8.3 oz)	100	3	12	1	1
Traditional Homestyle Chicken	1 cup (8.4 oz)	100	2	14	1	1
Traditional Italian Style Wedding	1 cup (8.4 oz)	100	4	12	1	1
Traditional Manhattan Clam Chowder	1 cup (8.4 oz)	100	2	17	4	2
Traditional New England Clam Chowder	1 cup (8.4 oz)	110	2	20	2	2
Traditional Potato Broccoli & Cheese	1 cup (8.8 oz)	180	10	18	2	2
Traditional Split Pea w/ Ham	1 cup (8.5 oz)	140	1	24	3	4
Traditional Turkey Noodle	1 cup (8.4 oz)	80	2	12	1	1
Vegetable Classics Creamy Mushroom	1 cup (8.1 oz)	130	3	9	2	1
Vegetable Classics French Onion	1 cup (8 oz)	50	2	8	3	tr
Vegetable Classics Hearty Black Bean w/ Bacon	1 cup (8.5 oz)	160	1	29	3	8
Vegetable Classics Hearty Tomato	1 cup (8.6 oz)	110	1	23	9	3

FOOD	PORTION	CAL	FAT	CARB	SUGAR	FIBER
Vegetable Classics Lentil	1 cup (8.5 oz)	150	2	28	1	5
Vegetable Classics Vegetable	1 cup (8.4 oz)	80	1	16	3	2
Snow's						
Clam Chowder	1 cup (8.4 oz)	200	15	13	3	1
Swanson						
50% Low Sodium Beef Broth	1 cup	15	0	1	1	0
Beef Broth	1 cup	15	0	1	0	0
Beef Stock	1 cup	30	0	3	3	0
Chicken Broth	1 cup	10	0	1	1	0
Chicken Stock	1 cup	20	0	1	1	0
Vegetable Broth	1 cup	15	0	3	2	tr
FROZEN						
Kettle Cuisine						
Angus Beef Steak Chili w/ Beans Gluten Free Dairy Free	1 pkg (10 oz)	250	12	17	9	4
Roasted Vegetable Gluten Free Dairy Free	1 pkg (10 oz)	140	6	19	4	5
Tabatchnick						
Minestrone	1 serv (7.5 oz)	100	2	18	3	4
Split Pea	1 serv (7.5 oz)	140	0	34	0	13
Vegetable	1 serv (7.5 oz)	90	2	17	3	4
MIX						
beef broth cube	1 cube	6	tr	1	–	–
chicken broth cube	1 cube (4.8 g)	9	tr	1	–	–
HamBeens						
15 Bean as prep	½ cup	120	1	20	1	9
15 Bean Beef as prep	½ cup	120	1	20	1	9
15 Bean Cajun as prep	½ cup	120	1	20	1	9
15 Bean Chicken as prep	½ cup	120	1	20	1	9

FOOD	PORTION	CAL	FAT	CARB	SUGAR	FIBER
Spanish American Black Bean as prep	½ cup	120	1	22	1	8
Health Valley						
Chicken Noodles w/ Vegetables	1 cup	110	0	24	1	3
Creamy Potato w/ Broccoli Fat Free	1 cup	80	0	17	2	3
Manischewitz						
Lentil as prep	1 cup	150	0	29	2	12
Matzo Ball Soup	1 cup	40	1	9	3	1
Southwestern Black Bean as prep	1 cup	90	1	16	2	4
Split Pea w/ Barley as prep	1 cup	110	0	21	2	3
Vegetable & Pasta as prep	1 cup	90	0	17	1	2
Silhouette Solution						
Mediterranean Tomato	1 pkg (1.16 oz)	110	3	8	4	1
Newbury Chicken Cream	1 pkg (1.3 oz)	110	3	8	1	1
Streit's						
Matzo Ball as prep	1 cup	50	0	12	4	0
Thai Kitchen						
Rice Noodle Bowl Lemongrass & Chili as prep	½ pkg	110	2	23	2	1
Rice Noodle Bowl Thai Ginger as prep	½ pkg	120	2	23	2	1
REFRIGERATED						
Moosewood						
Organic Creamy Potato & Corn Chowder	1 cup (8.4 oz)	170	6	28	5	3
Organic Hungarian Vegetable Noodle	1 cup (8.4 oz)	80	2	13	4	2

FOOD	PORTION	CAL	FAT	CARB	SUGAR	FIBER
Organic Savannah Sweet Potato Bisque	1 cup (8.4 oz)	200	11	20	6	2
Organic Texas Two Bean Chili	1 cup (8.4 oz)	200	4	34	9	8
Organic Tuscan White Bean & Vegetable	1 cup (8.4 oz)	130	2	24	5	5
Organic Classics						
French Onion w/ Croutons	1 cup	140	6	17	8	2
Seafood Chowder	1 cup	160	6	17	4	1
TAKE-OUT						
ban mien fish head	1 serv (10 oz)	277	10	27	2	4
beef stew soup	1 cup (8.8 oz)	221	5	20	–	–
bird's nest	1 cup (8.6 oz)	112	3	8	1	0
black bean turtle soup	1 cup	241	1	45	–	10
broccoli cheese	1 cup	165	9	15	7	2
brunswick stew soup	1 cup (8.5 oz)	232	6	17	–	–
caldo de res beef soup	1 cup	143	5	12	3	2
corn & cheese chowder	¾ cup	215	12	21	–	3
duck soup	1 cup (8.6 oz)	412	37	2	tr	tr
egg drop	1 cup	73	4	1	tr	0
gazpacho	1 cup	46	tr	5	–	–
greek lemon	¾ cup	63	2	7	–	2
hot & sour	1 serv (14 oz)	173	9	9	3	3
matzo ball soup	1 cup	118	5	10	tr	1
minestrone	1 cup	233	13	22	4	4
miso w/ tofu	1 cup	84	3	8	2	2
onion soup gratinee	1 serv	492	27	38	6	4
oxtail	1 cup	68	2	9	2	1
pasta e fagioli	1 cup (8.8 oz)	194	5	30	–	–
ratatouille	1 cup (7.5 oz)	266	25	12	–	–
shark fin	1 bowl (10 oz)	164	9	9	–	00
shrimp bisque	1 cup	263	14	13	10	tr

FOOD	PORTION	CAL	FAT	CARB	SUGAR	FIBER
sopa de albondigas	1 cup	171	11	9	3	1
thai lemon grass	1 bowl	100	4	5	–	–
vietnamese pho beef noodle	1 serv (7.8 oz)	480	12	78	2	1
wonton soup	1 cup	183	7	14	tr	1
zupa koprowa polish dill soup	1 bowl	54	2	6	–	–

SOUR CREAM

sour cream	1 tbsp (0.4 oz)	26	3	1	–	–
sour cream	1 cup (8 oz)	493	48	10	–	–
Breakstone's						
Sour Cream	2 tbsp (1 oz)	60	5	1	1	0
Cabot						
Light	2 tbsp	35	3	2	0	0
No Fat	2 tbsp	20	0	3	2	0
Sour Cream	2 tbsp	50	5	1	0	0
Friendship						
All Natural	2 tbsp (1 oz)	60	5	1	1	0
Light	1 tbsp (1 oz)	40	3	3	1	0
Nonfat	2 tbsp (1 oz)	25	0	4	2	0
Land O Lakes						
Fat Free	2 tbsp (1.1 oz)	20	0	3	2	0
Light	2 tbsp (1.1 oz)	40	3	2	2	0
Sour Cream	2 tbsp (1.1 oz)	60	6	2	2	0
Nancy's						
Organic	2 tbsp	60	6	2	1	0

SOUR CREAM SUBSTITUTES

nondairy	1 oz	59	6	2	–	–
nondairy	1 cup	479	45	15	–	–
Vegan Gourmet						
Alternative Sour Cream	2 tbsp (1 oz)	50	5	3	0	2

FOOD	PORTION	CAL	FAT	CARB	SUGAR	FIBER
SOURSOP						
fresh	1	416	2	105	–	–
fresh cut up	1 cup	150	1	38	–	–

SOY (*see also* CHEESE SUBSTITUTES, ICE CREAM AND FROZEN DESSERTS, MILK SUBSTITUTES, MISO, SMOOTHIES, SOY SAUCE, SOYBEANS, TEMPEH, TOFU, YOGURT FROZEN)

FOOD	PORTION	CAL	FAT	CARB	SUGAR	FIBER
I.M. Healthy						
SoyNut Butter Chocolate	2 tbsp	190	14	12	9	3
SoyNut Butter Honey Creamy	2 tbsp	170	11	10	4	3
SoyNut Butter Original Chunky	2 tbsp	170	11	10	3	3
SoyNut Butter Original Creamy	2 tbsp	170	11	10	3	3
SoyNut Butter Unsweetened Creamy	2 tbsp	190	15	6	1	5
KooLoos						
Soy Nuts & Flaxseed BBQ	1 pkg (1 oz)	130	4	16	1	3
Soy Nuts & Flaxseed Original	1 pkg (1 oz)	140	5	15	1	3
Simple Food						
Soynut Butter Chocolate	2 tbsp	190	12	8	8	2
Soynut Butter No Sugar No Salt	2 tbsp	200	14	8	2	2
South Beach						
Soy Nuts Dark Chocolate	1 pkg (0.7 oz)	100	6	9	6	2
Soy Wonder						
Creamy Spread	2 tbsp	170	11	10	3	1
SoyButter						
Spread	2 tbsp	200	15	8	4	2

SOY DRINKS (*see* MILK SUBSTITUTES, SMOOTHIES)

FOOD	PORTION	CAL	FAT	CARB	SUGAR	FIBER
SOY SAUCE						
shoyu	1 tbsp	9	tr	2	–	–
soy sauce	1 tbsp	7	tr	1	–	–
tamari	1 tbsp	11	tr	1	–	–
Angostura						
Lite Soy	1 tbsp (0.5 oz)	10	0	2	2	0
Soy Sauce	1 tbsp (0.5 oz)	10	0	1	1	0
Dave's Gourmet						
Soyabi Sauce	1 tbsp (0.6 oz)	30	2	4	3	–
La Choy						
Lite	1 tbsp (0.5 oz)	15	0	2	2	0
Mitsukan						
Ponzu Citrus Seasoned	1 tbsp (0.5 oz)	10	0	1	1	–
Soy Vay						
Wasabiyaki	1 tbsp	35	1	6	5	0
Tree Of Life						
Organic Shoyu	1 tbsp (0.5 oz)	15	0	1	1	0
Organic Tamari Wheat Free	1 tbsp (0.5 oz)	15	0	1	1	0
SOYBEANS						
dried cooked	1 cup	298	15	17	–	–
dry roasted	½ cup	387	19	28	–	–
green cooked	½ cup	127	6	10	–	4
roasted	½ cup	405	22	29	–	–
roasted & toasted	1 cup	490	26	33	–	–
roasted & toasted salted	1 cup	490	26	33	–	–
sprouts raw	½ cup	43	2	3	–	–
sprouts steamed	½ cup	38	2	3	–	–
sprouts stir fried	1 cup	125	7	9	–	–
Seapoint Farms						
Edamame Dry Roasted Goji Blend	¼ cup	120	3	15	5	7

FOOD	PORTION	CAL	FAT	CARB	SUGAR	FIBER
Edamame Dry Roasted Lightly Salted	¼ cup	130	4	10	1	8
Edamame Dry Roasted Wasabi	¼ cup	130	5	9	1	7
Edamame In Pods frzn	½ cup	100	3	9	1	4
Edamame In Pods Lightly Salted	½ cup	100	3	9	1	4
Edamame Shelled	½ cup	100	3	9	1	4
Organic Edamame In Pods	½ cup	100	3	9	1	4
Organic Edamame Shelled	½ cup	100	3	9	1	4

SPAGHETTI (see PASTA, PASTA DINNERS, PASTA SALAD, SPAGHETTI SAUCE)

SPAGHETTI SAUCE
JARRED

FOOD	PORTION	CAL	FAT	CARB	SUGAR	FIBER
marinara sauce	1 cup	171	8	25	–	–
spaghetti sauce	1 cup	272	12	40	–	–
Amy's						
Organic Family Marinara	½ cup (4.4 oz)	80	5	10	5	3
Organic Marinara Low Sodium	½ cup (4.4 oz)	40	1	7	5	1
Barilla						
Green & Black Olive	½ cup	80	3	10	5	4
Italian Baking Sauce	¼ cup (4.4 oz)	60	1	12	6	2
Mushroom & Garlic	½ cup	70	2	12	6	2
Dave's Gourmet						
Pasta Sauce Spicy Heirloom Marinara	½ cup (4.4 oz)	45	2	7	4	2
Pasta Sauce Wild Mushroom	½ cup (4.4 oz)	60	3	7	2	tr
Dei Fratelli						
Arrabbiata	½ cup (4.2 oz)	50	2	8	5	2
Pizza Sauce	¼ cup (2.2 oz)	30	2	5	4	1

FOOD	PORTION	CAL	FAT	CARB	SUGAR	FIBER
DelGrosso						
Garden Style	½ cup (4.4 oz)	70	2	12	7	2
Mushroom	½ cup (4.4 oz)	70	2	11	8	3
New York Style	¼ cup (2.1 oz)	35	1	6	4	1
Original Meat Flavored	½ cup (4.4 oz)	80	2	12	8	3
Pizza Sauce Pepperoni	¼ cup (2.2 oz)	40	1	6	4	2
Three Cheese	½ cup (4.4 oz)	80	2	13	8	3
Francesco Rinaldi						
Alfredo	¼ cup (2.1 oz)	80	6	3	1	0
Chunky Egglpant Parmesan	½ cup (4.4 oz)	90	5	11	9	tr
Chunky Mushroom & Pepper	½ cup (4.4 oz)	80	3	13	9	2
Hearty Mushroom Pepper & Onion	½ cup (4.4 oz)	80	3	12	8	2
Hearty Sweet & Tasty Tomato	½ cup (4.4 oz)	100	5	16	15	tr
Hearty Three Cheese	½ cup (4.4 oz)	80	2	15	14	tr
Organic Burgundy Marinara	½ cup (4.3 oz)	100	7	9	8	tr
Premium Vodka	¼ cup (2.1 oz)	60	4	4	4	0
Traditional Meat Flavored	½ cup (4.4 oz)	80	4	12	11	tr
Traditional No Salt Added	½ cup (4.4 oz)	70	3	12	6	2
Traditional Original	½ cup (4.4 oz)	80	3	12	11	tr
Lucini						
Rustic Tomato Basil	½ cup (4.4 oz)	80	5	8	6	2
Spicy Tuscan	½ cup (4.4 oz)	80	5	8	5	2
Muir Glen						
Organic Chunky Tomato	¼ cup	15	0	4	2	tr
Organic Garlic Roasted Garlic	½ cup	60	1	12	4	2

FOOD	PORTION	CAL	FAT	CARB	SUGAR	FIBER
Organic Pizza Sauce	¼ cup	40	2	6	3	1
Organic Tomato Sauce No Salt Added	¼ cup	25	0	5	3	1
Prego						
Heart Smart Traditional Italian	½ cup	100	3	15	9	3
Progresso						
Lobster Sauce	½ cup (4.3 oz)	100	7	6	3	2
Red Clam w/ Tomato & Basil	½ cup (4.4 oz)	60	1	8	4	1
White Clam w/ Garlic & Herb	½ cup (4.4 oz)	120	10	4	1	1
Ragu						
Old World Style Margherita	½ cup (4.4 oz)	70	2	10	6	2
Old World Style Sweet Tomato Basil	½ cup (4.4 oz)	60	2	10	6	3
S&W						
Tomato Sauce	¼ cup (2.1 oz)	20	0	4	2	1
Two Guys						
Jersey Tomato Sauce	½ cup (4.6 oz)	60	2	10	4	2
TAKE-OUT						
bolognese	5 oz	195	15	4	–	tr

SPANISH FOOD
FROZEN
Amy's

FOOD	PORTION	CAL	FAT	CARB	SUGAR	FIBER
Bowl Mexican Casserole	1 pkg (9.4 oz)	470	16	70	3	7
Burrito Black Bean	1 (6 oz)	280	8	44	4	4
Burrito Cheddar Cheese	1 (6 oz)	300	9	43	1	6
Burrito Southwestern	1 (5.5 oz)	300	10	43	2	6
Enchilada Black Bean Vegetable	1 (4.7 oz)	180	6	26	2	3

FOOD	PORTION	CAL	FAT	CARB	SUGAR	FIBER
Cedarlane						
Organic Burrito Low Fat Rice & Cheese	1 (6 oz)	260	1	48	2	7
Organic Enchilada Low Fat Black Bean & Tofu	1 (9 oz)	220	3	42	3	6
Roasted Chile Relleno	1 pkg (10 oz)	400	20	37	12	5
Zone Burrito Beans & Cheese	1 (6 oz)	350	13	37	3	8
El Monterey						
Burrito Bean & Cheese	1 (5 oz)	280	8	43	1	5
Burrito Beef & Bean	1 (5 oz)	370	17	42	2	4
Burrito Half Pound Spicy Red Hot Beef & Bean	1 (8 oz)	600	29	68	3	7
Burrito Supreme Breakfast Egg Cheese & Sausage	1 (4.5 oz)	300	13	34	1	1
Burrito Supreme Shredded Steak & Cheese	1 (5 oz)	290	9	41	1	1
Burrito XX Large Bean & Cheese	1 (10 oz)	590	17	88	2	5
Burrito XX Large Beef & Bean	1 (10 oz)	730	35	83	2	8
Cruncheros Cheese & Beef	3 (4.5 oz)	330	16	35	1	2
Cruncheros Taco Beef & Cheese	4 (5.6 oz)	460	29	38	2	2
Enchiladas Cheese w/ Sauce	1 serv (8 oz)	250	15	22	1	3
Enchiladas Shredded Beef w/ Sauce	1 serv (4 oz)	140	6	15	1	2

FOOD	PORTION	CAL	FAT	CARB	SUGAR	FIBER
Quesadillas Chicken & Cheese	2 (6 oz)	380	15	43	1	2
Quesadillas Steak & Cheese	2 (6 oz)	400	15	42	2	1
Tamales Chicken	1 (4.5 oz)	240	12	27	1	2
Tamales Shredded Beef	1 (4.5 oz)	310	19	27	1	3
Taquitos Southwest Chicken In A Seasoned Batter	2 (2.8 oz)	175	8	20	0	1
Taquitos Corn Shredded Beef	3 (4.5 oz)	300	13	31	1	1
Taquitos Flour Char-Broiled Chicken Breast	3 (5 oz)	380	19	36	1	1
Taquitos Flour Chicken & Cheese	3 (4.5 oz)	350	18	36	1	2
Tornados Apple Cinnamon	1 (3 oz)	180	5	31	8	0
Tornados Sausage Egg & Cheese	1 (3 oz)	230	13	23	1	1
Tornados Shredded Beef	1 (3 oz)	210	10	23	1	1
Tornados Steak Egg & Cheese	1 (3 oz)	170	6	22	1	0
Tornados XXL Southwest Chicken	1 (4.2 oz)	210	10	28	1	1
Health Is Wealth						
Vegetarian Hot Tamale Munchees	6 (3 oz)	160	3	26	0	3
Patio						
Burrito Bean & Cheese	1	280	8	44	4	5
Burrito Beef & Bean Mild	1	300	10	44	6	5
Enchilada Beef	1 meal	380	12	55	2	5
Enchilada Cheese	1 meal	390	13	58	2	10

FOOD	PORTION	CAL	FAT	CARB	SUGAR	FIBER
Enchilada Combo Dinner	1 meal	380	12	57	2	5
Enchilada & Beef Tamale	1 meal	460	14	69	2	5
READY-TO-EAT						
taco shell corn	1 (6.5 inch)	98	5	13	tr	2
taco shell flour	1 (7 inch)	173	9	19	tr	1
TAKE-OUT						
arroz con coco	1 cup	532	38	46	5	4
burrito w/ beans	1 med (5 oz)	295	8	45	1	7
burrito w/ beans & rice	1 (3.5 oz)	221	5	37	tr	4
burrito w/ beef	1 sm (3.4 oz)	297	13	25	tr	1
burrito w/ beef & beans	1 med (5 oz)	331	13	36	1	6
burrito w/ beef beans & cheese	1 med (5 oz)	379	19	30	1	5
burrito w/ chicken & beans	1 med (5 oz)	295	9	34	1	5
burrito w/ pork & beans	1 med (5 oz)	320	12	35	1	6
chiles rellenos meat & cheese filled	1 (5 oz)	213	16	9	3	2
chimichanga w/ bean cheese lettuce & tomato	1 (4.1 oz)	271	18	22	2	3
chimichanga w/ beef & rice	1 (10 oz)	634	36	58	5	5
chimichanga w/ beef beans lettuce & tomato	1 (4.1 oz)	254	15	22	2	3
chimichanga w/ beef cheese lettuce & tomato	1 (4.1 oz)	337	24	19	1	1
chimichanga w/ chicken sour cream lettuce & tomato	1 (4 oz)	277	20	17	1	1
empanada fruit filled	1 (3.8 oz)	452	25	55	25	2
empanada meat & vegetable	1 (7.8 oz)	881	61	66	1	3
empanada sweet potato	1 (7.8 oz)	546	23	76	22	4

FOOD	PORTION	CAL	FAT	CARB	SUGAR	FIBER
enchilada w/ beans	1 (4.1 oz)	179	6	27	2	6
enchilada w/ beans & cheese	1 (4.6 oz)	233	11	25	2	5
enchilada w/ beef	1 (4 oz)	214	10	21	2	3
enchilada w/ beef & beans	1 (4 oz)	195	8	25	2	4
frijoles	1 cup	278	2	49	6	9
frijoles w/ cheese	1 cup	225	8	29	–	–
nachos w/ beans & cheese	1 serv (9.4 oz)	616	33	57	2	13
nachos w/ beef beans cheese & sour cream	1 serv (19 oz)	1620	97	133	4	19
paella	1 serv (7 oz)	308	16	17	–	3
pupusa meat filled	1 (3.6 oz)	187	6	26	1	3
quesadilla w/ cheese	1 (5 oz)	498	28	40	1	3
quesadilla w/ meat & cheese	1 (6.5 oz)	605	35	40	1	2
taco de jueye w/ crab meat	1 (4.2 oz)	266	14	18	1	2
taco w/ beans lettuce tomato & salsa	1 (2.8 oz)	117	5	16	1	4
taco w/ chicken lettuce tomato & salsa	1 (2.5 oz)	114	5	10	1	1
taco w/ fish lettuce tomato & salsa	1 (2.7 oz)	101	4	10	1	1
tostada w/ beef lettuce tomato & salsa	1 (2.7 oz)	143	8	11	1	2

SPICES (see individual names, HERBS/SPICES)

SPINACH
CANNED

drained	1 cup	49	1	7	1	5

FOOD	PORTION	CAL	FAT	CARB	SUGAR	FIBER
Freshlike						
Cut Leaf	½ cup	45	1	5	0	3
Popeye						
Leaf Spinach	½ cup	30	0	4	tr	2
Leaf Spinach No Salt Added	½ cup	40	1	5	0	2
S&W						
Leaf	½ cup (4 oz)	30	0	4	0	2
FRESH						
baby raw	2 cups	20	0	5	0	3
cooked	1 cup	41	tr	7	1	4
malabar cooked	1 cup	10	tr	1	–	1
mustard cooked	1 cup	29	tr	5	–	4
new zealand cooked	1 cup	22	tr	4	–	–
raw	1 cup	7	tr	1	tr	1
Fresh Express						
Baby Spinach	3 cups	20	0	3	0	2
Organic Baby Spinach	3 cups	35	0	9	0	4
FROZEN						
chopped cooked	1 cup	30	tr	5	tr	4
Birds Eye						
Creamed	½ cup (4.4 oz)	90	4	9	3	4
Cascadian Farm						
Organic Cut	⅓ cup	25	0	3	tr	1
Cedarlane						
Organic Spanakopita Spinach & Feta Pie	½ pkg (5 oz)	260	8	38	3	2
Dr. Praeger's						
Spinach Bites	2 (2 oz)	110	3	17	3	2
Fillo Factory						
Spanakopita Spinach & Cheese Fillo Appetizers	3 (3 oz)	190	9	20	1	1

FOOD	PORTION	CAL	FAT	CARB	SUGAR	FIBER
Health Is Wealth						
Creamed	½ pkg (4.5 oz)	100	4	27	5	2
Spinach Munchees	6 (3oz)	180	7	25	1	3
TAKE-OUT						
indian saag	1 serv	28	2	2	–	1
spanakopita spinach pie	1 serv (3 oz)	148	11	8	1	1

SPINACH JUICE

juice	7 oz	14	0	2	–	–

SPORTS DRINKS (see ENERGY DRINKS)

SPOT

baked	3 oz	134	5	0	0	0

SPROUTS

kidney bean	½ cup	27	tr	4	–	–
lentil sprouts	½ cup	40	tr	8	–	–
mung bean	½ cup	16	tr	3	–	–
mung bean canned	½ cup	8	tr	1	–	–
mung bean cooked	½ cup	13	tr	3	–	–
pea	½ cup	77	tr	17	–	–
radish	½ cup	8	tr	1	–	–
La Choy						
Bean Sprouts	⅔ cup	15	0	3	tr	1
TAKE-OUT						
mung bean stir fried	½ cup	31	tr	7	–	–

SQUAB

boneless baked	1 (4 oz)	242	14	0	0	0

SQUASH (see also SQUASH SEEDS, ZUCCHINI)
CANNED

crookneck sliced	½ cup	14	tr	3	–	–
Sunshine						
Slice Yellow	½ cup	25	0	5	3	2

FOOD	PORTION	CAL	FAT	CARB	SUGAR	FIBER
FRESH						
acorn cooked mashed	½ cup	41	tr	11	–	3
acorn cubed baked	½ cup	57	tr	15	–	2
butternut baked	½ cup	41	tr	11	–	2
crookneck sliced cooked	½ cup	18	tr	4	–	1
hubbard baked	½ cup	51	tr	11	–	3
hubbard cooked mashed	½ cup	35	tr	8	–	3
scallop sliced cooked	½ cup	14	tr	3	–	1
spaghetti cooked	½ cup	23	tr	5	–	2
FROZEN						
butternut cooked mashed	½ cup	47	tr	12	–	3
crookneck sliced cooked	½ cup	24	tr	5	–	–
TAKE-OUT						
fritter	1 (0.8 oz)	81	5	8	1	1
squash pie	1 slice (5.4 oz)	291	12	40	24	2
SQUASH SEEDS						
roasted	1 oz	148	12	4	–	–
salted & roasted	1 oz	148	12	4	–	–
seeds dried	1 oz	154	13	5	–	–
seeds whole roasted	1 oz	127	6	15	–	–
SQUID						
baked	1 cup	192	6	5	0	0
canned in its own ink	1 can (4 oz)	122	2	4	0	0
dried	1 sm (1.5 oz)	147	2	5	0	0
pickled	1 oz	26	tr	1	tr	0
steamed	1 cup	147	2	5	0	0
TAKE-OUT						
arroz con calamares	1 cup	400	17	47	2	1
calamari breaded & fried	1 cup	296	12	17	1	1

FOOD	PORTION	CAL	FAT	CARB	SUGAR	FIBER
SQUIRREL						
roasted	3 oz	147	4	0	0	0
STARFRUIT						
fresh	1	42	tr	10	–	–
STRAWBERRIES						
canned in heavy syrup	½ cup	117	tr	30	28	2
fresh halves	1 cup	49	tr	12	7	3
fresh whole	1 pint	114	1	27	17	7
fresh whole	1 cup	46	tr	11	7	3
frzn sweetened sliced	½ cup	122	tr	33	31	2
frzn sweetened whole	1 cup	199	tr	54	48	5
frzn whole unsweetened	1 cup	77	tr	20	10	5
organic fresh whole	8 med	45	0	12	8	4
Chukar Cherries						
Dried	¼ cup	120	0	29	25	2
Emily's						
Dark Chocolate Covered	6 (1.4 oz)	170	8	28	22	2
FruitziO						
Freeze-Dried	1 pkg (0.9 oz)	100	0	22	17	1
LiteHouse						
Glaze Sugar Free	3 tbsp	35	0	8	0	0
Polar						
Strawberries In Syrup	½ cup	90	0	21	10	1
Stoneridge Orchards						
Dried	⅓ cup (1.4 oz)	140	0	35	32	0
STUFFING/DRESSING						
Zatarain's						
Creole Chicken as prep	½ cup	100	1	20	2	1
French Bread as prep	½ cup	100	1	20	2	1
TAKE-OUT						
bread	1 cup	352	17	44	5	2

FOOD	PORTION	CAL	FAT	CARB	SUGAR	FIBER
cornbread	½ cup	179	9	22	0	3
kishke stuffed derma	1 piece (1.3 oz)	166	12	13	tr	1
oyster	1 cup	304	18	29	3	2
sausage	½ cup	292	11	40	–	1
STURGEON						
broiled	3 oz	115	4	0	0	0
roe raw	1 oz	59	3	tr	–	–
smoked	1 oz	49	1	0	0	0
TAKE-OUT						
breaded & fried	4 oz	252	15	9	1	1
SUCKER						
white baked	3 oz	101	3	0	0	0
SUGAR (see also FRUCTOSE, SYRUP)						
brown organic	1 tsp	17	0	4	4	0
brown packed	1 cup (7.7 oz)	828	0	214	214	–
brown unpacked	1 cup (5.1 oz)	547	0	141	140	0
cinnamon sugar	1 tsp	16	tr	4	4	tr
cube	1 (2 g)	9	0	2	2	0
maple	1 piece (1 oz)	99	tr	25	24	0
powdered	1 tbsp (0.3 oz)	31	0	8	8	–
powdered unsifted	1 cup (4.2 oz)	467	tr	119	115	–
raw	1 pkg (5 g)	19	0	5	5	0
sugarcane stem	3 oz	54	0	14	–	3
white	1 packet (3 g)	12	0	3	3	0
white	1 tsp (4 g)	15	0	4	4	–
white	1 tbsp (0.4 oz)	49	0	13	13	0
white	1 cup (7 oz)	773	0	200	200	–
Domino						
Dark Brown	1 tsp (4 g)	15	0	4	4	–
Demerara Raw Cane	1 tsp	15	0	4	4	0

FOOD	PORTION	CAL	FAT	CARB	SUGAR	FIBER
Sugar In The Raw						
Turbinado Sugar	1 pkg (5 g)	20	0	5	5	–
Tree Of Life						
Date Sugar	1 tsp (4 g)	10	0	3	3	0
Organic Cane Juice Dehydrated	1 tsp (3.5 g)	15	0	3	3	0
Turbinado	1 tsp (4 g)	15	0	4	4	0
Wholesome Sweeteners						
Organic	1 tsp (4 g)	15	0	4	4	0
Organic Fair Trade Dark Brown Sugar	1 tsp (4 g)	15	0	4	4	0
Organic Fair Trade Powdered	¼ cup (1 oz)	120	0	30	30	0
Organic Fair Trade Sucanat	1 tsp (4 g)	15	0	4	4	0
Organic Turbinado	1 tsp (4 g)	15	0	4	4	0

SUGAR SUBSTITUTES

FOOD	PORTION	CAL	FAT	CARB	SUGAR	FIBER
Fructevia						
All Natural	1 tsp (4 g)	5	0	2	2	0
Fruit Sweetness						
Sugar Substitute	1 serv (0.9 oz)	0	0	0	0	0
Nevella						
No Calorie Sweetener	1 tsp	0	0	tr	0	0
Neway						
Sweet Sensation	¼ tsp	0	0	tr	0	0
PureVia						
All Natural	1 pkg (2 g)	0	0	2	tr	0
Splenda						
Brown Sugar Blend	½ tsp (2 g)	10	0	2	2	0
Cafe Sticks	1 pkg (1 g)	0	0	tr	0	0
Flavor Accents Sticks	1 pkg (1 g)	0	0	tr	0	0
Flavors For Coffee	1 pkg (1 g)	0	0	tr	0	0
No Calorie Granulated	1 tsp (0.5 g)	0	0	tr	0	0

FOOD	PORTION	CAL	FAT	CARB	SUGAR	FIBER
No Calorie Sweetener w/ Fiber	1 pkg	0	0	2	0	1
Sugar Blends	½ tsp (2 g)	10	0	2	2	-
Stevia Extract In The Raw						
100% Natural Sweetener	1 pkg (1 g)	0	0	0	0	0
Steviva						
Blend	1 tbsp (0.4 oz)	2	0	0	0	0
Sugar Twin						
Granulated Brown	1 tsp (0.4 g)	0	0	tr	0	0
Granulated White	1 tsp (0.4 g)	0	0	tr	0	0
Liquid	¼ tsp (1.3 g)	0	0	0	0	0
Packets	1 (0.8 g)	0	0	1	–	–
Susta						
Natural Sweetener	1 pkg (2 g)	5	0	2	tr	1
Sweet Fiber						
All Natural	1 pkg	0	0	tr	tr	tr
Sweete						
Sugar Free	1 pkg	0	0	tr	0	0
Truvia						
Calorie Free Sweetener	1 pkg (3.5 g)	0	0	3	0	0
Wholesome Sweeteners						
Organic Zero	1 pkg (6 g)	0	0	6	0	0
SUGAR-APPLE						
fresh	1	146	tr	37	–	–
fresh cut up	1 cup	236	1	59	–	–
SUNCHOKE						
fresh raw sliced	½ cup	57	tr	13	–	–
SUNFISH						
pumpkinseed baked	3 oz	97	1	0	0	0

FOOD	PORTION	CAL	FAT	CARB	SUGAR	FIBER
SUNFLOWER						
seeds dry roasted w/ salt	¼ cup	186	16	8	1	3
seeds dry roasted w/o salt	¼ cup	186	16	8	1	4
seeds w/ hulls dried	¼ cup	66	6	2	tr	1
Dakota Gourmet						
Seeds Honey Roasted	¼ cup (1 oz)	170	12	8	1	2
Lance						
Shelled Seeds	1 pkg (1.8 oz)	300	25	14	1	3
Tree Of Life						
Seeds Kernels Raw	¼ cup (1.3 oz)	210	18	7	1	2
SUSHI						
TAKE-OUT						
cucumber roll	1 (1.1 oz)	43	0	9	–	tr
inari	1 sm	46	1	9	–	0
prawn cooked	1 (1.1 oz)	36	0	8	–	1
roll california	1 (1.2 oz)	48	1	8	–	tr
roll fresh salmon	4 pieces	250	7	37	5	3
roll preserved radish	3 (1 oz)	27	0	6	–	tr
roll seaweed	1 (1.1 oz)	43	1	9	–	1
roll tuna	1 (1.1 oz)	37	0	6	–	tr
roll vegetable	1 (1.2 oz)	27	1	5	tr	–
roll yellowtain	1 (0.6 oz)	25	1	3	tr	–
saba	1 (0.8 oz)	33	1	5	–	tr
sashimi	1 serv (6 oz)	198	7	4	1	–
scallop cooked	1 (1 oz)	43	tr	8	–	tr
seasoned jellyfish	1 (1.2 oz)	58	1	11	–	tr
sweet beancurd	1 (1.2 oz)	64	2	10	–	1
unagi	1 (1 oz)	54	2	8	–	1
vinegared ginger	⅓ cup (1.6 oz)	48	tr	12	4	–
wasabi	2 tsp (0.3 oz)	5	tr	1	–	–

FOOD	PORTION	CAL	FAT	CARB	SUGAR	FIBER
SWAMP CABBAGE						
chopped cooked w/o salt	1 cup	20	tr	4	–	2
SWEET POTATO (see also YAM)						
baked w/ skin w/o salt	1 lg (6.3 oz)	162	tr	37	12	6
baked w/ skin w/o salt	1 med (4 oz)	103	tr	24	7	4
canned in syrup	½ cup	106	tr	25	6	3
canned mashed	½ cup	129	tr	30	7	2
leaves cooked w/o salt	1 cup	22	tr	5	3	1
paste dulce de calabaza	1 oz	82	tr	21	20	tr
Dr. Praeger's						
Sweet Potato Bites	2 (2 oz)	110	3	20	9	1
Green Giant						
Candied	¾ cup	240	7	41	20	3
Health Is Wealth						
Southern Style	½ pkg (5 oz)	190	5	36	8	2
Mann's						
Fresh Cubes	1 serv (3 oz)	60	0	15	3	3
Princella						
In Light Syrup	⅔ cup	160	0	39	20	3
Mashed	⅔ cup	120	0	28	15	3
Royal Prince						
Candied	½ cup	210	0	50	35	2
Trappey's						
Sugary Sam Cut Sweet	⅔ cup	160	0	39	20	3
Tree Of Life						
Organic Puree	½ cup (4.5 oz)	130	0	30	15	2
TAKE-OUT						
candied	1 serv (3.7 oz)	151	3	29	–	3
white fried batata blanca frita	1 serv (8 oz)	792	29	129	2	19

FOOD	PORTION	CAL	FAT	CARB	SUGAR	FIBER
SWEETBREAD (PANCREAS)						
beef braised	3 oz	230	15	0	0	0
lamb braised	3 oz	199	13	0	0	0
pork braised	3 oz	186	9	0	0	0
veal braised	3 oz	218	12	0	0	0
Rumba						
Beef	4 oz	260	23	0	0	0
SWISS CHARD						
cooked	½ cup	18	tr	4	–	–
raw chopped	½ cup	3	tr	1	–	–
SWORDFISH						
cooked	3 oz	132	4	0	0	0
raw	3 oz	103	3	0	0	0
SYRUP						
corn dark & light	¼ cup	240	tr	65	65	0
date syrup	1 tbsp	63	tr	15	–	0
maple	1 cup (11.1 oz)	824	1	212	191	–
maple	1 tbsp	52	0	13	12	–
raspberry	1 oz	76	0	19	–	–
rose hip	1 oz	9	0	2	2	0
sorghum	1 cup (11.6 oz)	957	0	247	247	–
sorghum	1 tbsp (0.7 oz)	61	0	16	16	–
sugar syrup	¼ cup	76	0	20	20	0
Cary's						
Maple	¼ cup	210	0	53	50	–
Sugar Free	¼ cup	30	0	12	0	tr
Hershey's						
Caramel	2 tbsp (1.4 oz)	110	0	27	21	–
Strawberry	2 tbsp (1.4 oz)	100	0	26	24	–
Strawberry Sugar Free	2 tbsp (1 oz)	10	0	4	–	–

FOOD	PORTION	CAL	FAT	CARB	SUGAR	FIBER
Nesquik						
Strawberry Calcium Fortified	2 tbsp (1.4 oz)	110	0	27	27	0
Neway						
Sweet Sensation Luo Han Guo Syrup	1 tsp	8	0	2	0	0
Tree Of Life						
Maple Grade A	¼ cup	200	0	53	53	–
Wholesome Sweeteners						
Organic Blue Agave	1 tbsp (0.7 oz)	60	0	16	16	0
Organic Blue Agave Cinnamon	2 tbsp (1 oz)	120	0	16	16	0
Organic Blue Agave Maple	2 tbsp (1 oz)	120	0	16	16	0
Organic Corn Syrup	2 tbsp (1 oz)	120	0	30	30	0

TAHINI (*see* SESAME)

TAMARIND

FOOD	PORTION	CAL	FAT	CARB	SUGAR	FIBER
dried sweetened pulpitas	1 piece (0.8 oz)	56	tr	15	14	1
dried sweetened pulpitas	½ cup	279	1	73	68	5
fresh	1 (2 g)	5	tr	1	0	tr
fresh cut up	1 cup	143	tr	38	34	3

TAMARIND JUICE

FOOD	PORTION	CAL	FAT	CARB	SUGAR	FIBER
nectar	1 cup	143	tr	37	32	1

TANGERINE

CANNED

FOOD	PORTION	CAL	FAT	CARB	SUGAR	FIBER
in light syrup	1 cup	154	tr	41	39	2
juice pack	1 cup	92	tr	24	22	2
FRESH						
fresh	1 med (3.1 oz)	47	tr	12	9	2

FOOD	PORTION	CAL	FAT	CARB	SUGAR	FIBER
fresh	1 lg (4.2 oz)	64	tr	16	13	2
fresh	1 sm (2.7 oz)	40	tr	10	8	1
sections	1 cup	103	1	26	21	4
Noble						
Florida Tangerines	1 (3.8 oz)	50	1	15	12	3

TANGERINE JUICE

canned sweetened	1 cup	124	1	30	29	1
fresh	1 cup	106	tr	25	24	1
Natalie's Orchid Island Juice						
100% Juice	8 oz	106	0	25	24	0
Santa Cruz						
Organic Sparkling	8 oz	110	0	26	26	0

TAPIOCA

pearl dry	¼ cup (1.3 oz)	136	tr	34	1	tr
starch	1 oz	98	tr	24	–	–

TARO

chips	10 (0.8 oz)	115	6	16	–	–
leaves cooked	½ cup	18	tr	3	–	–
raw sliced	½ cup	56	tr	14	–	–
shoots sliced cooked	½ cup	10	tr	2	–	–
sliced cooked	½ cup (2.3 oz)	94	tr	23	–	–
tahitian sliced cooked	½ cup	30	tr	5	–	–

TARPON

fresh	3 oz	87	2	0	0	0

TARRAGON

dried crumbled	1 tsp	2	tr	tr	–	0
ground	1 tsp	5	tr	1	–	tr

TEA/HERBAL TEA (*see also* ICED TEA)
HERBAL

chamomile brewed regular	1 cup	2	tr	tr	0	0
brewed tea	1 cup (6 oz)	2	0	1	–	0

FOOD	PORTION	CAL	FAT	CARB	SUGAR	FIBER
TAKE-OUT						
chai spiced latte decaf	1 cup	130	3	23	18	0
TEMPEH						
tempeh	½ cup	165	6	14	–	–
White Wave						
Five Grain	⅓ block (2.7 oz)	160	6	15	1	7
TESTICLES						
prairie oysters cooked	1 pair (6.8 oz)	241	6	0	0	0
THYME						
dried crumbled	1 tsp	3	tr	1	tr	tr
fresh	1 tsp	1	tr	tr	–	tr
ground	1 tsp	4	tr	1	tr	1
TILAPIA						
Gorton's						
Fillets Crunchy Breaded frzn	1 (3 oz)	80	3	tr	–	–
High Liner						
Loins	1 fillet (4 oz)	110	2	0	0	0
TAKE-OUT						
battered & fried	1 fillet (4 oz)	206	9	8	tr	tr
breaded & fried	1 fillet (4 oz)	300	14	16	2	1
broiled w/o fat	1 fillet (3.5 oz)	128	3	0	0	0
TILEFISH						
cooked	3 oz	125	4	0	0	0
cooked	½ fillet (5.3 oz)	220	7	0	0	0
raw	3 oz	81	2	0	0	0
TOFU						
firm	½ cup	183	11	5	–	2
firm	¼ block (3 oz)	118	7	3	–	1

FOOD	PORTION	CAL	FAT	CARB	SUGAR	FIBER
fresh fried	1 piece (0.5 oz)	35	3	1	–	tr
fuyu salted & fermented	1 block (⅓ oz)	13	1	1	–	tr
koyadofu dried frozen	1 piece (½ oz)	82	5	2	–	tr
okara	½ cup	47	1	8	–	1
regular	½ cup	94	6	2	–	1
regular	¼ block (4 oz)	88	6	2	–	1
Amy's						
Organic Tofu Scramble w/ Hash Browns & Veggies	1 pkg (8.9 oz)	320	19	19	4	4
House						
Atsu-Age Cutlet	1 (2.5 oz)	100	5	2	0	5
Cut-Age Shredded Fried	1 serv (0.5 oz)	50	4	0	0	0
Ganmodoki Fritter Small	3 (1.6 oz)	120	9	2	0	0
Medium Firm	3 oz	60	3	1	0	tr
Organic Extra Firm	3 oz	90	5	0	0	0
Organic Firm	3 oz	60	3	0	0	0
Soft Silken	3 oz	50	3	2	0	tr
Steak Cajun	1 (3 oz)	40	1	1	0	tr
Steak Grilled	1 (3 oz)	90	5	2	0	0
Sukui	3 oz	45	2	2	1	0
Tokusen Kinugoshi	1 piece (5 oz)	90	4	3	0	tr
Yaki Broiled	3 oz	90	5	2	0	0
TofuTown						
Tofu Tenders Havana Black Bean	½ pkg (5 oz)	210	8	18	13	2
Tofu Tenders Mediterranean Tahini	½ pkg (5 oz)	240	13	16	9	3
Tofu Tenders Sesame Ginger Teriyaki	½ pkg (5 oz)	240	9	24	16	3

FOOD	PORTION	CAL	FAT	CARB	SUGAR	FIBER
Tree Of Life						
Organic Firm	½ block (3.2 oz)	110	5	4	0	2
White Wave						
Baked Garlic Herb Italian	1 piece (2 oz)	90	5	2	0	1
Baked Sesame Peanut Thai	1 piece (2 oz)	90	5	2	1	1
Baked Zesty Lemon Pepper	1 piece (2 oz)	90	5	3	1	1
Extra Firm	⅕ block (3.2 oz)	110	6	3	0	1
Organic Extra Firm	⅕ block (3.2 oz)	110	6	3	0	1
Organic Firm	⅓ block (3.2 oz)	110	6	3	0	1
Organic Soft	⅕ block (3.2 oz)	110	6	3	0	1
Reduced Fat	⅕ block (3.2 oz)	90	4	4	1	2
TAKE-OUT						
breaded deep fried w/ soy sauce japanese style	1 piece (0.4 oz)	15	1	1	0	tr
soy sauce marinated & grilled	1 serv (4 oz)	181	11	6	–	1
TOMATILLO						
fresh	1 (1.2 oz)	11	tr	2	1	1
fresh chopped	½ cup (2.3 oz)	21	1	4	3	1
TOMATO						
CANNED						
green pickled	½ cup (2.5 oz)	26	tr	6	5	1
green whole pickled	1 (2.6 oz)	27	tr	6	5	1

FOOD	PORTION	CAL	FAT	CARB	SUGAR	FIBER
paste	¼ cup (2.3 oz)	54	tr	12	8	3
paste	1 can (6 oz)	139	1	32	21	7
paste no salt added	1 can (6 oz)	139	1	32	21	7
puree	1 cup (8.8 oz)	95	1	22	12	5
puree	1 can (28 oz)	312	2	74	40	16
puree w/o salt	1 can (28 oz)	312	2	74	40	16
sauce	1 cup (8.6 oz)	59	tr	13	10	4
sauce no salt added	1 cup (8.6 oz)	102	tr	21	13	4
stewed	1 cup (8.9 oz)	66	tr	16	9	3
Cento						
Paste	2 tbsp (1.2 oz)	30	0	7	5	2
Contadina						
Paste Italian Herbs	2 tbsp	35	1	7	4	1
Dei Fratelli						
Chopped Italian Tomatoes	½ cup (4.3 oz)	40	1	8	5	1
Hunt's						
Diced w/ Basil Garlic & Oregano	½ cup	35	0	7	5	2
Paste No Salt Added	2 tbsp (1.2 oz)	30	0	6	4	2
Muir Glen						
Organic Chunky Tomato & Herb	½ cup	60	1	11	5	2
Organic Diced Fire Roasted	½ cup	30	0	6	4	1
Organic Diced w/ Basil & Garlic	½ cup	30	0	6	4	1
Polar						
Grape	½ cup	50	0	12	11	2
Progresso						
Crushed w/ Added Puree	¼ cup (2.1 oz)	20	0	4	2	1
Diced	½ cup (4.4 oz)	25	0	5	3	1

FOOD	PORTION	CAL	FAT	CARB	SUGAR	FIBER
Puree	¼ cup (2.2 oz)	25	0	5	3	1
Whole Peeled w/ Basil	½ cup (4.2 oz)	20	0	4	3	1
Redpack						
Crushed In Puree	¼ cup	20	0	4	2	1
S&W						
Crushed	¼ cup (2.1 oz)	20	0	4	2	1
Paste	2 tbsp (1.2 oz)	30	0	6	3	1
Petite Cut	½ cup (4.4 oz)	25	0	6	4	2
Puree	¼ cup (2.2 oz)	30	0	6	3	2
Ready-Cut Italian Recipe	½ cup (4.2 oz)	25	0	4	4	tr
Ready-Cut No Salt Added	½ cup (4.4 oz)	25	0	6	4	2
Stewed No Salt Added	½ cup (4.4 oz)	35	0	9	7	2
Stewed Original	½ cup (4.3 oz)	35	0	7	5	2
Whole Peeled	½ cup (4.4 oz)	25	0	6	4	2
DRIED						
sun dried	¼ cup (0.5 oz)	35	tr	8	5	2
sun dried	1 piece (2 g)	5	tr	1	1	tr
sun dried in oil drained	¼ cup (1 oz)	59	4	6	–	2
sun dried in oil drained	1 piece (3 g)	6	tr	1	–	tr
tomato powder	1 oz	85	tr	21	12	5
FRESH						
bruschetta	¼ cup	50	3	6	4	tr
cherry	1 (0.6 oz)	3	tr	1	tr	tr
cherry	½ cup (2.6 oz)	13	tr	3	2	1
grape tomatoes	20	30	0	6	4	1
green	1 sm (3.2 oz)	21	tr	5	4	1
green	1 med (4.3 oz)	28	tr	6	5	1
green	1 lg (6.4 oz)	42	tr	9	7	2
green chopped	1 cup (6.3 oz)	41	tr	9	7	2
orange	1 (4 oz)	18	tr	4	–	1
orange chopped	1 cup (5.5 oz)	25	tr	5	–	1
plum	1 (2.2 oz)	11	tr	2	2	1

FOOD	PORTION	CAL	FAT	CARB	SUGAR	FIBER
red	1 lg (6.4 oz)	33	tr	7	5	2
red	1 sm (3.2 oz)	16	tr	4	2	1
red	1 med (4.3 oz)	22	tr	5	3	2
red chopped	½ cup (3.2 oz)	16	tr	4	2	1
red slice	1 lg (0.9 oz)	5	tr	1	1	tr
roma	1 (2.2 oz)	11	tr	2	2	1
yellow	1 (7.4 oz)	32	1	6	–	2
yellow chopped	½ cup (2.4 oz)	10	tr	2	–	1
TAKE-OUT						
aspic	½ cup (4 oz)	32	tr	6	5	tr
broiled slices	2 (2.9 oz)	18	tr	4	3	1
broiled whole	1 med (3.7 oz)	23	tr	5	3	2
bruschetta on toasted italian bread	1 slice	106	3	18	2	tr
fried slices	2 (2.5 oz)	122	9	8	2	1
scalloped	½ cup (4 oz)	99	5	12	5	1
stewed	½ cup (1.8 oz)	40	1	7	–	1
stuffed w/ rice	1 (5.2 oz)	110	3	20	3	2
stuffed w/ rice & meat	1 (5.2 oz)	142	6	15	3	2
TOMATO JUICE						
tomato juice	1 cup (8.5 oz)	41	tr	10	9	1
tomato juice w/o added salt	1 cup (8.5 oz)	41	tr	10	9	1
Dei Fratelli						
Tomato Juice	8 oz	40	0	10	0	1
Tree Of Life						
Organic 100% Juice	8 oz	50	0	10	10	–
TONGUE						
beef simmered	3 oz	241	19	0	0	0
lamb braised	3 oz	234	17	0	0	0
pork braised	3 oz	230	16	0	0	0
veal braised	3 oz	172	9	0	0	0

FOOD	PORTION	CAL	FAT	CARB	SUGAR	FIBER
Rumba						
Beef	4 oz	250	18	4	0	0
TORTILLA						
corn	1 (6 in diam)	56	1	12	–	1
corn w/o salt	1 (6 in diam)	56	1	12	–	1
flour w/o salt	1 (8 in diam)	114	3	20	–	1
French Meadow Bakery						
Fat Flush	1 (1 oz)	100	1	18	1	3
Gluten Free	1 (1.5 oz)	120	1	24	1	1
Hemp	1 (1.1 oz)	90	3	12	1	3
La Tortilla Factory						
Smart & Delicious Low Fat Low Sodium	1 (2.5 oz)	150	2	32	1	6
Salba Smart						
Whole Wheat Omega-3 Enriched	1 (1.5 oz)	120	3	21	1	2
TRAIL MIX						
Back To Nature						
Bar Harbor Blend	1 oz	130	7	17	14	2
Harvest Blend	1 oz	150	10	12	7	3
Nantucket Blend	1 oz	130	7	15	11	3
Pacific Heights Blend	1 oz	160	11	13	9	3
Kopali						
Organic Mix	½ pkg (1 oz)	130	6	15	7	4
Mrs. May's						
Coconut Almond Crunch	1 oz	183	15	10	6	2
TORTILLA CHIPS (see CHIPS)						
TREE FERN						
chopped cooked	½ cup	28	tr	8	–	–
TRIPE						
beef simmered	3 oz	80	3	2	0	0

FOOD	PORTION	CAL	FAT	CARB	SUGAR	FIBER
Rumba						
Beef Tripe	4 oz	110	5	0	0	0
TAKE-OUT						
mondongo w/ potatoes	1 cup	300	11	26	5	6
TRITICALE						
dry	½ cup (3.4 oz)	323	2	69	–	–
TROUT						
baked	3 oz	162	7	0	0	0
rainbow cooked	3 oz	129	4	0	0	0
seatrout baked	3 oz	113	4	0	0	0
TRUFFLES						
fresh	0.5 oz	4	tr	9	–	2
Aux Delices Des Bois						
Black Truffle Butter	0.5 oz	90	10	0	0	0
TUNA						
CANNED						
light in oil	3 oz	169	7	0	0	0
light in oil	1 can (6 oz)	399	14	0	0	0
light in water	1 can (5.8 oz)	192	1	0	0	0
light in water	3 oz	99	1	0	0	0
white in oil	1 can (6.2 oz)	331	14	0	0	0
white in oil	3 oz	158	7	0	0	0
white in water	1 can (6 oz)	234	4	0	0	0
white in water	3 oz	116	2	0	0	0
Bumble Bee						
Solid White Albacore In Water	¼ cup (2 oz)	60	1	0	0	0
Chicken Of The Sea						
Chunk White Albacore In Water	¼ cup (2 oz)	50	1	0	0	0

FOOD	PORTION	CAL	FAT	CARB	SUGAR	FIBER
Polar						
Albacore Solid White In Water	2 oz	70	1	0	0	0
Chunk Light In Water	2 oz	60	1	0	0	0
Progresso						
Albacore Solid White Olive Oil	¼ cup (2 oz)	90	3	0	0	0
Solid Light Olive Oil drained	¼ cup (2 oz)	120	6	0	0	0
StarKist						
Chunk Light In Water	¼ cup (2 oz)	60	5	0	0	0
Chunk Light In Water Flavor Pouch	1 pkg (3 oz)	90	1	0	0	0
Low Sodium Chunk White In Water	¼ cup (2 oz)	60	1	0	0	0
Solid Light In Water	2 oz	60	1	0	0	0
Solid White Albacore In Water	2 oz	70	1	0	0	0
Tuna Creations Hickory Smoked Flavor Pouch	2 oz	60	1	0	0	0
Tree Of Life						
Wild Light Tongol Chunk In Spring Water No Salt Added	¼ cup (2.4 oz)	50	0	0	0	0
FRESH						
bluefin cooked	3 oz	157	5	0	0	0
bluefin raw	3 oz	122	4	0	0	0
skipjack baked	3 oz	112	1	0	0	0
yellowfin baked	3 oz	118	1	0	0	0
MIX						
StarKist						
Lunch To-Go Chunk Light	1 pkg	310	9	27	8	2

FOOD	PORTION	CAL	FAT	CARB	SUGAR	FIBER
Tuna Helper						
Creamy Broccoli as prep	1 cup	310	11	39	2	2
Creamy Pasta as prep	1 cup	320	12	39	2	1
Tetrazzini as prep	1 cup	290	10	33	2	1
TAKE-OUT						
tuna salad	1 cup	383	19	19	–	–
TURBOT						
european baked	3 oz	104	3	0	0	0
TURKEY (see also JERKY, TURKEY DISHES)						
CANNED						
w/ broth	1 cup	220	9	0	0	0
Hormel						
Chunk White & Dark	2 oz	70	3	0	0	0
Premium Chunk White	2 oz	60	2	0	0	0
FRESH						
breast pre-basted w/ skin roasted	3.5 oz	126	3	0	0	0
breast roasted w/ skin	4 oz	212	8	0	0	0
breast roasted w/o skin	4 oz	212	4	0	0	0
dark meat w/o skin roasted	1 cup (5 oz)	262	10	0	0	0
dark meat w/o skin roasted	3 oz	170	7	0	0	0
ground cooked	3 oz	193	11	0	0	0
leg w/ skin roasted	1 (19 oz)	1136	54	0	0	0
light meat w/ skin roasted half turkey	2.3 lbs	2069	87	0	0	0
light meat w/o skin roasted	4 oz	183	4	0	0	0
neck simmered	1 (5.3 oz)	274	11	0	0	0
skin roasted	1 oz	141	13	0	0	0

FOOD	PORTION	CAL	FAT	CARB	SUGAR	FIBER
skin roasted from half turkey	8.7 oz	1096	98	0	0	0
tail cooked	1 (2 oz)	197	16	0	0	0
w/ skin roasted	1 serv (4.2 oz)	249	12	0	0	0
w/ skin roasted	½ turkey (4 lbs)	3857	181	0	0	0
w/o skin roasted	1 cup (5 oz)	238	7	0	0	0
w/o skin roasted	1 serv (3.7 oz)	177	5	0	0	0
wing w/ skin roasted	1 (6.5 oz)	426	23	0	0	0
wing w/o skin roasted	1	237	5	0	0	0
Butterball						
Burger Patties	1 (4 oz)	150	8	0	0	0
Cutlets	4 oz	120	1	0	0	0
Drumstick	4 oz	170	8	0	0	0
Ground 7% Fat	4 oz	150	8	0	0	0
Ground White	4 oz	130	4	0	0	0
Strips	4 oz	120	1	0	0	0
Thighs	4 oz	170	8	0	0	0
Wings	1 (6.3 oz)	380	25	0	0	0
Empire						
Gound White	4 oz	160	8	0	0	0
Perdue						
Breast Fillets Boneless Skinless cooked	3 oz	110	1	0	0	0
Drumsticks roasted	3 oz	140	7	0	0	0
Ground Breast cooked	3 oz	110	1	0	0	0
Patties cooked	1 (3 oz)	160	8	0	0	0
Whole Breast cooked	3 oz	170	8	0	0	0
Whole Dark Meat cooked	3 oz	190	11	0	0	0
Whole White Meat roasted	3 oz	150	7	0	0	0

FOOD	PORTION	CAL	FAT	CARB	SUGAR	FIBER
Shady Brook						
Tenderloin Zesty Italian Herb	4 oz	130	4	4	2	0
FROZEN						
roast boneless seasoned light & dark meat roasted	3.5 oz	155	6	3	0	0
sticks breaded fried	1 (2.2 oz)	179	11	11	–	–
Butterball						
Boneless Roast	4 oz	130	5	0	0	0
Breast Boneless Roast	4 oz	110	3	1	0	0
Breast Tenderloin Teriyaki	4 oz	110	1	4	3	–
Breast Whole	4 oz	110	3	1	1	0
Breast Whole Smoked Cooked	3 oz	120	5	1	1	0
Whole Turkey	1 serv (4 oz)	170	10	0	0	0
Whole Turkey Baked	3 oz	130	7	0	0	0
READY-TO-EAT						
bologna	1 slice (1 oz)	59	4	1	1	tr
breast	1 slice (0.7 oz)	22	tr	1	1	tr
ham	1 slice (1 oz)	35	1	1	tr	tr
pastrami	2 oz	70	2	2	2	tr
salami	1 slice (1 oz)	48	3	tr	tr	0
Applegate Farms						
Organic Herb	2 oz	50	1	0	0	0
Butterball						
Breast Honey Roasted Thick Sliced	1 slice (1 oz)	35	1	2	1	0
Breast Oven Roasted Extra Thin Slice	7 slices (2 oz)	70	2	3	2	0
Breast Smoked Thin Sliced	4 slices (1.9 oz)	70	2	4	2	0

FOOD	PORTION	CAL	FAT	CARB	SUGAR	FIBER
Breast Strips Oven Roasted	½ pkg (3 oz)	90	1	2	–	–
Deep Fried Original Thick Sliced	1 slice (1 oz)	30	1	1	0	0
Carl Buddig						
Honey Roasted Sliced	2 oz	90	5	2	–	–
Turkey Sliced	2 oz	90	5	tr	–	–
Healthy Ones						
Oven Roasted 97% Fat Free	7 slices (2 oz)	60	2	2	tr	–
Hormel						
Natural Choice Deli Turkey Honey	4 slices (2 oz)	60	1	3	3	0
Natural Choice Deli Turkey Oven Roasted	4 slices (2 oz)	60	1	3	3	0
Natural Choice Deli Turkey Smoked	4 slices (2 oz)	60	1	3	3	0
Oscar Mayer						
Breast Smoked Shaved	2 oz	50	1	2	0	0
Sara Lee						
Breast Cracked Pepper	4 slices (1.8 oz)	50	1	1	0	0

TURKEY DISHES
FROZEN

FOOD	PORTION	CAL	FAT	CARB	SUGAR	FIBER
gravy & turkey	1 cup (8.4 oz)	160	6	11	–	–

TAKE-OUT

FOOD	PORTION	CAL	FAT	CARB	SUGAR	FIBER
boneless breast w/ cranberry apple stuffing	1 serv (5 oz)	260	9	10	2	1
turkey tetrazzini	1 cup	369	18	29	2	2
turkey a la king	1 cup (8.5 oz)	465	34	16	4	1
turkey creole w/o rice	1 cup	189	4	9	5	2
turkey croquette	1 (2 oz)	158	9	8	2	tr
turkey divan	1 cup	321	14	9	2	3

FOOD	PORTION	CAL	FAT	CARB	SUGAR	FIBER
turkey fricassee	1 cup	322	18	8	tr	tr
turkey meatloaf	1 lg slice (5 oz)	243	9	11	3	1
turkey salad	1 cup	417	32	3	1	1

TURMERIC

ground	1 tsp	8	tr	1	tr	tr

TURNIPS

canned greens	½ cup	17	tr	3	–	–
cooked mashed	½ cup (4.2 oz)	47	tr	10	–	–
cubed cooked	½ cup (3 oz)	33	tr	7	–	–
fresh greens chopped cooked	½ cup	15	tr	3	–	2
frzn greens cooked	½ cup	24	tr	4	–	2
greens raw chopped	½ cup	7	tr	2	–	1
raw cubed	½ cup (2.4 oz)	25	tr	6	–	–
Allens						
Seasoned	½ cup	35	1	5	1	2

TURTLE

raw	3.5 oz	85	1	0	0	0

TUSK FISH

raw	3.5 oz	79	tr	0	0	0

VANILLA

vanilla extract	1 tsp (4.2 g)	12	0	1	1	0
vanilla extract	1 tbsp (0.5 oz)	37	tr	2	2	0
vanilla extract alcohol free	1 tsp (4.2 g)	2	0	1	1	0

VEAL (see also VEAL DISHES)

breast braised	3 oz	226	14	0	0	0
chop cooked	1 med (6.5 oz)	230	13	0	0	0

FOOD	PORTION	CAL	FAT	CARB	SUGAR	FIBER
chop breaded fried	1 med (6.5 oz)	290	12	13	0	tr
cubed braised	3 oz	160	4	0	0	0
cutlet cooked	3 oz	141	4	0	0	0
ground broiled	3 oz	146	6	0	0	0
leg roasted	3 oz	136	4	0	0	0
loin roasted	3 oz	184	10	0	0	0
patty breaded fried	1 (2.8 oz)	211	13	7	1	tr
shank braised	3 oz	162	5	0	0	0

VEAL DISHES
TAKE-OUT

FOOD	PORTION	CAL	FAT	CARB	SUGAR	FIBER
cordon bleu	1 serv (8 oz)	490	35	4	2	1
parmigiana	1 serv (6.4 oz)	362	21	15	3	2
scallopini	1 slice + sauce	238	17	2	1	tr
stew	1 serv (3.4 oz)	192	6	18	4	3
veal marengo	1 serv (8.8 oz)	274	9	7	3	1
veal marsala	1 slice + sauce (3.4 oz)	268	19	6	2	tr
veal paprikash	1 serv (8.6 oz)	280	12	5	1	1
veal picatta	1 piece + sauce	154	9	2	tr	tr

VEGETABLE JUICE

FOOD	PORTION	CAL	FAT	CARB	SUGAR	FIBER
low sodium tomato & vegetable juice	1 cup (3.5 oz)	53	tr	11	9	2
vegetable juice cocktail	8 oz	46	tr	11	8	2

FOOD	PORTION	CAL	FAT	CARB	SUGAR	FIBER
Dei Fratelli						
Vegetable Juice	8 oz	45	2	11	9	1
Green To Go						
100% Natural Organic as prep	1 pkg (0.3 oz)	32	tr	6	1	tr
Mott's						
100% Juice Veggie Blend	1 bottle (14 oz)	90	1	15	9	4
V8						
High Fiber	8 oz	60	0	13	8	5
Low Sodium	8 oz	50	0	10	8	2
Vegetable Juice	8 oz	50	0	10	–	2

VEGETABLES MIXED
CANNED

FOOD	PORTION	CAL	FAT	CARB	SUGAR	FIBER
mixed vegetables	½ cup	39	tr	8	–	–
peas & carrots	½ cup	48	tr	11	–	–
peas & onions	½ cup	30	tr	5	–	–
succotash	½ cup	102	1	23	–	–
McSweet						
Giardiniera	5 pieces (1 oz)	25	0	6	5	tr
S&W						
Mixed	½ cup (4.4 oz)	45	0	10	3	2
Peas & Pearl Onions	½ cup (4.3 oz)	40	0	11	1	3
The Gracious Gourmet						
Tapenade Fennel Blood Orange	2 tbsp (1 oz)	50	5	3	1	tr
Veg-All						
Original Mixed	½ cup	40	0	8	2	2
DRIED						
Fun-Yums						
Fresh Crispy Mixed Veggies	1 serv (0.9 oz)	114	4	18	2	1

FOOD	PORTION	CAL	FAT	CARB	SUGAR	FIBER
FRESH						
Mann's						
Broccoli & Cauliflower	1 serv (3 oz)	25	0	4	2	2
California Stir Fry	1 serv (3 oz)	30	0	6	3	2
Medley	1 serv (3 oz)	25	0	5	3	2
Veggies On The Go w/ Dip	1 cup + 1 tbsp dip	100	8	7	4	2
FROZEN						
mixed vegetables cooked	½ cup	54	tr	12	–	2
peas & carrots cooked	½ cup	38	tr	8	–	–
peas & onions cooked	½ cup	40	tr	8	–	–
succotash cooked	½ cup	79	1	17	–	–
Birds Eye						
Asparagus Gold & White Corn & Baby Carrots	⅔ cup	70	1	13	4	1
Steamfresh Asian Medley	1 cup (3.3 oz)	50	2	6	3	2
Steamfresh Broccoli Cauliflower & Carrots	¾ cup	30	0	5	2	2
Steamfresh Broccoli & Cauliflower	1 cup	30	0	4	2	2
Steamfresh Broccoli Carrots Sugar Snap Peas & Water Chestnuts	¾ cup (2.9 oz)	35	0	6	3	2
Steamfresh Mixed Vegetables	⅔ cup (3.2 oz)	40	0	12	4	2
Cascadian Farm						
Organic Peas & Carrots	⅔ cup	50	0	10	4	3
Organic Mixed Vegetables	⅔ cup	60	0	12	4	2

FOOD	PORTION	CAL	FAT	CARB	SUGAR	FIBER
French Meadow Bakery						
Vegetarian Sweet N' Spicy Cuban Style Veggies	1 pkg (12 oz)	250	9	39	9	7
Green Giant						
Garden Vegetable Medley as prep	½ cup	70	1	14	3	2
Mixed Vegetables as prep	½ cup	50	0	11	3	2
Szechuan Vegetables as prep	½ cup	50	1	9	5	2
Health Is Wealth						
Veggie Munchees Vegan	6 (3 oz)	150	4	26	2	3
La Choy						
Chop Suey Vegetables	½ cup (2.2 oz)	15	0	3	1	tr
Fancy Chinese Mixed Vegetables	½ cup (2.9 oz)	15	2	3	0	1
Stir Fry Vegetables	½ cup	15	0	3	1	2
Seapoint Farms						
Organic Veggie Blends w/ Edamame	¾ cup	60	2	7	tr	3
Eat Your Greens						
Veggie Blends w/ Edamame Garden	¾ cup	60	2	7	2	3
Veggie Blends w/ Edamame Oriental	¾ cup	60	1	8	2	3
TAKE-OUT						
buddha's delight	1 serv (16 oz)	174	5	17	8	3
pakoras	4 (1.7 oz)	57	2	7	1	2
ratatouille	1 serv (3.5 oz)	96	7	7	7	4
samosa	1 (2.4 oz)	206	11	22	1	2
stir fry mixed vegetables	1 serv (4 oz)	66	5	3	2	2
succotash	½ cup	111	1	23	–	–

FOOD	PORTION	CAL	FAT	CARB	SUGAR	FIBER
tapenade grilled vegetables	¼ cup	40	3	4	2	tr

VENISON (see also JERKY)

FOOD	PORTION	CAL	FAT	CARB	SUGAR	FIBER
roasted	4 oz	215	4	0	0	0

VINEGAR

FOOD	PORTION	CAL	FAT	CARB	SUGAR	FIBER
balsamic	1 tbsp	14	0	3	2	–
cider	1 tbsp	3	0	tr	tr	0
red wine	1 tbsp	3	0	tr	0	0
white	1 tbsp	3	0	tr	tr	0
Barengo						
Balsamic	1 tbsp (0.5 oz)	15	0	4	4	–
Red Wine	1 tbsp (0.5 oz)	0	0	0	0	0
Gedney						
Apple Cider	1 tbsp	3	0	0	0	0
Distilled White	1 tbsp	3	0	0	0	0
Gourme Mist						
Balsamic Of Modena	1 sec spray	1	0	0	0	0
Balsamic Vinegar + Raspberry	1 sec spray	1	0	0	0	0
Holland House						
Malt	1 tbsp (0.5 oz)	0	0	0	0	0
Red Wine	1 tbsp (0.5 oz)	0	0	0	0	0
Lucini						
Balsamic 10 Year Gran Reserve	1 tbsp (0.5 oz)	20	0	4	4	–
Balsamic Dark Cherry Infused	1 tbsp	30	0	7	7	–
Italian Wine Pinot Noir	1 tbsp (0.5 oz)	tr	0	0	0	0
Mitsukan						
Rice	1 tbsp (0.5 oz)	0	0	0	0	0
Rice Seasoned	1 tbsp (0.5 oz)	25	0	5	5	–

FOOD	PORTION	CAL	FAT	CARB	SUGAR	FIBER
Nakano						
Natural Rice	1 tbsp (0.5 oz)	0	0	0	0	0
Red Wine Italian Herb Seasoned	1 tbsp (0.5 oz)	20	0	5	5	–
Rice Pesto Seasoned	1 tbsp (0.5 oz)	20	0	5	5	–
Rice Red Pepper Seasoned	1 tbsp (0.5 oz)	20	0	5	5	–
Progresso						
Balsamic	2 tbsp (0.5 oz)	10	0	2	–	–
Tree Of Life						
Organic Apple Cider Raw Unfiltered	1 tbsp	0	0	tr	–	–
WAFFLES						
FROZEN						
Van's						
Belgian Multigrain	2 (2.7 oz)	190	8	25	3	4
Mini Homestyle	4 (2.8 oz)	210	8	32	6	1
Organic Flax	2 (2.7 oz)	190	9	24	3	3
Organic Homestyle	2 (2.7 oz)	200	9	25	3	2
Original 97% Fat Free	2 (2.7 oz)	140	2	26	4	3
Original Buttermilk	2 (2.7 oz)	220	9	31	6	1
Wheat Free Buckwheat	2 (3 oz)	230	9	36	5	2
Wheat Free Flax	2 (3 oz)	210	8	33	4	1
MIX						
plain as prep 7 in diam	1 (2.6 oz)	218	11	25	–	–
TAKE-OUT						
belgian	1 (4.7 oz)	412	13	65	6	3
blueberry 9 in sq	1 (7 oz)	556	16	90	12	5
round 10 in diam	1 (6.8 oz)	598	18	94	9	5
square	1 (7 oz) 9 in	620	19	98	9	5
whole wheat 9 in sq	1 (7 oz)	534	22	67	15	5

FOOD	PORTION	CAL	FAT	CARB	SUGAR	FIBER
WALNUTS						
black chopped	¼ cup	193	18	3	tr	2
english chopped	¼ cup	191	19	4	1	2
english ground	¼ cup	131	13	3	1	1
english halves	14 (1 oz)	185	18	4	1	2
english in shell	7 (1 oz)	183	18	4	1	2
honey roasted	¼ cup	172	16	7	4	2
Back To Nature						
Unroasted Unsalted	1 oz	190	18	4	1	2
WASABI (*see* HORSERADISH)						
WATER						
ice cubes	3	0	0	0	0	0
tap water	8 oz	0	0	0	0	0
Acquafibre						
Fiber Enhanced All Flavors	1 bottle (11.15 oz)	5	0	0	0	5
Adirondack						
Sparkling All Flavors	8 oz	0	0	0	0	0
Aqua Pacific						
Water	1 liter	0	0	0	0	0
Bot						
Fortified All Flavors	1 bottle (12 oz)	40	0	10	9	0
Dox						
Cardio Water	1 bottle (12 oz)	20	0	5	5	–
Evian						
Spring Water	1 liter	0	0	0	0	0
Fiji						
Natural Artesian	1 liter	0	0	0	0	0
Gerolsteiner						
Sparkling Mineral	8 oz	0	0	0	0	0

FOOD	PORTION	CAL	FAT	CARB	SUGAR	FIBER
H 10 O						
Citrus Sport For Men	1 bottle (15.9 oz)	0	0	0	0	0
Peach Mango Tea For Women	1 bottle (15.9 oz)	0	0	0	0	0
Hawaiian Springs						
Naturally Pure	1 liter	0	0	0	0	0
Highland Spring						
Spring Water	1 liter	0	0	0	0	0
Island Chill						
Artesian Water	1 liter	0	0	0	0	0
Jana						
Natural European Artesian	1 liter	0	0	0	0	0
Joint Juice						
Fitness Water All Flavors	1 bottle (18 oz)	10	0	1	–	–
Klear Splash						
Mini Sip	1 pkg (4 oz)	0	0	0	0	0
Life Water						
B-Strong	1 bottle (20 oz)	100	0	42	25	–
Enlighten	1 bottle (20 oz)	100	0	41	24	–
Zingseng	1 bottle (20 oz)	100	0	41	24	–
O Water						
Hydrate Black Raspberry	8 oz	25	0	7	7	0
Replenish Lemon Lime	8 oz	25	0	7	7	0
Vitalize Peach Mango	8 oz	25	0	7	7	0
San Benedetto						
Sparkling Mineral Water	1 liter	0	0	0	0	0

FOOD	PORTION	CAL	FAT	CARB	SUGAR	FIBER
Skinny Water						
Hi-Energy Acai Grape Blueberry	8 oz	0	0	0	0	0
Total-V Passionfruit Lemonade	8 oz	0	0	0	0	0
Snapple						
Antioxidant Water Awaken Dragonfruit	8 oz	50	0	12	12	–
Antioxidant Water Restore Agave Melon	8 oz	60	0	13	13	–
Lyte Water	8 oz	0	0	0	0	–
SoNu						
Water All Flavors	8 oz	45	0	13	13	0
Trim Water						
Purified	1 bottle (20 oz)	10	0	3	3	0
Twist						
Organics All Flavors	8 oz	10	0	2	2	0
Vitamin + Fiber Water						
All Fruit Flavors	8 oz	50	0	13	12	3
VitaminWater						
XXX Acai Blueberry Pomegranate	8 oz	50	0	13	13	–
WATER CHESTNUTS						
chinese sliced canned	½ cup	35	tr	9	–	–
fresh sliced	½ cup	66	tr	15	–	–
La Choy						
Sliced	½ cup	25	0	5	2	1
Polar						
Sliced	2 tbsp	10	0	3	1	1
WATERCRESS						
cooked w/o fat	1 cup	15	tr	2	tr	1
raw chopped	1 cup	4	tr	tr	tr	tr

FOOD	PORTION	CAL	FAT	CARB	SUGAR	FIBER
WATERMELON						
cut up	1 cup	46	tr	12	10	1
seeds dried	¼ cup	150	13	4	–	–
wedge	1 lg (20 oz)	172	1	43	35	2
wedge	1 med (10 oz)	86	tr	22	18	1
wedge	1 sm (2.5 oz)	21	tr	5	4	tr
whole melon	1 (9 lb)	1227	6	309	254	16
WATERMELON JUICE						
juice	8 oz	71	tr	18	15	1
WHALE						
beluga dried	1 oz	93	2	0	0	0
beluga raw	3.5 oz	111	1	0	0	0
WHEAT						
sprouted	1 cup (3.8 oz)	214	1	46	–	1
starch	3.5 oz	348	tr	86	–	–
Amazing Grass						
Organic Wheat Grass	1 tbsp (0.3 oz)	35	0	4	–	2
Near East						
Taboule Wheat Salad as prep	⅔ cup (3.5 oz)	120	3	24	1	5
White Wave						
Seitan Chicken Meat Of Wheat	3 oz	130	0	9	0	3
Seitan Traditional	3 oz	90	1	3	0	1
Seitan Vegetarian Stir Fry Strips	3 oz	110	2	2	0	1
WHEAT GERM						
plain	¼ cup	108	3	14	2	4
Kretschmer						
Original Toasted	¼ cup (0.6 oz)	35	1	10	–	7

FOOD	PORTION	CAL	FAT	CARB	SUGAR	FIBER
Tree Of Life						
Toasted	3 tbsp (0.8 oz)	100	3	12	3	3
WHEY						
acid dry	1 tbsp	10	tr	2	2	0
sweet dry	1 tbsp	26	tr	6	6	0
sweet fluid	½ cup	33	tr	6	6	0
whey cheese	1 oz	126	8	9	0	0
Action Whey						
Dream Shake All Flavors	1 scoop (0.8 oz)	90	3	3	2	1
WHIPPED TOPPINGS						
cream pressurized	1 cup (2.1 oz)	154	13	7	–	–
cream pressurized	1 tbsp (3 g)	8	tr	tr	–	–
nondairy frzn	1 tbsp	13	1	1	–	–
nondairy powdered as prep w/ whole milk	1 cup	151	10	13	–	–
nondairy pressurized	1 cup	184	16	11	–	–
nondairy pressurized	1 tbsp (4 g)	11	1	1	–	–
Cool Whip						
Chocolate	2 tbsp	25	2	2	2	–
Free	2 tbsp	15	0	3	1	–
Regular	2 tbsp	25	2	2	1	–
Strawberry	2 tbsp	25	2	2	1	–
TruWhip						
Whipped Topping	2 tbsp (0.4 oz)	130	2	3	2	0
WHITE BEANS						
canned	1 cup	306	1	58	–	–
dried regular cooked	1 cup	249	1	45	–	–
dried small cooked	1 cup	253	1	46	–	–

FOOD	PORTION	CAL	FAT	CARB	SUGAR	FIBER
WHITEFISH						
baked	3 oz	146	6	0	0	0
smoked	3 oz	92	1	0	0	0
smoked	1 oz	39	tr	0	0	0
WHITING						
broiled w/o fat	3 oz	99	1	0	0	0
fillet broiled w/o fat	1 (2.5 oz)	84	1	0	0	0
fillet steamed w/o fat	1 (2.6 oz)	84	1	0	0	0
hake raw	3.5 oz	84	1	0	0	0
TAKE-OUT						
fillet battered & fried	1 (3.1 oz)	157	7	6	tr	tr
fillet breaded & fried	1 (3.1 oz)	191	10	7	1	tr
WILD RICE						
cooked	1 cup (5.8 oz)	166	1	35	1	3
WINE						
chianti	1 serv (5 oz)	125	0	4	1	0
chinese cooking	1 bottle (15 oz)	559	0	3	0	0
cooking	¼ cup (2 oz)	29	0	4	1	0
haiku	1 serv	93	0	3	–	0
japanese plum	3 oz	139	tr	16	–	0
japanese sake	2 oz	78	0	3	0	0
kir	1 serv	78	0	3	–	0
madeira	3.5 oz	169	0	10	10	0
muscat	1 serv (5 oz)	123	0	8	–	–
nonalcoholic	1 serv (5 oz)	9	0	2	2	0
port	1 serv (3.5 oz)	165	0	14	8	0
red barbera	1 serv (5 oz)	125	0	4	–	–
red burgundy	1 serv (5 oz)	127	0	5	–	–
red cabernet franc	1 serv (5 oz)	122	0	4	–	–
red claret	1 serv (5 oz)	122	0	4	–	–
red gamay	1 serv (5 oz)	115	0	4	–	–

FOOD	PORTION	CAL	FAT	CARB	SUGAR	FIBER
red mouvedre	1 serv (5 oz)	129	0	4	–	–
red pinot noir	1 serv (5 oz)	121	0	3	–	–
red syrah	1 serv (5 oz)	122	0	4	–	–
red zinfandel	1 serv (5 oz)	129	0	4	–	–
sake screwdriver	1 serv	175	tr	23	–	tr
sangria	1 serv	88	tr	6	–	tr
sangria blanco	1 serv	155	tr	24	–	3
sherry	2 oz	84	0	5	–	–
vermouth dry	3.5 oz	105	0	1	–	–
vermouth sweet	3.5 oz	167	0	12	–	–
wassail wine	1 serv	142	tr	22	–	2
white	1 serv (5 oz)	121	0	4	1	0
white fume blanc	1 serv (5 oz)	121	0	3	–	–
white pinot blanc	1 serv (5 oz)	119	0	3	–	–
white pinot grigio	1 serv (5 oz)	122	0	3	–	–
white riesling	1 serv (5 oz)	118	0	6	–	–
white sauvignon blanc	1 serv (5 oz)	119	0	3	–	–
wine cooler	1 (7 oz)	116	tr	14	11	0
wine spritzer	1 serv (7 oz)	73	0	2	1	0
Almanden						
Merlot	5 oz	115	0	5	–	–
Bartles & Jaymes						
Wine Cooler Classic Original	1 bottle (12 oz)	190	0	29	–	–
Beringer						
Chardonnay	5 oz	125	0	0	–	–
Carlo Rossi						
Cabernet Sauvignon	5 oz	125	0	5	0	0
Franzia Vinter						
Select Merlot	5 oz	105	0	0	–	–
Holland House						
Cooking Wine Marsala	2 tbsp (1 oz)	45	0	4	4	–
Cooking Wine Red	2 tbsp (1 oz)	20	0	1	0	–

FOOD	PORTION	CAL	FAT	CARB	SUGAR	FIBER
Cooking Wine Sherry	2 tbsp (1 oz)	45	0	2	2	–
Cooking Wine Vermouth	2 tbsp (1 oz)	35	0	2	2	–
Cooking Wine White	2 tbsp (1 oz)	20	0	0	0	0
Twin Valley						
Cabernet Sauvignon	5 oz	120	0	5	–	–

WINGED BEANS

dried cooked w/o salt	1 cup	253	10	26	–	3

WRAPS (see BREAD, SANDWICHES)

YAM (see also SWEET POTATO)
CANNED
S&W

Candied	½ cup (4.9 oz)	170	0	46	21	4

FRESH

mountain yam hawaii cooked w/o salt	1 cup	119	tr	29	–	–
yam cooked w/o salt	1 cup	158	tr	38	1	5
House						
Black Ita Konnyaku Yam Cake	1 serv (2 oz)	5	0	1	0	tr

YARDLONG BEANS

sliced cooked w/o salt	1 cup	49	tr	10	–	–

YAUTIA (see MALANGA)

YEAST

baker's compressed	1 cake (0.6 oz)	18	tr	3	0	1
baker's dry	1 tbsp	35	1	5	0	3
baker's dry	1 pkg (7 g)	21	tr	3	0	2
brewer's dry	1 tbsp	35	1	5	0	3

YELLOW BEANS

fresh cooked w/o salt	1 cup	44	tr	10	2	4
fresh raw	1 cup	34	tr	8	–	4

FOOD	PORTION	CAL	FAT	CARB	SUGAR	FIBER
YELLOWTAIL						
baked	4 oz	199	7	0	0	0
YOGURT (*see also* YOGURT DRINKS, YOGURT FROZEN)						
plain lowfat	8 oz	143	4	16	16	0
plain nonfat	8 oz	127	tr	17	17	0
plain whole milk	8 oz	138	7	11	11	0
tofu yogurt	1 cup	246	5	42	3	1
Better Whey						
All Fruit Flavors	1 pkg (6 oz)	145	1	23	14	3
Plain	1 pkg (6 oz)	130	1	17	7	3
Breyers						
YoCrunch Blueberry w/ Granola	1 pkg	240	3	49	31	2
YoCrunch Cookie N' Cream w/ Oreo	1 pkg	240	6	41	30	0
YoCrunch Naturals Strawberry Banana w/ Granola	1 pkg	245	3	50	31	2
YoCrunch Naturals Strawberry w/ Dark Chocolate Chips	1 pkg	280	9	46	33	2
YoCrunch Raspberry w/ Granola	1 pkg	240	3	49	31	2
YoCrunch Strawberry w/ Granola	1 pkg	240	3	49	31	2
YoCrunch Vanilla Nestle	1 pkg	260	7	44	36	0
YoCrunch Vanilla w/ Butterfinger	1 pkg	260	7	45	34	0
YoCrunch Light Cookies N' Cream w/ Oreo	1 pkg	170	5	24	11	0
YoCrunch Light Strawberry w/ Granola	1 pkg	170	2	33	11	2

FOOD	PORTION	CAL	FAT	CARB	SUGAR	FIBER
Cabot						
Greek	1 pkg (6 oz)	210	17	9	6	0
Greek 2%	1 pkg (6 oz)	160	3	25	24	0
Non Fat Berry Banana	1 cup	130	0	24	19	0
Non Fat Black Cherry	1 cup	130	0	24	19	0
Non Fat French Vanilla	1 cup	130	0	24	19	–
Non Fat Plain	1 cup	100	0	19	13	0
Non Fat Raspberry	1 cup	130	0	24	19	0
Chobani						
Greek Yogurt Blueberry Nonfat	1 pkg (6 oz)	140	0	20	20	tr
Greek Yogurt Honey Nonfat	1 pkg (6 oz)	150	0	20	20	0
Greek Yogurt Peach Nonfat	1 pkg (6 oz)	140	0	20	19	tr
Greek Yogurt Pineapple	1 pkg (6 oz)	160	3	21	18	0
Greek Yogurt Plain Lowfat	1 pkg (6 oz)	130	4	7	7	0
Greek Yogurt Plain Nonfat	1 pkg (6 oz)	100	0	7	7	0
Greek Yogurt Pomegranate Nonfat	1 pkg (6 oz)	140	0	21	19	0
Greek Yogurt Raspberry Nonfat	1 pkg (6 oz)	120	0	22	19	1
Greek Yogurt Strawberry Banana	1 pkg (6 oz)	160	3	19	17	1
Greek Yogurt Strawberry Nonfat	1 pkg (6 oz)	140	0	20	19	tr
Greek Yogurt Vanilla Nonfat	1 pkg (6 oz)	120	0	13	13	0
Dannon						
Light & Fit 0% Fat Plus Vanilla	4 oz	50	0	10	7	–

FOOD	PORTION	CAL	FAT	CARB	SUGAR	FIBER
Fiber One						
Creamy Nonfat Vanilla	1 pkg (4 oz)	80	0	19	10	5
Friendship						
Plain	1 cup	150	3	18	17	1
Land O Lakes						
Strawberry Light	1 pkg (8 oz)	80	0	38	31	0
Strawberry Lowfat	1 pkg (8 oz)	190	2	36	29	0
Nancy's						
Lowfat Maple	1 pkg (8 oz)	180	3	26	26	0
Lowfat Plain	1 pkg (8 oz)	150	3	16	16	0
Lowfat Vanilla	1 pkg (8 oz)	140	3	15	15	0
Nonfat Fruit On The Top Cherry	1 pkg (8 oz)	140	1	25	20	1
Nonfat Plain	1 pkg (8 oz)	120	0	17	17	0
Nonfat Vanilla	1 pkg (8 oz)	220	0	40	39	0
Organic Soy Kiwi Lime	1 pkg (8 oz)	160	3	31	21	4
Organic Soy Plain	1 pkg (8 oz)	150	3	25	15	2
Organic Soy Vanilla	1 pkg (8 oz)	120	3	19	10	3
Whole Milk Fruit On The Top Peach	1 pkg (8 oz)	220	5	38	38	1
Whole Milk Honey	1 pkg (8 oz)	170	8	17	17	0
Oikos						
Organic Honey	1 pkg (5.3 oz)	120	0	18	17	0
Organic Plain	1 pkg (5.3 oz)	90	0	6	6	0
Organic Vanilla	1 pkg (5.3 oz)	110	0	12	11	0
Siggi's						
Icelandic Skyr Vanilla 0% Milkfat	1 pkg (6 oz)	120	0	12	10	0
Silk						
Soy Blueberry	1 pkg (6 oz)	150	2	29	21	1
Soy Key Lime	1 pkg (6 oz)	150	2	30	21	1
Soy Plain	1 cup (8 oz)	150	4	22	12	1
Soy Vanilla	1 pkg (6 oz)	150	3	25	18	1
Strawberry	1 pkg (6 oz)	160	2	31	22	1

FOOD	PORTION	CAL	FAT	CARB	SUGAR	FIBER
SoDelicious						
Coconut Milk Plain	1 pkg (6 oz)	130	7	16	12	3
Coconut Milk Vanilla	1 pkg (6 oz)	150	6	22	19	2
Dairy Free Cinnamon Bun	1 pkg (6 oz)	160	3	29	24	3
Dairy Free Raspberry	1 pkg (6 oz)	150	3	29	22	3
Straus						
Organic Maple Nonfat	1 pkg (8 oz)	170	0	30	22	0
Organic Maple Whole Milk	1 pkg (8 oz)	210	6	28	23	0
Organic Plain Lowfat	1 pkg (8 oz)	150	2	21	10	0
Organic Plain Nonfat	1 pkg (8 oz)	110	0	16	16	0
Organic Plain Whole Milk	1 pkg (8 oz)	160	7	13	9	1
The Greek Gods						
Honey	1 pkg (6 oz)	250	14	23	22	0
Plain Nonfat	1 pkg (6 oz)	60	0	10	7	2
Plain Traditional	1 pkg (4 oz)	130	11	5	5	0
Pomegranate	1 pkg (6 oz)	230	17	14	12	0
Vanilla Cinnamon Orange Reduced Fat	1 pkg (6 oz)	170	6	24	23	0
Yofarm						
YoSmooth Apricot	1 pkg	220	6	36	31	–
YoSmooth Peach	1 pkg	220	6	35	30	–
YoSmooth Raspberry	1 pkg	230	6	36	31	–
YOGURT DRINKS (see also SMOOTHIES)						
lassi	7 oz	78	5	8	8	0
Dahlicious						
Lassi Green Tea	1 bottle	110	0	21	19	2
Lassi Mango	1 bottle	130	0	27	24	2
Lassi Plain	1 bottle	110	0	21	19	2

FOOD	PORTION	CAL	FAT	CARB	SUGAR	FIBER
Promise						
Activ All Flavors	1 bottle (3.5 oz)	70	4	9	8	tr
Yo On The Go						
All Flavors	1 box (8 oz)	180	3	31	29	0
YOGURT FROZEN						
chocolate soft serve	1 cup	230	9	36	–	3
vanilla soft serve	1 cup	236	8	35	35	0
Dippin' Dots						
Strawberry Cheesecake	½ cup	100	0	21	17	1
Haagen-Dazs						
Lowfat Coffee	½ cup (3.7 oz)	200	5	31	20	0
Lowfat Tart Natural	½ cup (3.6 oz)	180	3	30	21	0
Lowfat Vanilla	½ cup (3.7 oz)	200	5	31	21	0
Lowfat Wildberry	½ cup (3.7 oz)	180	2	34	27	0
Turkey Hill						
Fudge Ripple	½ cup	100	0	21	16	0
Neapolitan	½ cup	90	0	19	14	1
Smoothie Orange Cream Swirl	½ cup	100	0	22	18	0
Smoothie Peach Mango	½ cup	90	0	21	17	0
Vanilla Bean	½ cup	100	0	19	14	0
ZUCCHINI						
baby raw	1 (0.5 oz)	3	tr	1	–	tr
canned italian style	1 cup	66	tr	16	–	–
fresh	1 sm (4.1 oz)	19	tr	4	2	1
pickled	¼ cup	16	tr	4	3	1
raw sliced	1 cup	19	tr	4	2	1
sliced cooked w/o salt	1 cup	29	tr	7	3	3

FOOD	PORTION	CAL	FAT	CARB	SUGAR	FIBER
TAKE-OUT						
breaded & fried	6 slices (3 oz)	141	11	10	3	1
indian pakora	1 serv	46	2	7	–	2
sticks breaded & fried	6 (2 oz)	90	7	6	2	1

PART TWO

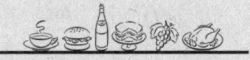

Restaurant Chains

A CUP OF JOE TO GO?

Drinking coffee, decaffeinated or regular, lowers the risk for type 2 diabetes. Research has shown those who drank 4 cups of coffee a day had a 25% lower risk for diabetes than those who drank between zero and 2 cups daily.

FOOD	PORTION	CAL	FAT	CARB	SUGAR	FIBER
A&W						
BEVERAGES						
Coke	1 sm (11 oz)	145	0	37	37	0
Diet Coke	1 sm (11 oz)	0	0	0	0	0
Diet Root Beer	1 sm (15 oz)	0	0	0	0	0
Float Diet Root Beer	1 sm (14 oz)	170	5	30	17	0
Float Root Beer	1 sm (14 oz)	330	5	70	57	0
Milkshake Chocolate	1 med	700	29	100	60	2
Milkshake Strawberry	1 med	670	29	90	52	0
Milkshake Vanilla	1 med	720	31	97	57	0
Root Beer	1 sm (15 oz)	220	0	57	29	0
DESSERTS						
Cone Vanilla	1 med	260	7	41	29	1
Freeze A&W Root Beer	1 med	480	10	89	42	0
Polar Swirl M&M	1 med	710	25	107	93	2
Polar Swirl Oreo	1 med	690	24	107	79	3
Polar Swirl Reese's	1 med	740	31	97	85	3
Sundae Caramel	1 med	340	9	57	13	0
Sundae Chocolate	1 med	320	8	53	15	0
Sundae Hot Fudge	1 med	350	11	54	15	4
Sundae Strawberry	1 med	300	8	47	12	0
Sundae Vanilla	1 med	310	8	52	18	0
MAIN MENU SELECTIONS						
Cheese Curds	1 serv	570	40	27	3	2
Cheese Dog	1	320	20	25	4	1
Cheeseburger Original Bacon	1	570	33	41	9	2
Cheeseburger Original Bacon Double	1	800	48	47	10	2
Cheeseburger Original Double	1	720	42	46	10	2
Chicken Strips	3	500	29	32	2	7
Chili Bowl	1 serv	190	6	22	9	5
Coney Chili Dog	1	310	18	24	5	2

FOOD	PORTION	CAL	FAT	CARB	SUGAR	FIBER
Coney Chili Dog Cheese	1	350	21	27	5	2
Fries	1 lg	430	18	61	1	6
Fries Cheese	1 serv	380	19	50	0	4
Fries Chili	1 serv	370	16	49	2	5
Fries Chili & Cheese	1 serv	400	19	51	2	5
Hot Dog Plain	1	280	17	22	4	1
Onion Rings	1 serv	350	18	45	3	2
Papa Burger	1	720	42	46	10	2
Sandwich Crispy Chicken	1	590	29	54	8	3
Sandwich Grilled Chicken	1	440	19	54	9	2
SAUCES						
Dipping Sauce BBQ	1 serv (1 oz)	40	0	10	6	0
Dipping Sauce Honey Mustard	1 serv (1 oz)	100	6	12	6	0
Dipping Sauce Ranch	1 serv (1 oz)	160	17	2	1	0
Dipping Sauce Sweet & Sour	1 serv (1 oz)	45	0	12	7	0

AU BON PAIN
BAKED SELECTIONS

FOOD	PORTION	CAL	FAT	CARB	SUGAR	FIBER
Bagel Asiago Cheese	1	360	4	64	4	3
Bagel Cinnamon Raisin	1	320	1	67	4	3
Bagel Everything	1	350	5	64	4	3
Bagel Honey 9 Grain	1	330	2	68	4	6
Bagel Jalapeno Double Cheddar	1	350	10	55	4	2
Bagel Onion Dill	1	350	1	72	5	4
Bagel Plain	1	290	1	59	4	2
Bagel Poppy Seed	1	290	1	59	4	2
Bagel Sesame Seed	1	330	5	61	4	3
Baguette Artisan Honey Multigrain Salad Size	1 (3.5 oz)	240	3	47	1	4

FOOD	PORTION	CAL	FAT	CARB	SUGAR	FIBER
Baguette Artisan Honey Multigrain Sandwich Size	1 (4.7 oz)	310	3	62	1	6
Baguette Artisan Salad Size	1 (3.5 oz)	210	1	44	1	2
Baguette Artisan Sandwich Size	1 (4.7 oz)	290	1	59	1	2
Blondie	1	330	19	61	25	3
Bread Artisan Multigrain	1 serv (4 oz)	260	3	51	0	4
Bread Artisan Sundried Tomato	1 serv (4 oz)	240	1	49	2	2
Bread Cheese	1 serv (4.8 oz)	290	8	55	1	3
Bread Country White	1 serv (4 oz)	240	1	50	1	2
Bread Bowl	1 (9.24 oz)	640	3	127	3	6
Bread Stick Rosemary Garlic	1 (2.3 oz)	200	5	33	2	2
Brownie Chocolate Chip	1	380	17	62	41	1
Brownie Hazelnut Mocha	1	430	21	58	31	3
Brownie Rocky Road	1	410	17	62	31	2
Ciabatta	1 sm	180	1	37	2	2
Cinnamon Roll	1	350	12	53	21	2
Cookie Chocolate Chip	1 (2 oz)	260	12	37	22	1
Cookie Confetti	1 (2.4 oz)	310	14	42	25	1
Cookie English Toffee	1 (2 oz)	210	11	26	15	1
Cookie Gingerbread	1 (2.7 oz)	300	9	50	21	1
Cookie Hazelnut Fudge	1 (2.25 oz)	290	16	34	25	3
Cookie Oatmeal Raisin	1 (2 oz)	230	8	36	23	2
Cookie Shortbread	1 (2.3 oz)	310	9	34	10	1
Creme De Fleur	1 serv	550	26	71	32	1
Croissant Almond	1	560	36	52	16	4
Croissant Apple	1	230	10	31	11	2
Croissant Chocolate	1	330	17	42	16	3
Croissant Plain	1 (2.8 oz)	260	15	28	3	1

FOOD	PORTION	CAL	FAT	CARB	SUGAR	FIBER
Croissant Raspberry Cheese	1	330	16	41	16	1
Croissant Sweet Cheese	1	320	16	39	15	1
Danish Cherry	1	370	19	44	15	1
Danish Sweet Cheese	1	380	20	44	16	1
Focaccia	1 piece (4.4 oz)	310	4	57	2	3
Lahvash	1 (4 oz)	320	1	62	1	2
Macaroon Chocolate Dipped Cranberry Almond	1	320	16	42	33	3
Mini Loaf Bacon & Cheese	1 (4.8 oz)	540	31	50	20	1
Muffin Blueberry	1	510	19	76	33	5
Muffin Carrot Walnut	1	520	25	66	38	4
Muffin Corn	1	460	16	69	29	2
Muffin Cranberry Walnut	1	500	24	61	26	5
Muffin Double Chocolate Chunk	1	590	20	83	46	5
Muffin Pumpkin	1	490	17	75	35	2
Muffin Raisin Bran	1	410	9	74	40	9
Muffin Low Fat Triple Berry	1	290	2	61	31	2
Pastry Hazelnut Creme	1	540	34	50	20	3
Poundcake Cappuccino	1 slice (5.2 oz)	530	26	68	43	1
Poundcake Chocolate	1 slice (4.7 oz)	500	29	58	35	3
Poundcake Lemon	1 slice (4.9 oz)	520	27	64	40	0
Poundcake Marble	1 slice (4.7 oz)	490	27	59	35	1
Roll Pecan	1	630	32	80	38	3

FOOD	PORTION	CAL	FAT	CARB	SUGAR	FIBER
Roll Soft	1 (4.7 oz)	410	11	65	9	3
Scone Cinnamon	1	430	24	48	16	1
Scone Orange	1	410	20	51	16	2
Shortbread Chocolate Dipped	1	350	20	38	14	1
Toasts Basil Pesto Cheese	3 pieces (2 oz)	140	2	26	1	1
Tulip Blueberry	1	370	20	44	25	1
Tulip Chocolate Raspberry	1	430	21	55	34	1
Tulip Key Lime	1	440	22	55	33	1
BEVERAGES						
Blast Caramel	1 med (16 oz)	540	17	104	99	0
Blast Coffee	1 med (16 oz)	440	21	71	67	0
Blast Mocha	1 med (16 oz)	440	17	80	74	2
Blast Vanilla	1 med (12 oz)	540	17	104	99	0
Caffe Americano	1 sm (12 oz)	5	0	1	1	0
Cappuccino	1 sm (12 oz)	120	7	10	10	0
Caramel Macchiato	1 sm (12 oz)	350	10	53	50	0
Chocolate Milk	1 (12 oz)	320	9	54	51	3
Hot Chocolate	1 sm (12 oz)	350	11	58	54	3
Iced Caramel Macchiato	1 sm (12 oz)	290	7	49	46	0
Iced Tea Peach	1 med (22 oz)	120	0	30	30	0
Latte Caffe	1 sm (12 oz)	200	11	17	17	0
Latte Chai	1 sm (12 oz)	290	11	38	26	0
Latte Iced Caffe	1 sm (12 oz)	110	6	19	10	0
Latte Iced Chai	1 sm (12 oz)	190	5	31	18	0
Latte Iced Mocha	1 sm (12 oz)	210	11	27	26	1
Latte Iced Vanilla	1 sm (12 oz)	240	5	44	44	0
Latte Iced White Chocolate	1 sm (12 oz)	250	11	35	32	0
Latte Mocha	1 sm (12 oz)	300	16	35	33	1
Latte Vanilla	1 sm (12 oz)	320	9	50	50	0
Latte White Chocolate	1 sm (12 oz)	310	14	41	38	0

FOOD	PORTION	CAL	FAT	CARB	SUGAR	FIBER
Lemonade	1 med (22 oz)	300	0	72	72	0
Orange Juice	1 (8 oz)	110	0	26	26	1
Smoothie Peach	1 med (16 oz)	310	1	69	41	4
Smoothie Strawberry	1 med (16 oz)	310	1	66	43	3
MAIN MENU SELECTIONS						
Fruit Cup	1 sm (6 oz)	70	0	16	15	1
Harvest Rice Bowl Cajun Shrimp	1 (20 oz)	520	17	69	8	2
Harvest Rice Bowl Cajun Shrimp w/ Brown Rice	1 (20 oz)	560	20	73	8	5
Harvest Rice Bowl Mayan Chicken	1 (19.25 oz)	490	14	67	5	4
Harvest Rice Bowl Mayan Chicken w/ Brown Rice	1 (19.25 oz)	540	16	71	5	7
Harvest Rice Bowl Steak Teriyaki	1 (19.25 oz)	530	15	72	11	2
Harvest Rice Bowl Steak Teriyaki w/ Brown Rice	1 (19.25 oz)	570	18	76	11	5
Macaroni & Cheese	1 med (12 oz)	440	26	31	4	2
Stew Beef	1 med (12 oz)	300	16	25	4	3
Stew Chicken Vegetable	1 med (12 oz)	290	17	26	5	3
SALAD DRESSINGS AND SPREADS						
Artichoke Aioli	1 serv (1 oz)	130	14	1	0	0
Basil Pesto	1 serv (1 oz)	140	15	1	0	0
Chili Dijon	1 serv (1 oz)	120	12	3	2	1
Cream Cheese Honey Pecan	1 serv (2 oz)	120	10	5	4	0
Cream Cheese Honey Walnut	1 serv (2 oz)	140	9	12	12	0
Cream Cheese Lite	1 serv (2 oz)	120	9	5	3	0
Cream Cheese Plain	1 serv (2 oz)	170	16	4	3	0
Cream Cheese Strawberry	1 serv (2 oz)	180	15	9	8	0

FOOD	PORTION	CAL	FAT	CARB	SUGAR	FIBER
Cream Cheese Sundried Tomato	1 serv (2 oz)	120	10	5	4	0
Cream Cheese Vegetable	1 serv (2 oz)	170	16	3	2	0
Dressing Balsamic Vinaigrette	1 serv (2.25 oz)	190	16	11	10	0
Dressing Blue Cheese	1 serv (1.75 oz)	230	24	2	1	0
Dressing Caesar	1 serv (2 oz)	280	28	4	3	0
Dressing Fat Free Raspberry Vinaigrette	1 serv (2.25 oz)	70	0	17	16	0
Dressing Light Honey Mustard	1 serv (2.25 oz)	180	11	21	19	1
Dressing Light Olive Oil Vinaigrette	1 serv (2.25 oz)	130	10	9	7	0
Dressing Light Ranch	1 serv (2.25 oz)	150	15	3	2	0
Dressing Thai Peanut	1 serv (2.25 oz)	230	13	24	22	1
Guacamole	1 serv (1 oz)	60	6	2	0	2
Honey Mustard	1 serv (2.5 oz)	210	13	23	21	1
Hummus Roasted Red Pepper	1 serv (2 oz)	80	5	6	0	2
Mayonnaise	1 serv (1 oz)	200	22	0	0	0
Mayonnaise Herb	1 serv (1 oz)	210	23	1	1	0
Mayonnaise Jalapeno	1 serv (1 oz)	140	15	0	0	0
Mayonnaise Tarragon Sauce	1 serv (2 oz)	420	45	2	2	0
Mustard	1 tsp	0	0	0	0	0
Spread Herb Bagel	1 serv (2 oz)	130	11	5	4	0
Spread Sundried Tomato	1 serv (0.53 oz)	70	6	4	1	0
SALADS						
Caesar Asiago	1 serv	210	12	18	4	3

FOOD	PORTION	CAL	FAT	CARB	SUGAR	FIBER
Caesar Asiago Grilled Chicken	1 (8.5 oz)	340	13	19	4	3
Caesar Asiago Side	1 (3.2 oz)	120	6	12	2	2
Chef's	1 serv	230	14	7	5	3
Garden	1 (7 oz)	80	2	14	3	4
Garden Side	1 (3.6 oz)	50	1	10	2	3
Mediterranean Chicken	1 (9.75 oz)	330	16	12	1	2
Riviera	1 (9.5 oz)	260	7	46	31	5
Thai Peanut Chicken	1 (11 oz)	250	8	22	7	4
Tuna Garden	1 (10.5 oz)	350	25	14	4	4
Turkey Medallion Cobb	1 (11 oz)	340	19	15	3	3
Turkey Spinach Sonoma	1 (12.3 oz)	310	13	22	9	5
SANDWICHES						
Arizona Chicken	1 (12 oz)	750	29	61	6	4
Baguette Turkey & Swiss	1 (12.3 oz)	770	38	65	4	3
Baja Turkey	1 (13 oz)	700	32	61	6	4
Breakfast Asiago Bagel Prosciutto & Egg	1 (9.6 oz)	660	25	67	4	3
Breakfast Asiago Bagel Sausage Egg & Cheddar	1 (10.2 oz)	770	45	55	4	0
Breakfast Bagel & Bacon	1 (4.2 oz)	340	6	56	4	0
Breakfast Egg On A Bagel	1 (6.8 oz)	370	4	62	5	2
Breakfast Egg On A Bagel w/ Bacon	1 (7.2 oz)	410	8	58	4	0
Breakfast Egg On A Bagel w/ Bacon Cheese	1 (7.9 oz)	500	15	59	4	0
Breakfast Egg On A Bagel w/ Cheese	1 (7.6 oz)	450	10	62	5	2
Breakfast Onion Dill Bagel Smoked Salmon & Wasabi	1 (7.1 oz)	490	11	77	6	3
Caprese	1 (11.8 oz)	700	35	65	3	4
Chicken Mozzarella	1 (14.5 oz)	800	27	71	6	2

FOOD	PORTION	CAL	FAT	CARB	SUGAR	FIBER
Chicken Pesto	1 (12.5 oz)	700	23	62	5	2
Chicken Tarragon	1 (11 oz)	720	29	61	5	1
Ciabatta Bacon & Egg Melt	1 (7 oz)	400	15	40	2	2
Ciabatta Ham & Cheddar	1 (12 oz)	650	20	80	19	4
Club Smoked Turkey	1 (11.6 oz)	780	43	56	4	2
Croissant Ham & Cheese	1 (4.2 oz)	350	18	34	4	1
Croissant Spinach & Cheese	1	250	14	25	3	2
Hot BBQ Chicken On Farmhouse Roll	1 (14.3 oz)	970	44	78	14	4
Hot Eggplant & Mozzarella	1 (12.4 oz)	710	37	68	5	6
Hot Steakhouse On Ciabatta	1 (13 oz)	800	41	70	8	4
Melt Tuna	1 (12.5 oz)	760	41	60	6	4
Melt Turkey	1 (12.2 oz)	890	47	70	18	3
Portobello & Goat Cheese	1 (10 oz)	610	33	61	4	6
Portobello Egg & Cheddar	1 (8.5 oz)	590	37	42	2	3
Prosciutto Mozzarella	1 (12.7 oz)	880	49	71	5	4
Spicy Tuna	1 (10.3 oz)	640	34	57	3	6
The Montana	1 (12.5 oz)	560	23	62	5	4
Turkey & Cranberry Chutney	1 (10.9 oz)	680	24	63	25	3
Wrap Chicken Caesar Asiago	1	700	25	69	6	3
Wrap Chopped Turkey Club	1 (12 oz)	660	27	70	5	4
Wrap Mediterranean	1 (12.8 oz)	670	28	80	5	7
Wrap Southwest Tuna	1 (14 oz)	900	51	72	6	5
Wrap Thai Peanut Chicken	1 (14.5 oz)	660	19	84	10	4

FOOD	PORTION	CAL	FAT	CARB	SUGAR	FIBER
Wrap Turkey Spinach Sonoma	1 (12 oz)	630	19	80	12	5
Wrap Hot Cajun Shrimp	1 (14.9 oz)	700	24	95	8	4
Wrap Hot Mayan Chicken	1 (13.5 oz)	630	19	92	6	5
Wrap Hot Steak Teriyaki	1 (13.5 oz)	660	19	93	9	5
SOUPS						
Baked Stuffed Potato	1 med (12 oz)	350	21	30	6	2
Broccoli Cheddar	1 med (12 oz)	310	21	20	7	2
Carrot Ginger	1 med (12 oz)	130	5	21	10	3
Chicken Florentine	1 med (12 oz)	240	13	25	4	1
Chicken & Dumplings	1 med (12 oz)	210	7	28	6	2
Chicken Noodle	1 med (12 oz)	130	3	20	2	2
Clam Chowder	1 med (12 oz)	320	18	27	8	1
Corn & Green Chili Bisque	1 med (12 oz)	250	14	29	6	3
Corn Chowder	1 med (12 oz)	350	18	40	10	3
Curried Rice & Lentil	1 med (12 oz)	150	2	30	4	8
French Moroccan Tomato Lentil	1 med (12 oz)	180	2	32	7	8
French Onion	1 med (12 oz)	130	5	19	6	2
Garden Vegetable	1 med (12 oz)	80	2	14	5	3
Harvest Pumpkin	1 med (12 oz)	190	10	26	6	2
Hearty Cabbage	1 med (12 oz)	110	5	14	4	3
Italian Wedding	1 med (12 oz)	170	7	10	4	2
Jamaican Black Bean	1 med (12 oz)	180	1	45	4	25
Mediterranean Pepper	1 med (12 oz)	100	3	18	3	5
Old Fashioned Tomato Rice	1 med (12 oz)	120	1	24	7	3
Pasta E Fagioli	1 med (12 oz)	240	8	36	3	9
Portuguese Kale	1 med (12 oz)	120	5	15	2	3
Potato Cheese	1 med (12 oz)	250	14	25	4	2
Potato Leek	1 med (12 oz)	300	20	28	2	2

FOOD	PORTION	CAL	FAT	CARB	SUGAR	FIBER
Red Beans Italian Sausage & Rice	1 med (12 oz)	200	5	28	3	16
Southern Black Eyed Pea	1 med (12 oz)	180	2	31	4	12
Southwest Tortilla	1 med (12 oz)	200	11	24	5	4
Southwest Vegetable	1 med (12 oz)	160	3	17	3	3
Split Pea	1 med (12 oz)	210	2	42	3	15
Thai Coconut Curry	1 med (12 oz)	150	7	20	4	2
Tomato Basil Bisque	1 med (12 oz)	210	8	29	18	5
Tomato Cheddar	1 med (12 oz)	240	15	17	7	2
Tomato Florentine	1 med (12 oz)	120	3	19	6	2
Tuscan Vegetable	1 med (12 oz)	170	5	24	3	3
Vegetable Beef Barley	1 med (12 oz)	140	3	21	4	4
Vegetarian Chili	1 med (12 oz)	230	3	40	7	11
Vegetarian Lentil	1 med (12 oz)	140	2	32	4	11
Vegetarian Minestrone	1 med (12 oz)	120	2	21	6	4
Wild Mushroom Bisque	1 med (12 oz)	190	9	23	6	2
YOGURT						
Blueberry w/ Fruit	1 sm (7.5 oz)	220	2	44	37	0
Blueberry w/ Granola & Fruit	1 sm (8.5 oz)	310	6	56	36	2
Strawberry w/ Blueberries	1 sm (7.5 oz)	220	2	44	37	0
Strawberry w/ Granola & Blueberries	1 sm (8.5 oz)	310	6	56	36	2
Vanilla w/ Blueberries	1 sm (7.5 oz)	190	2	32	30	0
Vanilla w/ Granola & Blueberries	1 sm (8.5 oz)	310	6	56	36	2

BAHAMA BREEZE
BEVERAGES

FOOD	PORTION	CAL	FAT	CARB	SUGAR	FIBER
Beer Light	1 serv (12 oz)	103	0	6	–	–
Beer Regular	1 serv (12 oz)	153	0	13	–	–
Berries In Paradise	1 serv	110	0	24	–	–
Captain Berry Island	1 serv	110	0	24	–	–

FOOD	PORTION	CAL	FAT	CARB	SUGAR	FIBER
Island Refresher	1 serv	370	7	73	–	–
Lemon Breeze	1 serv	410	0	103	–	–
Mango Beach	1 serv	300	8	56	–	–
Mango Mango Man	1 serv	300	8	56	–	–
Raspberry Surfer	1 serv	210	0	52	–	–
Shake Banana	1 serv	590	30	69	–	–
Shake Chocolate	1 serv	700	32	92	–	–
Shake Chocolate Banana	1 serv	760	31	108	–	–
Shake Mango	1 serv	450	25	47	–	–
Shake Raspberry	1 serv	560	29	64	–	–
Shake Strawberry	1 serv	530	32	50	–	–
Shake Strawberry Banana	1 serv	600	28	77	–	–
Shake Vanilla	1 serv	560	30	62	–	–
Slushies Kiwi	1 serv	120	0	29	–	–
Slushies Mango	1 serv	180	0	45	–	–
Slushies Strawberry	1 serv	240	0	58	–	–
Strawberry Beach	1 serv	370	7	74	–	–
Virgin Bahama Rita	1 serv	160	0	39	–	–
Virgin Ultimate Pina Colada	1 serv	340	9	65	–	–
Wine	1 serv (5 oz)	122	0	4	–	–
CHILDREN'S MENU SELECTIONS						
Bowtie Mac N' Cheese	1 serv	790	46	74	–	–
Cheese Pizza	1 sm	750	23	101	–	–
Crispy Chicken	1 serv	420	24	23	–	–
French Fries	1 serv	265	13	34	–	–
Fresh Fruit Salad	1 serv	40	0	10	–	–
DESSERTS						
Bananas Supreme	1 serv	940	45	122	–	–
Chocolate Island	1 serv	1380	83	142	–	–
Dulce De Leche Cheesecake	1 serv	940	56	94	–	–
Rebecca's Key Lime Pie	1 serv	990	34	154	–	–

FOOD	PORTION	CAL	FAT	CARB	SUGAR	FIBER
Warm Chocolate Pineapple Upside Down Cake	1 serv	1140	58	144	–	–
MAIN MENU SELECTIONS						
Bahamian Grilled Chicken Kabobs w/ Yellow Rice	1 serv	770	11	98	–	–
Breeze Wood Grilled Chicken Breast w/ Citrus Butter Sauce	1 serv	680	39	18	–	–
Breeze Wood Grilled Chicken Breast w/ Citrus Butter Sauce Lighter Portion	1 serv	390	23	11	–	–
Broccoli	1 serv	120	9	6	–	–
Burger Wood Grilled Angus	1 serv	680	39	39	–	–
Chicken Santiago	1 serv	1180	58	85	–	–
Chicken Santiago Lighter Portion	1 serv	1020	55	85	–	–
Cinnamon Mashed Sweet Potatoes	1 serv	260	9	44	–	–
Coconut Shrimp Dinner	1 serv	794	50	60	–	–
Crab Claws St. Thomas	1 serv	710	64	13	–	–
Crab Shrimp & Avocado Stack w/ Honey Red Pepper Drizzle	1 serv	250	6	20	–	–
Creole Baked Goat Cheese	1 serv	380	33	0	–	–
Crispy Yuca	1 serv	620	36	73	–	–
Filet Mignon w/ Onion Rings	1 serv	450	23	10	–	–
Fire Roasted Jerk Shrimp	1 serv	260	14	2	–	–
French Fries	1 serv	530	26	67	–	–

FOOD	PORTION	CAL	FAT	CARB	SUGAR	FIBER
Garlic Mashed Potatoes	1 serv	290	20	24	–	–
Herb Cheese Toast	1 slice	120	5	15	–	–
Island Flatbread Grilled Chicken	1	515	22	43	–	–
Island Flatbread Shrimp	1	480	20	43	–	–
Island Flatbread Vine Ripened Tomato	1	430	20	43	–	–
Island Onion Rings	1 serv	1910	116	186	–	–
Jamaican Grilled Chicken Breast	1 serv	310	4	2	–	–
Jamaican Grilled Chicken Breast Lighter Portion	1 serv	160	2	1	–	–
Linguine Calypso Shrimp Lighter Portion	1 serv	790	43	58	–	–
Margarita Chicken w/ Roasted Corn Salsa	1 serv	470	6	30	–	–
Margarita Chicken w/ Roasted Corn Salsa Lighter Portion	1 serv	310	5	24	–	–
Pasta Jerk Chicken	1 serv	1430	87	107	–	–
Pasta Jerk Chicken Lighter Portion	1 serv	780	39	72	–	–
Pasta Lobster & Shrimp	1 serv	1080	42	82	–	–
Pasta Pan-Seared Salmon	1 serv	1550	99	96	–	–
Pasta Pan-Seared Salmon Lighter Portion	1 serv	910	55	68	–	–
Plantains	1 serv	270	6	53	–	–
Quesadilla Fresh Vegetable	1	435	48	70	–	–
Quesadilla Fresh Vegetable & Chicken	1	480	24	11	–	–
Roasted Cuban Bread	1 serv	590	23	77	–	–

FOOD	PORTION	CAL	FAT	CARB	SUGAR	FIBER
Sandwich Cuban	1	1130	59	69	–	–
Sandwich Oak Grilled Chicken	1	530	19	45	–	–
Sandwich Sun Drenched Portobello & Veg	1	670	22	90	–	–
Seafood Paella	1 serv	800	23	54	–	–
Smothered Pork Tenderloin w/ Lemon Butter	1 serv	900	59	9	–	–
Spinach Dip w/ Island Chips	1 serv	680	60	17	–	–
Tacos Key West Fish	1 serv	550	26	30	–	–
Tostones w/ Chicken	1 serv	1250	63	121	–	–
West Indies Patties	1 serv	1150	68	102	–	–
West Indies Ribs	1 serv	810	55	7	–	–
Wings Habanero	1 serv	920	53	11	–	–
Wings Jamaican Grilled	1 serv	960	60	2	–	–
Wood Grilled Top Sirloin w/ Cheese & Peppers	1 serv	440	21	4	–	–
Yellow Rice	1 serv	220	3	44	–	–
Yellow Rice & Black Beans	1 serv	280	3	55	–	–
SALAD DRESSINGS AND TOPPINGS						
Citrus Mustard	1 serv	95	4	16	–	–
Dip Cilantro Vinaigrette	1 serv	110	6	12	–	–
Dipping Sauce Tangy	1 serv	50	1	12	–	–
Dressing Blue Cheese	1 serv	175	18	15	–	–
Dressing Caesar	1 serv	200	21	1	–	–
Dressing Ranch	1 serv	130	14	2	–	–
Dressing Tropical Island Vinaigrette	1 serv	60	4	15	–	–
Guava BBQ Sauce	1 serv	50	0	12	–	–
Homemade Croutons	12	500	29	47	–	–

FOOD	PORTION	CAL	FAT	CARB	SUGAR	FIBER
Salsa Apple Mango	1 serv	20	0	5	–	–
Salsa Black Bean & Corn	1 serv	70	2	10	–	–
Salsa Mango Pineapple	1 serv	60	0	15	–	–
Salsa Tomato	1 serv	30	1	4	–	–
Sauce Chili Horseradish	1 serv	130	11	8	–	–
Sour Cream	1 serv	90	8	3	–	–
Sour Cream Ancho Chili	1 serv	70	6	4	–	–
Tomato Salsa	1 serv	30	1	4	–	–
SALADS						
Breeze No Dressing	1 serv	90	5	6	–	–
Caesar No Dressing	1 serv	70	3	6	–	–
Crispy Chicken Club w/ BBQ Drizzle	1 serv	880	52	47	–	–
Fresh Fruit	1 serv	130	0	32	–	–
Grilled Chicken Ceasar w/ Croutons w/o Dressing	1 serv	490	20	22	–	–
Grilled Chicken Cobb	1 serv	600	38	4	–	–
Grilled Fresh Salmon Tostada w/ Chimichurri Sauce w/o Dressing	1 serv	1045	57	52	–	–
Tropical Fruit & Grilled Chicken On Greens w/o Dressing	1 serv	430	11	40	–	–
Vine Ripened Tomato	1 serv	60	1	12	–	–
SOUPS						
Bahamian Seafood Chowder	1 serv	600	47	27	–	–
Chicken Tortilla	1 serv	290	12	26	–	–
Cuban Black Bean	1 serv	320	4	52	–	–

FOOD	PORTION	CAL	FAT	CARB	SUGAR	FIBER
BAJA FRESH						
CHILDREN'S MENU SELECTIONS						
Kid's Mini Burrito Bean & Cheese	1 serv	540	14	84	–	11
Kid's Mini Burrito Bean & Cheese w/ Chicken	1 serv	590	15	84	–	12
Kid's Mini Quesadilla Cheese	1 serv	610	26	72	–	5
Kid's Mini Quesadilla Cheese w/ Chicken	1 serv	650	27	72	–	5
Kid's Taquitos Chicken	1 serv	630	33	60	–	4
MAIN MENU SELECTIONS						
Black Beans	1 serv	360	3	61	–	26
Burrito Baja Breaded Fish	1 serv	850	44	78	–	7
Burrito Baja Carnitas	1 serv	830	45	67	–	8
Burrito Baja Chicken	1 serv	790	38	65	–	8
Burrito Baja Mahi Mahi	1 serv	780	38	66	–	7
Burrito Baja Shrimp	1 serv	760	37	66	–	7
Burrito Baja Steak	1 serv	850	46	67	–	7
Burrito Bare Carnitas	1 serv	600	14	99	–	20
Burrito Bare Chicken	1 serv	640	7	97	–	20
Burrito Bare Steak	1 serv	700	15	99	–	19
Burrito Bare Veggie & Cheese	1 serv	580	10	101	–	20
Burrito Bean & Cheese Breaded Fish	1 serv	1030	41	108	–	20
Burrito Bean & Cheese Carnitas	1 serv	1010	42	98	–	21
Burrito Bean & Cheese Chicken	1 serv	970	35	96	–	21
Burrito Bean & Cheese Mahi Mahi	1 serv	960	35	96	–	20

FOOD	PORTION	CAL	FAT	CARB	SUGAR	FIBER
Burrito Bean & Cheese No Meat	1 serv	840	33	96	–	20
Burrito Bean & Cheese Shrimp	1 serv	950	34	96	–	20
Burrito Bean & Cheese Steak	1 serv	1030	43	97	–	20
Burrito Dos Manos Breaded Fish	1 serv	890	33	107	–	13
Burrito Dos Manos Carnitas	1 serv	780	30	95	–	14
Burrito Dos Manos Chicken	½ serv	760	26	94	–	14
Burrito Dos Manos Mahi Mahi	1 serv	780	26	95	–	13
Burrito Dos Manos Shrimp	1 serv	780	26	95	–	13
Burrito Dos Manos Steak	½ serv	795	30	95	–	13
Burrito Grilled Veggie	1 serv	506	33	94	–	16
Burrito Mexicano Breaded Fish	1 serv	850	19	129	–	18
Burrito Mexicano Carnitas	1 serv	830	20	119	–	19
Burrito Mexicano Chicken	1 serv	790	13	117	–	20
Burrito Mexicano Mahi Mahi	1 serv	790	13	117	–	18
Burrito Mexicano Shrimp	1 serv	770	13	117	–	18
Burrito Mexicano Steak	1 serv	860	21	118	–	18
Burrito Ultimo Breaded Fish	1 serv	940	42	96	–	8
Burrito Ultimo Carnitas	1 serv	920	44	86	–	9
Burrito Ultimo Chicken	1 serv	880	36	84	–	9

FOOD	PORTION	CAL	FAT	CARB	SUGAR	FIBER
Burrito Ultimo Mahi Mahi	1 serv	880	36	84	–	8
Burrito Ultimo Shrimp	1 serv	860	36	85	–	8
Burrito Ultimo Steak	1 serv	950	44	85	–	8
Chips & Guacamole	1 serv	1340	83	141	–	20
Chips & Salsa Baja	1 serv	810	37	98	–	14
Fajitas Corn Tortillas Breaded Fish	1 serv	1060	37	130	–	22
Fajitas Corn Tortillas Carnitas	1 serv	920	34	108	–	23
Fajitas Corn Tortillas Chicken	1 serv	860	24	105	–	24
Fajitas Corn Tortillas Mahi Mahi	1 serv	840	23	105	–	22
Fajitas Corn Tortillas Shrimp	1 serv	840	23	106	–	22
Fajitas Corn Tortillas Steak	1 serv	960	36	107	–	22
Fajitas Flour Tortillas Breaded Fish	1 serv	1340	46	172	–	25
Fajitas Flour Tortillas Carnitas	1 serv	1190	43	150	–	26
Fajitas Flour Tortillas Chicken	1 serv	1140	33	147	–	27
Fajitas Flour Tortillas Mahi Mahi	1 serv	1120	32	147	–	25
Fajitas Flour Tortillas Shrimp	1 serv	1120	32	148	–	25
Fajitas Flour Tortillas Steak	1 serv	960	36	170	–	22
Guacamole Side	1 (3 oz)	110	13	5	–	2
Nachos Breaded Fish	1 serv	2090	116	176	–	31
Nachos Carnitas	1 serv	2060	117	166	–	32
Nachos Cheese	1 serv	1890	108	163	–	31

FOOD	PORTION	CAL	FAT	CARB	SUGAR	FIBER
Nachos Chicken	1 serv	2020	110	164	–	32
Nachos Mahi Mahi	1 serv	2020	110	164	–	31
Nachos Shrimp	1 serv	2000	110	164	–	31
Nachos Steak	1 serv	2120	118	163	–	31
Pico De Gallo Side	1 serv (8 oz)	50	1	12	–	3
Pinto Beans	1 serv	320	1	56	–	21
Pronto Guacamole Side	1 serv (6 oz)	560	34	60	–	8
Quesadilla Breaded Fish	1 serv	1400	86	96	–	8
Quesadilla Carnitas	1 serv	1370	87	86	–	9
Quesadilla Cheese	1 serv	1200	78	84	–	8
Quesadilla Chicken	1 serv	1330	80	84	–	9
Quesadilla Mahi Mahi	1 serv	1330	79	84	–	8
Quesadilla Shrimp	1 serv	1310	79	84	–	8
Quesadilla Steak	1 serv	1430	87	84	–	8
Quesadilla Veggie	1 serv	1260	78	96	–	11
Rice	1 serv	280	4	55	–	4
Rice & Beans Plate	1 serv	420	5	72	–	18
Salsa Baja Side	1 serv (8 oz)	70	3	7	–	4
Salsa Roja Side	1 serv (8 oz)	70	1	13	–	4
Salsa Verde Side	1 serv (8 oz)	50	0	11	–	3
Soup Tortilla w/ Chicken	1 serv (13.6 oz)	320	14	29	–	4
Soup Tortilla w/o Chicken	1 serv (12.4 oz)	270	14	29	–	4
Taco Grilled Mahi Mahi	1 serv	230	9	26	–	4
Taco Baja Breaded Fish	1 serv	250	13	27	–	2
Taco Baja Chicken	1 serv	210	5	28	–	2
Taco Baja Shrimp	1 serv	200	5	28	–	2
Taco Baja Steak	1 serv	230	8	28	–	2
Taco Soft Breaded Fish	1 serv	240	11	23	–	2
Taco Soft Carnitas	1 serv	250	12	21	–	2
Taco Soft Chicken	1 serv	230	10	20	–	2
Taco Soft Mahi Mahi	1 serv	240	10	20	–	2
Taco Soft Shrimp	1 serv	230	10	21	–	2

FOOD	PORTION	CAL	FAT	CARB	SUGAR	FIBER
Taco Soft Steak	1 serv	260	13	21	–	2
Taquitos Chicken w/ Beans	3	780	40	68	–	17
Taquitos Chicken w/ Rice	3	740	40	66	–	8
Veggie Mix	1 serv	110	0	24	–	6
SALAD DRESSINGS						
Chipotle Vinaigrette	1 serv (2.5 oz)	110	9	0	0	0
Fat Free Salsa Verde	1 serv (2.5 oz)	15	0	3	–	1
Olive Oil Vinaigrette	1 serv (2.5 oz)	290	31	2	–	0
Ranch	1 serv (2.5 oz)	260	26	4	–	0
SALADS						
Baja Ensalada Chicken	1 serv	310	7	18	–	7
Baja Ensalada Shrimp	1 serv	230	6	18	–	6
Baja Ensalada Steak	1 serv	450	18	18	–	6
Chipotle w/ Carnitas	1 serv	640	30	56	–	10
Chipotle w/ Chicken	1 serv	590	22	54	–	11
Chipotle w/ Steak	1 serv	700	31	54	–	9
Side By Side Carnitas	1 serv	570	40	16	–	8
Side By Side Chicken	1 serv	500	27	12	–	9
Side By Side Steak	1 serv	620	42	14	–	6
Side Salad	1 (6.5 oz)	130	6	16	–	4
Tostada Breaded Fish	1 serv	1200	61	111	–	25
Tostada Carnitas	1 serv	1180	62	100	–	26
Tostada Chicken	1 serv	1140	55	98	–	27
Tostada Mahi Mahi	1 serv	1130	55	99	–	25
Tostada No Meat	1 serv	1010	53	98	–	25
Tostada Shrimp	1 serv	1120	55	99	–	25
Tostada Steak	1 serv	1230	63	98	–	25

FOOD	PORTION	CAL	FAT	CARB	SUGAR	FIBER
BASKIN-ROBBINS						
BEVERAGES						
Cappuccino Blast w/ Whipped Cream	1 sm (16 oz)	330	14	48	42	0
Shake Chocolate Chip	1 sm (16 oz)	660	32	78	74	1
Shake Chocolate Chip Cookie Dough	1 sm (16 oz)	750	31	99	88	1
Shake Mint Chocolate Chip	1 sm (16 oz)	680	33	83	79	1
Shake Vanilla	1 sm (16 oz)	670	33	80	73	0
FROZEN YOGURT						
Cheeries Julilee	1 scoop (4 oz)	240	12	30	26	1
Vanilla Fat Free	1 scoop (4 oz)	150	0	32	31	0
ICE CREAM						
Butter Almond Crunch Reduced Fat No Sugar Added	1 scoop (4 oz)	220	11	31	7	4
Butter Pecan	1 scoop (4 oz)	280	18	24	24	1
Cabana Berry Banana Reduced Fat No Sugar Added	1 scoop (4 oz)	150	6	27	7	3
Chocolate	1 scoop (4 oz)	260	14	33	31	0
Chocolate Chip	1 scoop (4 oz)	270	16	28	26	1
Chocolate Chip Cookie Dough	1 scoop (4 oz)	310	15	36	30	0
Chocolate Overload Reduced Fat No Sugar Added	1 scoop (4 oz)	190	8	37	7	5
Gold Medal Ribbon	1 scoop (4 oz)	260	13	34	33	0
Mint Chocolate Chip	1 scoop (4 oz)	270	16	28	26	1
Nutty Coconut	1 scoop (4 oz)	300	20	28	27	1
Oreo Cookies 'N Cream	1 scoop (4 oz)	280	15	32	27	1
Peanut Butter 'N Chocolate	1 scoop (4 oz)	320	20	31	28	1

FOOD	PORTION	CAL	FAT	CARB	SUGAR	FIBER
Pistachio Almond	1 scoop (4 oz)	290	19	25	23	1
Pralines'N Cream	1 scoop (4 oz)	280	14	35	31	1
Reese's Peanut Butter Cup	1 scoop (4 oz)	300	18	31	29	1
Rocky Road	1 scoop (4 oz)	290	15	36	32	5
Sundae Caramel Soft Serve	1 (10 oz)	580	21	89	78	1
Sundae Hot Fudge Soft Serve	1 (10 oz)	610	25	86	75	1
Sundae Strawberry Soft Serve	1 (10 oz)	450	18	59	57	1
Tax Crunch	1 scoop (4 oz)	330	20	32	28	1
Vanilla	1 scoop (4 oz)	260	16	26	26	0
Vanilla Soft Serve	1 serv (6 oz)	280	11	37	36	0
Very Berry Strawberry	1 scoop (4 oz)	320	11	28	27	0
ICES						
Sherbet Rainbow	1 scoop (4 oz)	160	2	34	34	0
Sorbet Lemon	1 scoop (4 oz)	130	0	33	33	0
Sorbet Mango	1 scoop (4 oz)	120	0	32	30	0
Sorbet Strawberry	1 scoop (4 oz)	130	0	34	34	0

BILLY'S BURGER HUT

BEVERAGES

FOOD	PORTION	CAL	FAT	CARB	SUGAR	FIBER
Shake Chocolate	1 (20 oz)	420	10	63	50	0
Shake Vanilla	1 (20 oz)	320	10	49	44	0
MAIN MENU SELECTIONS						
Big Billy's Roast Beef Sub	1	843	54	62	12	3
Billyburger	1	426	22	35	6	3
Billyburger w/ Cheese	1	498	35	35	8	4
Billy's Best Red Potato Salad	1 serv	190	9	12	4	3
Billy's Biggest Burger ½ Pounder w/ Everything	1	852	58	61	15	4

FOOD	PORTION	CAL	FAT	CARB	SUGAR	FIBER
Billy's Famous 7 Layer Salad	1 serv	558	49	18	9	2
Billy's Seafood Sandwich	1	399	18	43	9	3
Caesar Side Salad	1 serv	360	28	12	1	4
Chili w/ Cheese & Onion	1 serv	380	12	35	8	7
Cowboy Cobb Salad	1 serv	735	45	25	10	9
Cowboy Coleslaw	1 serv	180	9	11	4	3
French Fries	1 reg	230	12	25	7	1
Onion Rings	1 serv	250	10	37	6	1
Super Billy Burger w/ Bacon	1	663	41	39	9	4

BLIMPIE
DESSERTS

FOOD	PORTION	CAL	FAT	CARB	SUGAR	FIBER
Cookie Chocolate Chunk	1 (1.5 oz)	200	10	25	16	0
Cookie Oatmeal Raisin	1 (1.5 oz)	180	7	27	16	tr
Cookie Peanut Butter	1 (1.5 oz)	210	13	21	13	tr
Cookie Sugar	1 (2.5 oz)	320	16	42	23	0
Cookie White Chocolate Macadamia Nut	1 (1.5 oz)	200	11	25	16	0

SALAD DRESSINGS AND SAUCES

FOOD	PORTION	CAL	FAT	CARB	SUGAR	FIBER
Dressing Blue Cheese	1 serv (1.5 oz)	230	24	2	2	–
Dressing Buttermilk Ranch	1 serv (1.5 oz)	230	24	2	1	–
Dressing Buttermilk Ranch Light	1 serv (1.5 oz)	70	4	8	3	–
Dressing Creamy Caesar	1 serv (1.5 oz)	210	21	2	1	–
Dressing Creamy Italian	1 serv (1.5 oz)	180	18	4	3	0
Dressing Dijon Honey Mustard	1 serv (1.5 oz)	180	17	8	7	–
Dressing Italian Fat Free	1 serv (1.5 oz)	25	0	5	3	0
Dressing Italian Light	1 serv (1.5 oz)	20	1	2	2	–
Dressing Peppercorn	1 serv (1.5 oz)	240	26	1	1	0
Dressing Thousand Island	1 serv (1.5 oz)	210	20	6	6	0

FOOD	PORTION	CAL	FAT	CARB	SUGAR	FIBER
Guacamole	1 serv (1 oz)	45	4	2	0	1
Mayonnaise	1 serv (1 oz)	200	22	0	0	0
Mustard Yellow Deli	1 serv (0.5 oz)	15	0	0	0	0
Oil Blend	1 serv (0.5 oz)	130	14	0	0	0
Sauce Blimpie Special	1 serv (0.5 oz)	40	5	0	–	–
Sauce Red Hot Original	1 serv (1 oz)	10	0	2	0	0
SALADS						
Antipasto	1 serv (11.6 oz)	254	14	12	6	4
Buffalo Chicken	1 serv (7.7 oz)	220	9	10	5	4
Chicken Caesar	1 serv (9.4 oz)	190	8	6	3	3
Cole Slaw	1 side (4 oz)	160	9	20	17	2
Garden	1 serv (6.5 oz)	30	0	6	3	3
Macaroni	1 side (5 oz)	330	22	28	8	2
Northwest Potato	1 side (5 oz)	260	17	22	3	3
Potato	1 side (4.7 oz)	230	12	28	8	3
Tuna	1 serv (9.4 oz)	270	19	6	3	3
Ultimate Club	1 serv (10.1 oz)	280	14	10	5	3
SANDWICHES						
6 Inch Sub Blimpie Best	1 (10.4 oz)	450	17	49	10	3
6 Inch Sub Blimpie Best Super Stacked	1 (12.8 oz)	550	22	52	12	3
6 Inch Sub Blimpie Trio Super Stacked	1 (13.5 oz)	510	15	51	11	3
6 Inch Sub BLT	1 (7.2 oz)	430	22	43	6	2
6 Inch Sub BLT Super Stacked	1 (8.4 oz)	640	41	43	6	2
6 Inch Sub Chicken Cheddar Bacon Ranch	1 (12.1 oz)	600	29	48	8	3
6 Inch Sub Chicken Teriyaki	1 (8.7 oz)	450	12	52	13	2
6 Inch Sub Club	1 (10.2 oz)	410	13	49	9	3
6 Inch Sub Cuban	1 (8.2 oz)	410	11	43	6	1

FOOD	PORTION	CAL	FAT	CARB	SUGAR	FIBER
6 Inch Sub French Dip	1 (13.4 oz)	410	11	46	3	1
6 Inch Sub Ham & Swiss	1 (10 oz)	420	14	49	10	3
6 Inch Sub Hot Pastrami	1 (7.2 oz)	430	16	42	5	1
6 Inch Sub Meatball	1 (10 oz)	580	31	50	6	4
6 Inch Sub Reuben	1 (9.2 oz)	530	20	52	7	3
6 Inch Sub Roast Beef & Provolone	1 (10.8 oz)	430	14	46	7	3
6 Inch Sub Roast Beef & Provolone On Wheat	1 (11.3 oz)	430	16	44	6	6
6 Inch Sub Super Staked Hot Pastrami	1 (10.1 oz)	570	23	43	7	1
6 Inch Sub Tuna	1 (8.9 oz)	470	21	43	5	2
6 Inch Sub Turkey & Provolone	1 (10.8 oz)	410	13	49	8	3
6 Inch Sub Turkey & Provolone On Wheat	1 (11.3 oz)	420	14	47	8	6
6 Inch Sub VegiMax	1 (10.2 oz)	520	20	56	8	5
Blimpie Burger	1 (6 oz)	460	24	42	4	1
Blimpie Dog	1 (6.3 oz)	510	29	45	7	1
Ciabatta Buffalo Chicken	1 (11.3 oz)	540	23	49	5	3
Ciabatta French Dip	1 (13.8 oz)	430	11	49	2	2
Ciabatta Grilled Chicken Caesar	1 (10.1 oz)	580	20	62	4	3
Ciabatta Mediterranean	1 (10.1 oz)	450	8	65	6	3
Ciabatta Roast Beef Turkey & Cheddar	1 (10 oz)	520	24	51	6	3
Ciabatta Sicilian	1 (10 oz)	590	22	66	9	3
Ciabatta Spicy Chicken & Pepperoni	1 (10.1 oz)	710	34	65	4	3
Ciabatta Tuscan	1 (9.9 oz)	570	20	65	6	3
Ciabatta Ultimate Club	1 (7.4 oz)	520	24	47	5	2
Wrap Chicken Caesar	1 (9.7 oz)	220	8	56	5	4
Wrap Southwestern	1 (10 oz)	530	22	61	10	4

FOOD	PORTION	CAL	FAT	CARB	SUGAR	FIBER
SOUPS						
Bean w/ Ham	1 serv (8.6 oz)	140	1	23	2	11
Chicken Noodle	1 serv (8.6 oz)	130	4	18	5	2
Chicken w/ White & Wild Rice	1 serv (8.6 oz)	250	10	15	4	4
Cream Of Broccoli w/ Cheese	1 serv (8.6 oz)	250	19	13	2	tr
Cream Of Potato	1 serv (8.6 oz)	190	9	24	3	3
Garden Vegetable	1 serv (8.6 oz)	80	1	14	5	3
Grande Chili w/ Bean & Beef	1 serv (8.6 oz)	310	9	31	9	9
Tomato Basil w/ Raviolini	1 serv (8.6 oz)	110	1	22	5	0
Vegetable Beef	1 serv (8.6 oz)	80	2	13	3	2
BOB EVANS						
BREAKFAST SELECTIONS						
Bacon	1 piece	36	4	0	0	0
Benedict Ham & Cheese	1 serv	826	52	44	8	0
Country Benedict Sausage	1 serv	936	66	40	6	0
Country Benedict Spinach Bacon & Tomato	1 serv	729	48	42	8	1
Country Biscuit Breakfast	1 serv	659	45	40	6	1
Egg Hardcooked	1	60	4	1	0	0
Egg Over Easy	1	101	8	1	1	0
Egg Scrambled	1 serv	255	17	2	0	0
Egg Beaters	1 serv	173	12	3	2	0
French Toast	1 slice	131	2	13	3	1
French Toast Stuffed Plain	1 serv	599	20	53	21	3
Fruit & Yogurt Plate	1 serv	403	2	93	80	9

FOOD	PORTION	CAL	FAT	CARB	SUGAR	FIBER
Grits	1 serv	178	7	28	0	2
Ham Smoked	1 slice	87	2	2	1	0
Hotcake Blueberry	1	328	9	55	17	2
Hotcake Buttermilk	1	318	9	53	16	2
Hotcake Cinnamon	1	417	15	66	27	2
Hotcake Multigrain	1	322	10	52	16	3
Mush	1 serv	79	3	11	5	2
Oatmeal	1 serv	172	3	32	1	4
Omelette Bacon & Cheese	1 serv	825	66	6	2	1
Omelette Border Scramble	1	756	58	15	6	3
Omelette Egg Beaters Bacon & Cheese	1 serv	615	47	7	4	1
Omelette Egg Beaters Border Scramble	1 serv	517	37	16	8	3
Omelette Egg Beaters Farmer's Market	1 serv	569	41	14	7	2
Omelette Egg Beaters Garden Harvest	1 serv	444	31	14	7	2
Omelette Egg Beaters Ham & Cheddar	1 serv	426	29	5	3	1
Omelette Egg Beaters Sausage & Cheddar	1 serv	502	40	4	2	1
Omelette Egg Beaters Three Cheese	1 serv	435	34	5	3	1
Omelette Farmer's Market	1	778	60	13	5	2
Omelette Garden Harvest	1 serv	654	50	13	5	2
Omelette Ham & Cheddar	1 serv	634	48	3	0	1
Omelette Sausage & Cheddar	1 serv	741	61	3	0	1

FOOD	PORTION	CAL	FAT	CARB	SUGAR	FIBER
Omelette Three Cheese	1 serv	645	52	4	0	1
Omelette Western	1 serv	654	48	8	3	2
Pot Roast Hash	1 serv	652	39	34	5	4
Sausage Gravy Bowl	1 serv	268	17	21	1	0
Sausage Link	1	125	11	0	0	0
Skillet Sunshine	1 serv	842	60	36	2	4
Waffles Sweet Cream	1 serv	598	12	100	30	3
CHILDREN'S MENU SELECTIONS						
Fruit & Yogurt Dippers	1 serv	275	2	61	54	5
Hotcakes	1 serv	501	17	79	26	2
Kid's Macaroni & Cheese	1 serv	320	11	45	11	2
Kid's Pasta	1 serv	113	5	15	4	1
Mini Cheeseburgers	1 serv	306	19	21	4	1
Smiley Face Potatoes	1 serv	524	31	57	2	3
Sundae Fudge Blast	1 serv	244	11	33	25	0
Sundae Reese's I'm Smiling	1 serv	330	17	41	32	1
MAIN MENU SELECTIONS						
Seniors Chicken Parmesan	1 serv	522	26	33	7	3
Seniors Garden Vegetable Alfredo	1 serv	363	23	29	7	5
Seniors Garden Vegetable Alfredo Chicken	1 serv	452	26	29	7	5
Seniors Steak Tips & Noodles	1 serv	422	22	23	3	2
Seniors Stir-Fry Chicken	1 serv	368	13	44	16	5
SOUPS						
Bean	1 cup	144	3	19	1	3
Cheddar Baked Potato	1 cup	294	20	19	3	1
Sausage Chili	1 cup	268	17	18	2	7
Vegetable Beef	1 cup	135	5	17	2	3

FOOD	PORTION	CAL	FAT	CARB	SUGAR	FIBER
BRUEGGER'S BAGELS						
BAGELS						
Asiago Parmesan	1	330	4	62	8	4
Baked Apple	1	370	3	77	19	5
Blueberry	1	330	2	67	14	4
Chocolate Chip	1	350	5	64	14	4
Cinnamon Sugar	1	330	2	69	17	4
Cranberry Orange	1	330	2	68	17	4
Everything	1	320	2	64	8	4
Garlic	1	320	2	65	8	4
Honey Grain	1	330	3	65	10	5
Jalapeno Bagel	1	320	2	64	8	4
Multi-Grain	1	350	4	68	10	6
Onion	1	320	2	64	8	4
Plain	1	320	2	64	8	4
Poppy	1	320	3	64	8	4
Pumpernickel	1	330	3	67	11	12
Pumpkin	1	330	2	68	13	6
Rosemary Olive Oil	1	350	7	64	10	4
Salt	1	320	2	64	8	4
Sesame	1	360	3	68	11	4
Sourdough	1	340	2	68	8	4
Square Asiago Parmesan	1	360	5	66	11	4
Square Everything	1	320	2	64	8	4
Square Plain	1	350	3	70	11	4
Square Sesame	1	360	3	68	11	4
Sun Dried Tomato	1	320	2	64	11	4
Whole Wheat	1	390	6	73	8	9
DESSERTS						
Brownie Chocolate Chunk	1	330	18	40	27	2
Cake Lemon Pound	1 slice	320	13	48	25	tr
Cookie Chocolate Chip	1	500	22	71	43	3
Cookie Oatmeal Raisin	1	460	19	71	39	3

FOOD	PORTION	CAL	FAT	CARB	SUGAR	FIBER
Cookie Peanut Butter	1	480	23	63	38	2
Cookie Triple Chocolate Chunk	1	560	28	71	44	3
Cookie White Chocolate Macadamia	1	580	31	70	46	1
Luscious Lemon Bar	1	300	16	36	24	0
Marshmallow Chew	1	280	6	55	29	0
Muffin Blueberry	1	450	19	64	29	3
Muffin Chocolate	1	460	24	57	38	3
Oreo Dream Bar	1	470	28	49	35	2
Pecan Chocolate Chunk	1 slice	310	19	32	16	1
Raspberry Sammies	1 slice	340	16	44	21	1
Seven Layer Bar	1	650	43	58	42	5
Toffee Almond Bar	1	400	19	53	34	1
SALADS						
Caesar w/ Dressing	1 serv	270	17	22	5	2
Tossed Chicken Caesar w/ Dressing	1 serv	370	20	23	5	2
Tossed Mandarin Medley	1 serv	340	17	36	27	4
Tossed Sesame Chicken	1 serv	480	28	30	18	2
SANDWICHES						
BLT w/ Mayo	1	570	23	72	10	5
Chicken Fajita	1	530	11	81	16	6
Cranberry Gobbler	1	620	21	78	17	5
Cuban Chicken	1	680	25	74	10	4
Denver Egg	1	460	18	74	11	5
Egg Cheese	1	420	18	71	9	4
Egg Cheese Bacon	1	460	23	65	9	4
Egg Cheese Ham	1	460	18	73	11	4
Egg Cheese Sausage	1	640	38	72	10	5
Leonardo Da Veggie	1	480	12	74	11	5
Radishy Roast Beef	1	560	18	73	11	5
Roadhouse Chicken	1	710	19	84	22	4

FOOD	PORTION	CAL	FAT	CARB	SUGAR	FIBER
Roast Beef	1	730	36	71	10	5
Santa Fe Turkey	1	490	9	75	12	5
Smoked Salmon	1	490	10	74	10	5
Softwich BLT w/ Mayo	1	600	25	73	14	5
Softwich Chicken Breast	1	630	11	81	21	5
Softwich Chicken Fajita	1	570	10	81	18	6
Softwich Chicken Salad	1	670	27	76	15	5
Softwich Cranberry Gobbler	1	730	28	80	20	5
Softwich Cuban Chicken	1	810	32	77	15	4
Softwich Garden Veggie	1	380	3	76	15	6
Softwich Ham	1	510	6	85	25	5
Softwich Herby Turkey	1	580	14	80	13	5
Softwich Hummus	1	540	13	85	13	11
Softwich Leonardo De Veggie	1	550	15	79	16	6
Softwich Mediterranean	1	790	33	90	13	11
Softwich Peanut Chicken	1	590	12	82	18	5
Softwich Radishy Roast Beef	1	670	26	75	14	5
Softwich Roadhouse Chicken	1	670	19	74	13	4
Softwich Roast Beef	1	750	40	72	10	5
Softwich Roasted Turkey	1	550	15	74	13	5
Softwich Smoked Salmon	1	520	11	76	14	5
Softwich Supreme Club w/o Mayo	1	880	39	79	18	5
Softwich Tuna Salad	1	720	34	76	14	5
Softwich Western Wheat	1	820	58	76	14	8
Supreme Club w/o Mayo	1	470	9	72	11	5
Tuna Salad	1	620	27	73	10	5
Turkey	1	510	14	70	9	5
Wrap Classic w/ Bacon	1	520	45	52	4	4

FOOD	PORTION	CAL	FAT	CARB	SUGAR	FIBER
Wrap Classic w/ Ham	1	510	41	54	5	4
Wrap Classic w/ Sausage	1	660	60	52	3	4
Wrap Rio Grande Bacon	1	560	49	55	6	4
Wrap Rio Grande Ham	1	630	34	55	7	4
Wrap Rio Grande Sausage	1	510	47	53	4	4
Wrap Sesame Chicken Salad	1	770	36	80	18	5
Wrap Tossed Chicken Caesar	1	660	28	73	5	5
Wrap Tossed Mandarin Medley Salad	1	630	25	87	26	7
SOUPS						
Chicken Pot Pie	1 cup	250	19	12	2	2
Chicken Spaetzle	1 cup	120	5	12	2	1
Chicken Wild Rice	1 cup	260	19	16	2	1
Creamy Tomato	1 cup	150	9	16	11	3
Hearty Mushroom Barley	1 cup	110	2	18	3	4
Italian Wedding	1 cup	160	8	15	2	2
Minestrone	1 cup	120	2	21	3	5
Moroccan Stew	1 cup	140	3	26	8	4
New England Clam	1 cup	300	18	23	tr	1
Sweet Potato Cheddar	1 cup	200	11	20	6	2
SPREADS						
Cream Cheese Cucumber Dill	1 scoop (1.5 oz)	140	13	3	1	0
Cream Cheese Garden Veggie	1 scoop (1.5 oz)	130	11	5	2	1
Cream Cheese Honey Walnut	1 scoop (1.5 oz)	150	12	8	3	tr
Cream Cheese Jalapeno	1 scoop (1.5 oz)	140	13	4	2	0

FOOD	PORTION	CAL	FAT	CARB	SUGAR	FIBER
Cream Cheese Light Garden Veggie	1 scoop (1.5 oz)	90	6	3	2	0
Cream Cheese Light Herb Garlic	1 scoop (1.5 oz)	100	6	4	2	0
Cream Cheese Light Plain	1 scoop (1.5 oz)	100	6	4	3	tr
Cream Cheese Olive Pimento	1 scoop (1.5 oz)	140	13	3	1	0
Cream Cheese Onion & Chive	1 scoop (1.5 oz)	140	13	3	2	0
Cream Cheese Plain	1 scoop (1.5 oz)	130	11	6	2	tr
Cream Cheese Pumpkin	1 scoop (1.5 oz)	120	11	4	3	0
Cream Cheese Strawberry	1 scoop (1.5 oz)	140	13	4	2	0
Cream Cheese Wildberry	1 scoop (1.5 oz)	140	12	5	3	0
Hummus	1 scoop (2 oz)	110	6	10	0	0

BURGER KING
BEVERAGES

FOOD	PORTION	CAL	FAT	CARB	SUGAR	FIBER
Apple Juice	1 (6.67 oz)	90	0	23	21	–
BK Joe Regular	1 sm	5	0	1	0	–
BK Joe Turbo	1 sm (12 oz)	10	0	1	0	–
Chocolate Milk 1% Low Fat	1 (9 oz)	180	3	31	29	1
Coke Classic	1 sm (16 oz)	140	0	39	39	–
Diet Coke	1 sm (16 oz)	0	0	0	0	0
Dr Pepper	1 sm (16 oz)	140	0	39	39	–
Frozen Coke	1 sm (16 oz)	110	0	31	31	–
Iced Coffee Mocha BK Joe	1 (16 oz)	380	10	66	63	1
Iced Minute Maid Cherry	1 sm (16 oz)	110	0	31	31	–

FOOD	PORTION	CAL	FAT	CARB	SUGAR	FIBER
Milk 1% Low Fat	1	110	3	13	12	0
Minute Maid Orange Juice	8 oz	140	0	33	30	–
Shake Chocolate	1 sm (16 oz)	470	14	75	72	1
Shake Oreo Sundae Chocolate	1 sm (16 oz)	680	24	105	95	2
Shake Oreo Sundae Strawberry	1 sm (16 oz)	660	23	103	94	1
Shake Oreo Sundae Vanilla	1 sm (16 oz)	610	24	87	78	1
Shake Strawberry	1 sm (16 oz)	460	14	73	71	0
Shake Vanilla	1 sm (16 oz)	400	15	57	55	0
Sprite	1 sm (16 oz)	140	0	39	39	–
Water Nestle Pure Life	1 bottle (16 oz)	0	0	0	0	0
BREAKFAST SELECTIONS						
Biscuit Bacon Egg & Cheese	1	410	25	31	4	1
Biscuit Ham Egg & Cheese	1	390	22	31	4	1
Biscuit Sausage	1	390	26	28	2	1
Biscuit Sausage Egg & Cheese	1	530	37	31	4	1
Croissan'wich Bacon Egg & Cheese	1	340	20	26	5	tr
Croissan'wich Double w/ Bacon Egg & Cheese	1	430	27	27	6	tr
Croissan'wich Double w/ Ham Bacon Egg & Cheese	1	420	24	27	7	1
Croissan'wich Double w/ Ham Egg & Cheese	1	420	23	27	7	1
Croissan'wich Double w/ Ham Sausage Egg & Cheese	1	550	37	27	6	1

FOOD	PORTION	CAL	FAT	CARB	SUGAR	FIBER
Croissan'wich Double w/ Sausage Bacon Egg & Cheese	1	550	39	27	6	1
Croissan'wich Double w/ Sausage Egg & Cheese	1	680	51	26	6	1
Croissan'wich Egg & Cheese	1	300	17	26	5	tr
Croissan'wich Ham Egg & Cheese	1	340	18	26	6	1
Croissan'wich Sausage & Cheese	1	370	25	23	4	tr
Croissan'wich Sausage Egg & Cheese	1	470	32	26	5	tr
French Toast Sticks	3 pieces	240	13	26	6	1
Hash Browns	1 sm	260	17	25	0	2
Hash Browns	1 lg	620	40	60	1	6
Omelet Sandwich Enormous	1	730	45	44	8	2
Omelet Sandwich Ham	1	290	13	33	8	1
DESSERTS						
Cini-minis	1 serv	390	18	51	19	2
Dutch Apple Pie	1 serv	300	13	45	23	1
Hershey Sundae Pie	1	310	19	32	22	1
MAIN MENU SELECTIONS						
BK Chicken Fries	6 pieces	260	15	18	1	2
BK Stacker Double	1	610	39	32	5	1
BK Stacker Quad	1	1000	68	34	6	1
BK Stacker Triple	1	800	54	33	5	1
BK Veggie Burger	1	420	16	46	8	7
Cheeseburger	1	330	16	31	6	1
Cheeseburger Double	1	500	29	31	6	1
Chicken Sandwich Original	1	660	40	52	5	4

FOOD	PORTION	CAL	FAT	CARB	SUGAR	FIBER
Chicken Sandwich Tendercrisp	1	790	44	68	9	5
Chicken Sandwich Tendergrill	1	510	19	49	7	4
Chicken Tenders	5 pieces	210	12	13	0	0
Chick'n Crisp Spicy Sandwich	1	480	31	36	4	1
Double Cheeseburger	1	410	21	30	6	1
French Fries No Salt Added	1 sm	230	13	26	1	2
French Fries Salted	1 sm	230	13	26	1	2
French Fries Salted	1 lg	500	28	57	1	5
Hamburger	1	290	12	30	6	1
Onion Rings	1 sm	140	7	18	2	2
Onion Rings	1 lg	440	22	53	6	5
Sandwich BK Big Fish	1	640	32	67	9	3
The Angus Steak Burger	1	640	33	55	10	3
Whopper	1	670	39	51	11	3
Whopper w/ Cheese	1	760	47	52	11	3
Whopper Double	1	900	57	51	11	3
Whopper Double w/ Cheese	1	990	64	52	11	3
Whopper Jr.	1	370	21	31	6	2
Whopper Jr. w/ Cheese	1	410	24	32	6	2
Whopper Triple	1	1130	74	51	11	3
Whopper Triple w/ Cheese	1	1230	82	52	11	3
SALAD DRESSINGS AND TOPPINGS						
Breakfast Syrup	1 serv (1 oz)	80	0	21	14	0
Croutons Garlic Parmesan	1 serv	60	2	9	1	0
Dipping Sauce Barbecue	1 serv (1 oz)	40	0	11	10	0
Dipping Sauce Honey Mustard	1 serv (1 oz)	90	6	8	7	0

FOOD	PORTION	CAL	FAT	CARB	SUGAR	FIBER
Dipping Sauce Ranch	1 serv (1 oz)	140	15	1	1	0
Dipping Sauce Sweet And Sour	1 serv (1 oz)	40	0	11	10	0
Dressing Ken's Creamy Caesar	1 serv (2 oz)	210	21	4	3	0
Dressing Ken's Fat Free Ranch	1 serv (2 oz)	60	0	15	5	2
Dressing Ken's Honey Mustard	1 serv (2 oz)	270	23	15	14	0
Dressing Ken's Ranch	1 serv (2 oz)	190	20	2	1	0
Jam Grape	1 serv	30	0	7	6	0
Jam Strawberry	1 serv	30	0	7	6	0
Ketchup	1 pkg	10	0	3	2	0
Mayonnaise	1 pkg	80	9	1	0	0
SALADS						
Chicken Garden Tendercrisp	1	410	22	26	5	5
Chicken Garden Tendergrill w/o Dressing or Croutons	1	240	9	8	3	4
Side Garden w/o Dressing	1	15	0	3	1	1

BURGERVILLE
BEVERAGES

FOOD	PORTION	CAL	FAT	CARB	SUGAR	FIBER
Barq's Root Beer	1 (20 oz)	180	0	49	–	0
Coca Cola	1 (20 oz)	161	0	44	–	0
Diet Coke	1 (20 oz)	0	0	0	–	0
Hot Chocolate Ghirardelli	1 (12 oz)	230	0	38	–	2
House Coffee	1 (10 oz)	5	0	1	–	0
Iced Tea	1 (20 oz)	0	0	0	–	0

FOOD	PORTION	CAL	FAT	CARB	SUGAR	FIBER
Iced Tea Nestea Raspberry	1 (20 oz)	127	0	34	–	0
Lemonade Odwalla	1 (20 oz)	240	0	65	–	0
Milk 2%	1 (8 oz)	121	5	12	–	0
Orange Juice Odwalla	1 (10 oz)	138	0	31	–	1
Pibb Xtra	1 (20 oz)	163	0	42	–	0
Sprite	1 (20 oz)	158	0	42	–	0
BREAKFAST SELECTIONS						
Bagel	1	310	1	63	–	2
Bagel Bacon And Egg	1	490	16	64	–	2
Bagel Ham And Egg	1	490	13	65	–	2
Bagel Sausage And Egg	1	640	31	64	–	2
Breakfast Platter w/ Bacon	1 serv	730	49	55	–	1
Breakfast Platter w/ Ham	1 serv	725	46	56	–	1
Breakfast Platter w/ Sausage	1 serv	880	64	56	–	1
Hash Browns	1 serv	230	15	22	–	0
Toaster Biscuit	1	320	9	31	–	1
Toaster Biscuit Bacon And Egg	1	450	29	32	–	1
Toaster Biscuit Ham And Egg	1	440	26	33	–	1
Toaster Biscuit Sausage And Egg	1	600	44	32	–	1
DESSERTS						
Cone Vanilla	1	250	11	32	–	0
Cone YoCream Frozen Yogurt	1	190	0	39	–	0
Cookie Chocolate Chunk	1	320	14	48	–	0
Cookie Oatmeal Raisin	1	290	8	50	–	1
Cookie Sugar	1	305	15	39	–	1

FOOD	PORTION	CAL	FAT	CARB	SUGAR	FIBER
Cookie White Chocolate Macadamia	1	340	16	46	–	0
Strawberry Shortcake	1 serv	440	15	72	–	3
Sundae Caramel	1	380	15	56	–	0
Sundae Fresh Strawberry	1	340	14	48	–	1
Sundae Hot Fudge	1	380	18	51	–	0
Sundae Triple Berry	1	340	14	46	–	0
Sundae YoCream Caramel	1	260	1	56	–	0
Sundae YoCream Hot Fudge	1	260	4	51	–	0
Sundae YoCream Strawberry	1	220	0	48	–	1
Sundae YoCream Triple Berry	1	200	0	43	–	0
MAIN MENU SELECTIONS						
Apple Slices	1 serv	29	0	9	–	2
Cheeseburger	1	350	19	29	–	2
Cheeseburger Colossal	1	520	30	31	–	5
Cheeseburger Double Beef	1	430	25	29	–	2
Cheeseburger Tillamook	1	630	40	31	–	5
Cheeseburger Tillamook Pepper Bacon	1	690	46	28	–	5
Chicken Strips	5	320	14	26	–	0
French Fries	1 serv	410	18	57	–	6
Gardenburger Spicy Black Bean	1	550	32	45	–	10
Gardenburger The Original	1	450	19	52	–	8
Halibut	3 pieces	320	16	24	–	0
Hamburger	1	300	15	29	–	2

FOOD	PORTION	CAL	FAT	CARB	SUGAR	FIBER
Hamburger Burgerville Classic	1	510	30	30	–	5
Onion Rings Walla Walla	1 serv	810	48	83	–	1
Sandwich Crispy Chicken	1	490	19	59	–	3
Sandwich Deluxe Crispy Chicken	1	590	30	56	–	3
Sandwich Halibut	1	480	27	41	–	2
Sandwich Low Fat Grilled Chicken	1	320	5	44	–	3
Sandwich Nine Grain Turkey Club	1	550	32	38	–	3
Sweet Potato Fries	1 serv	530	29	60	–	3
Turkey Burger Seasoned	1	540	29	33	–	5
Yukon Golds	1 serv	450	21	59	–	5
SALAD DRESSINGS AND TOPPINGS						
Burgerville Spread Cups	1	280	30	4	–	0
Cream Cheese	1 serv	100	10	1	–	0
Cream Cheese Light	1 serv	70	5	2	–	0
Dip BBQ Sauce	1 serv	60	1	13	–	0
Dressing Blue Cheese	1 serv	240	24	3	–	0
Dressing Caesar	1 serv	220	22	2	–	0
Dressing Honey Mustard	1 serv	210	20	6	–	0
Dressing Ranch	1 serv	195	21	2	–	0
Sauce Sweet And Sour	1 serv	90	4	12	–	0
Tartar Cups	1	260	28	2	–	0
Vinaigrette Honey Lime	1 serv	250	23	10	–	0
Vinaigrette Raspberry	1 serv	45	2	6	–	0
SALADS						
Grilled Chicken	1	430	27	16	–	7
Rogue River Smokey Blue	1	290	11	38	–	4
Side Salad	1	50	3	4	–	2

FOOD	PORTION	CAL	FAT	CARB	SUGAR	FIBER
Wild Smoked Salmon & Hazelnuts	1	440	28	19	–	7

CARL'S JR.
BEVERAGES
Malt Chocolate	1 (15 oz)	780	35	98	79	1
Malt Oreo Cookie	1 (15 oz)	790	39	91	72	1
Malt Strawberry	1 (15 oz)	770	35	97	83	0
Malt Vanilla	1 (15 oz)	760	35	99	84	0
Shake Chocolate	1 (14 oz)	710	33	85	71	1
Shake Oreo Cookie	1 (14 oz)	720	37	79	64	1
Shake Strawberry	1 (14 oz)	700	33	84	75	0
Shake Vanilla	1 (14 oz)	710	33	86	76	0

BREAKFAST SELECTIONS
Breakfast Burger	1	830	47	65	13	3
Burrito Bacon & Egg	1	570	33	37	1	1
Burrito Loaded Breakfast	1	820	51	52	3	2
Burrito Steak & Egg	1	660	36	44	4	2
French Toast Dips w/o Syrup	5	430	18	58	15	1
Hash Brown Nuggets	1 serv	330	21	32	1	3
Sandwich Sourdough Breakfast	1 serv	460	21	39	4	2
Sunrise Croissant Sandwich	1	560	41	27	5	1

DESSERTS
Cheesecake Strawberry Swirl	1 serv	290	17	30	20	0
Chocolate Cake	1 serv	300	12	48	37	1
Cookie Chocolate Chip	1	350	18	46	27	1

MAIN MENU SELECTIONS
Burger Jalapeno	1	720	45	50	10	3
Burger Teriyaki	1	660	34	61	19	3

FOOD	PORTION	CAL	FAT	CARB	SUGAR	FIBER
Cheeseburger Double Western Bacon	1	970	52	71	15	3
Cheeseburger Western Bacon	1	710	33	70	15	3
Chicken Breast Strips	3	420	25	28	1	1
Chicken Stars	4	170	11	10	0	1
CrissCut Fries	1 serv	410	24	43	0	4
Famous Star w/ Cheese	1	660	39	53	10	3
Fish & Chips	1 serv	630	28	68	4	3
French Fries	1 sm	290	14	37	0	3
Fried Zucchini	1 serv	320	19	31	0	0
Hamburger Big	1	470	17	54	13	3
Hamburger Kid's	1	460	17	53	13	2
Onion Rings	1 serv	430	21	53	5	2
Sandwich Bacon Swiss Crispy Chicken	1	720	35	64	9	3
Sandwich Carl's Catch Fish	1	660	31	75	14	3
Sandwich Charbroiled BBQ Chicken	1	360	5	48	12	4
Sandwich Charbroiled Chicken Club	1	550	25	43	9	4
Sandwich Charbroiled Santa Fe Chicken	1	610	32	43	10	4
Sandwich Spicy Chicken	1	560	30	59	7	2
Six Dollar Burger The Bacon Cheese	1	1070	76	50	10	3
Six Dollar Burger The Guacamole Bacon	1	1140	86	54	11	6
Six Dollar Burger The Jalapeno	1	1030	74	52	11	3
Six Dollar Burger The Low Carb	1	490	37	6	4	2

FOOD	PORTION	CAL	FAT	CARB	SUGAR	FIBER
Six Dollar Burger The Original	1	1010	68	60	18	3
Six Dollar Burger The Western Bacon	1	1130	66	83	19	4
Super Star w/ Cheese	1	930	59	54	10	3
SALAD DRESSINGS						
Blue Cheese	1 serv (2 oz)	320	34	1	1	0
House	1 serv (2 oz)	220	22	2	2	0
Italian Fat Free	1 serv (2 oz)	15	0	4	2	0
Low Fat Balsamic	1 serv (2 oz)	35	15	5	3	0
Thousand Island	1 serv (2 oz)	240	23	7	3	0
SALADS						
Charbroiled Chicken	1	260	7	16	8	5
Side	1	50	3	5	3	2

CARVEL

FOOD	PORTION	CAL	FAT	CARB	SUGAR	FIBER
Brown Bonnet	1	370	21	40	29	0
Cake Ice Cream	1 slice	270	14	33	23	1
Carvelanche Cake Mix	1 reg (16 oz)	720	27	106	74	0
Carvelanche Cookies & Cream	1 reg (16 oz)	550	30	64	49	0
Carvelanche Triple Fudge Cake Mix	1 reg (16 oz)	900	41	134	101	4
Chipsters	1	330	16	44	25	4
Cone Cake Chocolate	1 sm	260	13	32	25	1
Cone Cake Chocolate	1 lg	600	30	71	59	3
Cone Cake Vanilla	1 sm	280	16	31	24	0
Cone Cake Vanilla	1 lg	650	36	68	57	0
Cone Sugar Chocolate	1 sm	300	13	40	29	1
Cone Sugar Vanilla	1 sm	320	15	39	28	0
Cone Waffle Chocolate	1 sm	330	13	47	31	2
Cone Waffle Chocolate	1 lg	660	30	86	65	3
Cone Waffle Vanilla	1 sm	350	16	46	30	1
Cone Waffle Vanilla	1 lg	710	36	83	63	1

FOOD	PORTION	CAL	FAT	CARB	SUGAR	FIBER
Dashers Banana Barge	1	940	46	121	86	7
Dashers Bananas Foster	1	600	24	90	60	2
Dashers Fudge Brownie	1	810	42	98	80	4
Dashers Mint Chocolate Chip	1	720	39	85	63	2
Dashers Peanut Butter Cup	1	1090	63	97	79	4
Dashers Strawberry Shortcake	1	590	29	78	59	2
Flying Saucer 98% Fat Free Chocolate	1	180	3	34	19	1
Flying Saucer 98% Fat Free Vanilla	1	180	3	35	20	1
Flying Saucer Chocolate	1	230	10	33	20	1
Flying Saucer Deluxe Sprinkles	1	330	15	47	26	1
Flying Saucer Vanilla	1	240	11	33	19	1
Ice Cream Chocolate	1 sm (4 oz)	250	13	29	25	0
Ice Cream Vanilla	1 sm (4 oz)	240	14	25	21	0
Ice Cream No Fat Chocolate	1 sm (4 oz)	160	0	37	33	0
Ice Cream No Fat Vanilla	1 sm (4 oz)	160	0	33	29	0
Sherbet All Flavors	1 sm (4 oz)	180	2	39	30	0
Sinful Love Bar	1	460	29	47	28	5
Sprinkle Cup	1	230	15	28	20	1
Sundae Bittersweet Fudge	1 reg	690	38	77	64	1
Sundae Caramel	1 reg	670	34	81	60	0
Sundae Hot Fudge	1 reg	670	38	73	62	1
Sundae Strawberry	1 reg	580	33	63	54	1
Sundae Mini Chocolate Syrup	1	200	9	27	20	0
Thick Shake Chocolate	1 reg (16 oz)	650	27	93	69	2
Thick Shake Vanilla	1 reg (16 oz)	610	28	81	74	0

FOOD	PORTION	CAL	FAT	CARB	SUGAR	FIBER
Thinny Thin Classic Sundae No Fat Fudge	1 reg	380	2	81	46	0
Thinny Thin Classic Sundae No Fat Strawberry	1 reg	320	0	69	59	1
Thinny Thin Miniature Sundae No Fat	1	190	0	45	20	0
Thinny Thin Miniature Sundae No Sugar Added	1	200	3	42	6	0
Thinny Thin No Fat Carvelanche Strawberry	1 (16 oz)	430	0	91	81	1
Thinny Thin No Fat Chocolate	1 sm	160	0	37	33	0
Thinny Thin No Fat Vanilla	1 sm	160	0	33	29	0
Thinny Thin No Sugar Added Vanilla	1 sm	180	3	34	10	0
Thinny Thin Parfait No Fat	1	190	0	42	20	0
Thinny Thin Shake No Fat Chocolate	1 (16 oz)	440	0	104	59	0
Thinny Thin Shake No Fat Mocha	1 (16 oz)	440	0	97	52	0
Thinny Thin Shake No Fat Vanilla	1 (16 oz)	300	0	62	55	0

CHIPOTLE

FOOD	PORTION	CAL	FAT	CARB	SUGAR	FIBER
Barbacoa	1 serv (4 oz)	228	13	1	0	0
Black Beans	1 serv (4 oz)	130	1	22	3	12
Carnitas	1 serv (4 oz)	227	12	0	0	0
Cheese	1 serv (1 oz)	110	9	tr	0	0
Chicken	1 serv (4 oz)	219	11	0	0	0
Chips	1 serv (4 oz)	490	19	71	1	5

FOOD	PORTION	CAL	FAT	CARB	SUGAR	FIBER
Crispy Taco Shells	3	180	7	26	0	2
Fajita Vegetables	1 serv (3 oz)	100	8	6	3	1
Flour Tortilla	1 (13 inch)	330	8	55	1	5
Flour Tortilla	1 (6 inch)	300	8	48	0	6
Guacamole	1 serv (4 oz)	170	15	8	1	5
Lettuce	1 serv (1 oz)	5	0	tr	0	tr
Pinto Beans	1 serv (4 oz)	138	1	23	3	10
Rice	1 serv (3.5 oz)	168	5	28	0	tr
Salsa Corn	1 serv (4 oz)	100	1	22	3	3
Salsa Tomato	1 serv (4 oz)	25	0	6	3	1
Sour Cream	1 serv (2 oz)	120	10	2	2	0
Steak	1 serv (4 oz)	230	12	2	0	0
Tomatillo Green	1 serv (2 oz)	15	tr	3	2	1
Tomatillo Red	1 serv (2 oz)	28	1	4	1	1
Vinaigrette	1 serv (2 oz)	282	26	11	25	0

CHURCH'S CHICKEN

DESSERTS

FOOD	PORTION	CAL	FAT	CARB	SUGAR	FIBER
Pie Apple	1 pie (3 oz)	280	11	39	15	1
Pie Edward's Double Lemon	1 pie (3 oz)	300	14	39	29	0
Pie Edward's Strawberry Cream Cheese	1 pie (2.8 oz)	280	15	32	22	2

MAIN MENU SELECTIONS

FOOD	PORTION	CAL	FAT	CARB	SUGAR	FIBER
Biscuit Honey Butter	1	240	12	28	4	1
Cajun Rice	1 reg	130	7	16	0	tr
Chicken Fried Steak w/ White Gravy	1 serv (7.5 oz)	610	43	31	2	2
Cole Slaw	1 reg	150	10	15	7	2
Corn On The Cob	1 ear	140	3	24	2	9
Country Fried Steak w/ White Gravy	1 serv (5.8 oz)	470	28	36	4	1
Crunchy Tenders	1 (2 oz)	120	6	6	0	tr
French Fries	1 reg	290	14	38	1	4

FOOD	PORTION	CAL	FAT	CARB	SUGAR	FIBER
Jalapeno Cheese Bombers	4 (4 oz)	240	10	29	5	3
Macaroni & Cheese	1 reg	210	11	23	6	1
Mashed Potatoes & Gravy	1 reg	70	2	12	2	1
Okra	1 reg	350	22	36	3	5
Original Breast	1	200	11	3	0	1
Original Leg	1	110	6	3	0	0
Original Thigh	1	330	23	8	0	1
Original Wing	1	300	19	7	0	3
Sandwich Bigger Better Chicken w/ Cheese	1	510	27	46	4	4
Sandwich Country Fried Steak	1	490	32	38	4	2
Sandwich Spicy Fish	1	320	20	25	3	2
Spicy Breast	1	320	20	12	0	1
Spicy Crunchy Tenders	1 (2 oz)	135	7	7	0	4
Spicy Fish Fillet	1 piece (2.3 oz)	160	9	13	1	1
Spicy Leg	1	180	11	8	0	1
Spicy Thigh	1	480	35	20	0	2
Spicy Wing	1	430	27	17	0	2
Sweet Corn Nuggets	1 reg	600	29	72	14	5
Whole Jalapeno Peppers	2	10	0	2	tr	1
SAUCES						
BBQ	1 pkg	30	0	7	2	0
Creamy Jalapeno	1 pkg	100	11	1	0	0
Honey	1 pkg	27	0	7	7	0
Honey Mustard	1 pkg	110	11	4	1	0
Hot Sauce	1 pkg	0	0	0	0	0
Ketchup	1 pkg	18	0	5	4	0
Purple Pepper	1 pkg	45	0	12	6	0
Ranch	1 pkg	130	13	1	0	0
Sweet & Sour	1 pkg	30	0	8	2	0

FOOD	PORTION	CAL	FAT	CARB	SUGAR	FIBER
CINNABON						
BAKED SELECTIONS						
Caramel Pecanbon	1	1100	56	141	47	8
Cinnabon Bites	6	520	16	78	25	2
Cinnabon Classic	1	813	32	117	55	4
Cinnabon Stix	1	379	21	41	14	1
Cinnamon Filled Churro	1	281	11	39	–	–
Minibon	1	339	13	49	22	2
BEVERAGES						
Caramelatta Chill	1 (16 oz)	520	19	76	73	0
Chillatta Cappuccino	1 (16 oz)	330	11	56	51	1
Chillatta Caramel	1 (16 oz)	480	18	72	68	0
Chillatta Chocolate Mocha	1 (16 oz)	460	14	72	61	3
Chillatta Mango	1 (16 oz)	340	11	57	47	0
Chillatta Strawberry	1 (16 oz)	330	11	54	46	0
Chillatta Strawberry Banana	1 (16 oz)	350	11	58	49	0
Chillatta Tropical Blast	1 (16 oz)	330	7	69	48	–
Mochalatta Chill	1 (16 oz)	450	18	66	62	1
CORNER BAKERY						
BREAKFAST SELECTIONS						
Baked French Toast	1 serv	570	15	86	–	1
Buckhead Cheese Grits	1 serv	350	22	19	–	2
Oatmeal	1 serv	280	7	41	–	3
Oatmeal Crunchy Honey Banana	1 serv	380	3	78	–	5
Oatmeal Swiss	1 serv	330	1	79	–	6
Panini Ham & Cheddar	1	720	34	57	–	2
Panini Smoked Bacon & Cheddar	1	680	34	56	–	2
Scrambler All American w/o Potatoes & Bread	1 serv	310	22	3	–	0

FOOD	PORTION	CAL	FAT	CARB	SUGAR	FIBER
Scrambler Anaheim w/o Potatoes & Bread	1 serv	490	36	10	–	4
Scrambler Farmer's w/o Potatoes & Bread	1 serv	430	31	6	–	1
The Commuter Croissant	1	720	46	44	–	2
PASTA						
Chicken Carbonara	1 serv	740	28	70	–	4
Half Moon Cheese Ravioli	1 serv	550	21	63	–	4
Penne w/ Marinara	1 serv	550	11	92	–	14
Pesto Cavatappi	1 serv	930	40	93	–	13
SALAD DRESSINGS						
Caesar	1 serv	310	32	2	–	0
House	1 serv	280	27	8	–	0
Ranch	1 serv	160	16	2	–	0
Vinaigrette Balsamic	1 serv	300	31	4	–	0
SALADS						
Caesar	1 serv	520	44	19	–	5
Caesar w/ Roasted Chicken & Croutons	1 serv	640	49	8	–	5
Chopped w/o Bread	1 serv	810	61	27	–	10
Harvest	1 serv	860	68	53	–	10
Harvest w/ Roasted Chicken	1 serv	980	72	53	–	10
Santa Fe Ranch	1 serv	680	44	56	–	10
Santa Fe Ranch w/ Roasted Chicken	1 serv	800	49	56	–	10
Side Cucumber Tomato	1 (6 oz)	120	9	9	–	2
Side Egg	1 (6 oz)	570	53	2	–	0
Side Roasted Potato Bacon	1 (6 oz)	370	23	29	–	3
Side Seasonal Fruit Medley	1 (6 oz)	90	0	22	–	2

FOOD	PORTION	CAL	FAT	CARB	SUGAR	FIBER
Side Tomato Mozzarella Pasta	1 (6 oz)	205	8	24	–	4
Side Tuna	1 (6 oz)	310	16	3	–	1
SANDWICHES						
Bavarian w/ Ham	1	720	25	78	–	4
Bavarian w/ Turkey	1	690	22	78	–	4
Chicken Pesto	1	840	41	75	–	5
Panini California Grille	1	700	41	59	–	8
Panini Chicken Pomodori	1	890	45	74	–	5
Panini Club	1	900	48	72	–	4
Panini Corned Beef Reuben	1	930	48	76	–	2
Panini Grilled Ham & Swiss	1	880	44	75	–	4
Southwest Roast Beef	1	840	37	78	–	5
Tomato Mozzarella	1	670	26	73	–	5
Tuna Salad On Olive Bread	1	450	16	42	–	3
Turkey Derby	1	650	29	60	–	5
Turkey Frisco	1	850	38	79	–	9
Uptown Turkey	1	660	29	61	–	9
SOUPS						
Big Al's Chili w/ Cheddar Cheese	1 (10 oz)	380	17	29	–	8
Bread Bowl	1	420	30	21	–	2
Cheddar	1 (10 oz)	310	23	16	–	2
Chicken Wild Mushroom Brie Stew	1 (10 oz)	260	14	20	–	2
Loaded Baked Potato w/ Garnish	1 (10 oz)	420	29	29	–	2
Mom's Chicken Noodle	1 (10 oz)	170	4	23	–	1
Old Fashioned Beef Stew	1 (10 oz)	260	13	20	–	2

FOOD	PORTION	CAL	FAT	CARB	SUGAR	FIBER
Roasted Poblano Corn Chowder	1 (10 oz)	330	21	34	–	4
Roasted Tomato Basil w/o Garnish	1 (10 oz)	170	5	27	–	4
Zesty Chicken Tortilla w/ Tortilla Strips	1 (10 oz)	230	11	26	–	5

D'ANGELO

CHILDREN'S MENU SELECTIONS

FOOD	PORTION	CAL	FAT	CARB	SUGAR	FIBER
D'Lite Turkey	1	217	3	30	2	3
Sub Cheeseburger	1	294	13	28	2	3
Sub Ham & Cheese	1	227	5	32	3	1
Sub Kidz Tuna	1	438	29	30	2	1
Sub Meatball	1	330	15	37	5	4

SALAD DRESSINGS

FOOD	PORTION	CAL	FAT	CARB	SUGAR	FIBER
Bleu Cheese	1 serv	152	15	3	2	0
Caesar	1 serv	397	43	6	6	0
Caesar Fat Free	1 serv	57	0	9	9	0
Creamy Italian	1 serv	340	37	9	6	0
Greek w/ Feta Cheese	1 serv	227	26	6	3	0
Honey Mustard	1 serv	150	142	7	6	0
Olive Oil Vinaigrette	1 serv	170	17	9	6	0
Ranch Lite	1 serv	240	19	6	4	1

SALADS

FOOD	PORTION	CAL	FAT	CARB	SUGAR	FIBER
Antipasto	1 serv	284	18	17	7	6
Caesar w/ Dressing	1 serv	474	39	25	7	4
Chicken Caesar w/ Dressing	1 serv	533	38	19	8	4
Chicken Stir Fry w/o Dressing	1 serv	168	3	11	6	4
Cobb w/o Dressing	1 serv	292	17	11	5	4
Greek	1 serv	290	23	17	8	4
Lobster w/o Dressing	1 serv	376	26	12	6	4
Roast Beef w/o Dressing	1 serv	131	3	10	5	4

FOOD	PORTION	CAL	FAT	CARB	SUGAR	FIBER
Steak Tip Caesar	1 serv	661	50	21	9	3
Tossed Garden w/o Dressing	1 serv	49	1	11	5	4
Turkey w/o Dressing	1 serv	157	2	10	5	4
SANDWICHES						
D'Lite Chicken Caesar Salad	1	374	7	43	9	4
D'Lite Chicken Stir Fry	1	426	6	57	8	7
D'Lite Classic Veggie	1	362	7	63	10	8
D'Lite Fresh Veggie	1	348	7	62	14	7
D'Lite Grilled Chicken Breast	1	388	7	52	5	6
D'Lite Roast Beef	1	338	5	51	5	6
D'Lite Turkey	1	347	4	51	5	6
D'Lite Turkey Cranberry	1	444	4	75	22	6
Pokket Big Papi	1	469	11	53	6	3
Pokket BLT & Cheese	1	397	17	38	5	3
Pokket Caesar Salad	1	616	39	54	7	3
Pokket Capicola & Cheese	1	362	13	35	2	2
Pokket Cheese	1	519	27	41	6	2
Pokket Cheeseburger	1	459	25	31	3	2
Pokket Chicken Caesar Salad	1	674	39	47	7	3
Pokket Chicken Club	1	526	28	36	3	2
Pokket Chicken Honey Dijon	1	508	20	40	6	2
Pokket Chicken Salad	1	623	42	34	3	2
Pokket Chicken Stir Fry	1	380	9	39	5	2
Pokket Classic Vegetable	1	368	13	46	8	4
Pokket Classic Veggie No Cheese	1	212	1	44	7	4
Pokket Greek	1	790	61	49	8	4
Pokket Grilled Chicken	1	303	5	35	3	2

FOOD	PORTION	CAL	FAT	CARB	SUGAR	FIBER
Pokket Ham	1	229	3	35	3	2
Pokket Ham & Cheese	1	326	10	38	5	2
Pokket Ham & Salami	1	386	17	34	3	12
Pokket Hamburger	1	399	20	29	2	2
Pokket Italian	1	525	30	36	4	2
Pokket Lobster	1	530	31	34	2	2
Pokket Meatball	1	574	31	52	10	4
Pokket Mortadella & Cheese	1	410	21	35	2	2
Pokket Number 9	1	407	18	31	4	2
Pokket Pastrami	1	438	25	33	1	1
Pokket Pepperoni	1	407	20	35	3	3
Pokket Roast Beef	1	247	3	33	2	2
Pokket Salad	1	196	1	40	6	4
Pokket Salami & Cheese	1	509	30	33	2	2
Pokket Seafood Salad	1	449	22	50	7	3
Pokket Steak	1	305	12	24	1	1
Pokket Steak & Cheese	1	377	17	26	2	1
Pokket Steak Bomb	1	631	32	44	4	3
Pokket Steak Tip	1	452	16	45	12	2
Pokket Tuna	1	664	49	33	2	2
Pokket Turkey	1	256	2	33	2	2
Pokket Turkey Club	1	332	7	32	4	2
Sub Big Papi	1 sm	525	15	60	7	7
Sub BLT & Cheese	1 sm	463	19	51	7	6
Sub Capicola & Cheese	1 sm	408	13	48	4	5
Sub Cheese	1 sm	589	28	55	8	5
Sub Cheeseburger	1 sm	526	26	44	5	5
Sub Chicken Club	1	593	29	49	5	5
Sub Chicken Honey Dijon	1	575	22	53	8	5
Sub Chicken Salad	1 sm	692	44	48	5	5
Sub Chicken Stir Fry	1 sm	449	11	53	7	6
Sub Classic Veggie	1 sm	462	15	64	10	8

FOOD	PORTION	CAL	FAT	CARB	SUGAR	FIBER
Sub Grilled Chicken	1 sm	369	7	48	4	5
Sub Ham	1 sm	302	5	49	6	2
Sub Ham & Cheese	1 sm	395	11	52	7	2
Sub Ham & Salami	1 sm	456	19	48	5	2
Sub Hamburger	1 sm	466	22	42	4	5
Sub Italian	1 sm	614	31	54	6	3
Sub Lobster	1 sm	598	33	48	4	5
Sub Meatball	1 sm	644	33	66	12	7
Sub Meatballs & Cheese	1 sm	750	41	67	13	7
Sub Mortadella & Cheese	1 sm	479	23	49	4	5
Sub Number 9	1 sm	450	19	41	5	4
Sub Pastrami	1 sm	613	34	47	3	5
Sub Pepperoni	1 sm	603	33	49	6	7
Sub Roast Beef	1 sm	320	5	48	5	5
Sub Salad	1 sm	281	3	57	11	8
Sub Salami & Cheese	1 sm	579	32	47	4	5
Sub Seafood Salad	1 sm	498	23	61	8	6
Sub Steak	1 sm	373	14	37	2	4
Sub Steak & Cheese	1 sm	446	19	40	4	4
Sub Steak Bomb	1 sm	670	33	52	6	6
Sub Steak Tip	1 sm	545	18	63	14	3
Sub Tuna	1	685	46	47	4	2
Sub Turkey Club	1 sm	401	9	49	6	3
Sub Toasted Italian Bistro	1 sm	585	31	49	5	5
Sub Toasted Pastrami Reuben	1 sm	750	47	55	7	7
Sub Toasted Roast Beef & Cheddar	1 sm	564	26	51	8	5
Sub Toasted Spicy Meatball	1 sm	933	57	71	17	9
Sub Toasted Tuna & Swiss	1 sm	796	54	49	6	5

FOOD	PORTION	CAL	FAT	CARB	SUGAR	FIBER
Sub Toasted Turkey Thanksgiving	1 sm	705	20	80	11	6
Sub Toasted Turkey & Ham	1 sm	532	24	49	5	5
Wrap Big Papi	1	593	23	56	3	4
Wrap BLT & Cheese	1	544	26	54	4	4
Wrap Buffalo Chicken Salad	1	823	44	67	7	4
Wrap Caesar Salad	1	711	44	65	7	5
Wrap Capicola & Cheese	1	494	20	53	2	4
Wrap Cheese	1	675	35	59	6	4
Wrap Cheeseburger	1	609	33	48	3	3
Wrap Chicken Caesar Salad	1	830	47	65	7	5
Wrap Chicken Cobb	1	931	55	71	17	6
Wrap Chicken Filet & Bacon	1	639	28	58	4	2
Wrap Chicken Honey Dijon	1	672	29	43	8	5
Wrap Chicken Salad	1	782	51	53	3	4
Wrap Chicken Stir Fry	1	535	17	57	5	4
Wrap Classic Veggie	1	486	13	68	9	5
Wrap Greek	1	765	61	44	7	4
Wrap Grilled Chicken	1	422	6	59	4	4
Wrap Ham & Cheese	1	435	10	60	6	3
Wrap Ham & Salami	1	513	18	57	4	3
Wrap Hamburger	1	509	21	50	3	3
Wrap Italian	1	631	29	59	5	3
Wrap Lobster	1	749	43	57	3	3
Wrap Meatball	1	687	31	75	11	5
Wrap Mortadella & Cheese	1	522	21	58	3	3
Wrap Number 9	1	517	24	44	4	3
Wrap Pastrami	1	550	25	55	2	2

FOOD	PORTION	CAL	FAT	CARB	SUGAR	FIBER
Wrap Peppercorn Steak	1	702	40	45	4	3
Wrap Pepperoni	1	519	21	57	4	4
Wrap Roast Beef	1	448	13	58	2	4
Wrap Salad	1	324	2	66	10	6
Wrap Salami & Cheese	1	605	29	56	3	3
Wrap Seafood Salad	1	541	22	69	7	3
Wrap Steak	1	392	13	41	2	2
Wrap Steak & Cheese	1	464	18	43	3	2
Wrap Steak Bomb	1	670	33	52	6	6
Wrap Steak Tip	1	432	16	41	12	2
Wrap Tuna	1	731	44	56	4	3
Wrap Turkey	1	369	3	55	3	3
Wrap Turkey Club	1	415	8	52	4	3
SOUPS						
Beef Stew	1 sm	220	8	23	6	2
Broccoli & Cheddar Cheese	1 sm	270	21	11	3	2
Chicken Noodle	1 sm	110	3	14	4	1
Hearty Vegetable	1 sm	40	0	7	4	2
Italian Wedding	1 sm	120	6	11	3	2
Lobster Bisque	1 sm	360	29	16	3	1
New England Clam Chowder	1 sm	320	18	31	1	1
Portuguese Kale	1 sm	130	4	16	5	3

DUNKIN' DONUTS
BAGELS

FOOD	PORTION	CAL	FAT	CARB	SUGAR	FIBER
Blueberry	1	330	3	65	10	5
Cinnamon Raisin	1	330	4	65	13	5
Everything	1	350	5	66	5	5
Garlic	1	340	3	68	5	6
Multigrain	1	390	8	65	7	9
Onion	1	310	2	63	3	3
Plain	1	320	3	63	5	5

FOOD	PORTION	CAL	FAT	CARB	SUGAR	FIBER
Poppy Seed	1	350	6	64	5	5
Salt	1	320	3	63	5	5
Sesame	1	360	6	63	5	5
Wheat	1	320	4	61	4	5
BAKED SELECTIONS						
Apple Fritter	1	400	15	63	22	2
Biscuit	1	280	14	32	2	1
Bismark Chocolate Iced	1	350	14	53	22	1
Coffee Roll	1	370	18	49	17	2
Coffee Roll Chocolate Frosted	1	380	19	50	18	2
Coffee Roll Maple Frosted	1	380	18	50	19	2
Coffee Roll Vanilla Frosted	1	380	18	50	19	2
Cookie Chocolate Chunk	1	540	23	80	48	3
Cookie Oatmeal Raisin	1	480	14	83	51	5
Danish Apple Cheese	1	330	16	41	18	1
Danish Cheese	1	330	17	39	17	1
Danish Strawberry Cheese	1	320	16	40	18	1
Donut Apple Crumb	1	460	14	80	49	2
Donut Apple N' Spice	1	240	11	32	8	1
Donut Bavarian Kreme	1	250	12	31	9	1
Donut Blueberry Cake	1	330	18	38	19	1
Donut Blueberry Crumb	1	470	14	84	52	2
Donut Boston Kreme	1	280	12	38	16	1
Donut Bow Tie	1	310	15	39	15	1
Donut Chocolate Coconut	1	340	18	42	24	2
Donut Chocolate Frosted	1	340	19	38	19	1
Donut Chocolate Glazed Cake	1	280	15	33	16	1

FOOD	PORTION	CAL	FAT	CARB	SUGAR	FIBER
Donut Chocolate Kreme Filled	1	310	16	37	17	1
Donut Cinnamon	1	290	18	30	12	1
Donut Double Chocolate Cake	1	290	16	34	17	1
Donut Glazed Cake	1	320	18	37	18	1
Donut Jelly Filled	1	260	11	36	6	1
Donut Maple Frosted	1	230	10	33	14	1
Donut Marble Frosted	1	230	10	32	13	1
Donut Old Fashioned	1	280	18	27	9	1
Donut Powdered	1	300	18	30	12	1
Donut Strawberry Frosted	1	230	10	33	14	1
Donut Sugar Raised	1	190	9	22	4	1
Donut Vanilla Kreme Filled	1	320	17	37	18	1
Eclair	1	350	14	53	22	1
English Muffin	1	160	2	31	2	2
Fritter Glazed	1	400	15	63	22	2
Muffin Blueberry	1	510	16	87	51	2
Muffin Blueberry Reduced Fat	1	450	10	86	45	2
Muffin Chocolate Chip	1	630	23	98	59	3
Muffin Coffee Cake	1	660	26	98	57	1
Muffin Corn	1	510	17	84	36	1
Muffin Cranberry Orange Low Fat	1	390	3	83	42	4
Muffin Honey Bran Raisin	1	500	14	86	48	5
Munchkins Cinnamon Cake	1	60	3	6	2	0
Munchkins Glazed	1	50	3	7	3	0
Munchkins Glazed Chocolate Cake	1	60	3	8	4	0

FOOD	PORTION	CAL	FAT	CARB	SUGAR	FIBER
Munchkins Jelly Filled	1	60	3	8	1	0
Munchkins Plain Cake	1	50	3	5	2	0
Munchkins Powdered Cake	1	60	4	6	3	0
Munchkins Sugar Raised	1	40	3	5	1	0
Stick Cinnamon Cake	1	310	20	30	12	1
Stick Glazed Cake	1	340	20	38	20	1
Stick Glazed Chocolate Cake	1	390	25	40	17	2
Stick Jelly	1	400	20	54	20	1
Stick Plain Cake	1	300	20	26	9	1
Stick Powdered Cake	1	320	20	31	13	1
BEVERAGES						
Coffee Blueberry	1 sm (10 oz)	15	0	2	0	0
Coffee Caramel	1 sm (10 oz)	10	0	2	0	0
Coffee Cinnamon	1 sm (10 oz)	15	0	2	0	0
Coffee Coconut	1 sm (10 oz)	10	0	1	0	0
Coffee Regular	1 med (14 oz)	10	0	1	0	0
Coffee Regular	1 lg (20 oz)	10	0	2	0	0
Coffee Regular	1 extra lg	15	0	2	0	0
Coffee Regular	1 sm (10 oz)	5	0	1	0	0
Coffee Toasted Almond	1 sm (10 oz)	10	0	1	0	0
Coffee White Chocolate	1 sm (10 oz)	110	0	25	19	0
Coffee w/ Cream	1 (10 oz)	60	6	2	0	0
Coffee w/ Cream & Sugar	1 sm (10 oz)	120	6	19	17	0
Coffee w/ Milk	1 sm (10 oz)	35	1	2	1	0
Coffee w/ Milk & Sugar	1 sm (10 oz)	80	1	20	19	0
Coffee w/ Skim Milk	1 sm (10 oz)	15	0	3	2	0
Coffee w/ Skim Milk & Sugar	1 sm (10 oz)	70	0	20	19	0
Coffee w/ Sugar	1 sm (10 oz)	60	0	18	17	0
Coolatta Tropicana Orange	1 sm (16 oz)	220	0	52	50	0

FOOD	PORTION	CAL	FAT	CARB	SUGAR	FIBER
Dunkaccino	1 sm (10 oz)	230	11	35	24	1
Espresso	1 (1.75 oz)	0	0	0	0	0
Espresso w/ Sugar	1 (1.75 oz)	30	0	7	7	0
Hot Chocolate	1 sm (10 oz)	210	7	39	30	2
Iced Coffee	1 sm (16 oz)	10	0	2	0	0
Iced Coffee w/ Cream	1 sm (16 oz)	70	6	3	0	0
Iced Coffee w/ Cream & Sugar	1 sm (16 oz)	120	6	20	17	0
Iced Coffee w/ Milk	1 sm (16 oz)	30	1	3	1	0
Iced Coffee w/ Milk & Sugar	1 sm (16 oz)	90	1	21	19	0
Iced Coffee w/ Skim Milk	1 sm (16 oz)	20	0	2	2	0
Iced Coffee w/ Skim Milk & Sugar	1 sm (16 oz)	80	0	21	19	0
Iced Coffee w/ Sugar	1 sm (16 oz)	70	0	19	17	0
Iced Latte	1 sm (16 oz)	120	6	10	10	0
Iced Latte Caramel Swirl	1 sm (16 oz)	220	6	35	34	0
Iced Latte Caramel Swirl w/ Skim Milk	1 sm (16 oz)	180	0	36	35	0
Iced Latte Lite	1 med (24 oz)	120	0	19	15	0
Iced Latte Mocha Swirl	1 sm (16 oz)	220	6	35	32	1
Iced Latte Mocha Swirl w/ Skim Milk	1 sm (16 oz)	180	0	36	32	1
Iced Latte w/ Skim Milk	1 sm (16 oz)	70	0	11	10	0
Iced Latte w/ Skim Milk & Sugar	1 sm (16 oz)	130	0	28	27	0
Iced Latte w/ Sugar	1 sm (16 oz)	170	7	27	27	0
Latte	1 sm (10 oz)	120	6	10	10	0
Tea Regular Or Decaffeinated	1 (10 oz)	0	0	0	0	0
Tea w/ Milk	1 (10 oz)	20	1	1	1	0
Tea w/ Milk & Sugar	1 (10 oz)	80	1	19	19	0
Tea w/ Skim Milk	1 (10 oz)	10	0	2	2	0

FOOD	PORTION	CAL	FAT	CARB	SUGAR	FIBER
Tea w/ Skim Milk & Sugar	1 (10 oz)	70	0	19	19	0
Tea w/ Sugar	1 (10 oz)	60	0	17	17	0
Turbo Shot	1 sm (1.75 oz)	0	0	0	0	0
CREAM CHEESE						
Blueberry Reduced Fat	1 serv (1.75 oz)	150	9	15	11	0
Onion & Chive Reduced Fat	1 serv (1.75 oz)	130	11	6	3	0
Plain	1 serv (1.75 oz)	150	15	3	3	0
Plain Reduced Fat	1 serv (1.75 oz)	100	8	5	2	0
Salmon Reduced Fat	1 serv (1.75 oz)	140	11	6	3	0
Strawberry Reduced Fat	1 serv (1.75 oz)	150	10	15	11	0
Veggie Reduced Fat	1 serv (1.75 oz)	120	10	6	2	0
SANDWICHES						
Bagel Egg Cheese	1	470	14	66	7	5
Bagel Ham Egg Cheese	1	510	16	67	7	5
Bagel Sausage Egg Cheese	1	640	29	67	7	5
Biscuit Egg Cheese	1	430	26	36	4	1
Biscuit Sausage Egg Cheese	1	610	40	36	4	1
Croissant Bacon Egg Cheese	1	510	31	39	6	2
Croissant Egg Cheese	1	470	28	39	6	2
Croissant Ham Egg Cheese Cheese	1	510	30	39	6	2
English Muffin Bacon Egg Cheese	1	360	16	34	3	2

FOOD	PORTION	CAL	FAT	CARB	SUGAR	FIBER
English Muffin Egg Cheese	1	320	13	34	3	2
English Muffin Ham Egg Cheese	1	360	15	35	3	2
English Muffin Sausage Egg Cheese	1	490	28	35	3	2
Flatbread Egg White Turkey	1	280	6	37	5	3
Flatbread Egg White Veggie	1	290	9	39	4	3

EL POLLO LOCO

DESSERTS

FOOD	PORTION	CAL	FAT	CARB	SUGAR	FIBER
Caramel Flan	1 serv (5.5 oz)	290	12	41	39	0
Churros	2	300	18	32	10	2
Cone Vanilla	1	330	8	55	47	0
Soft Serve Vanilla	1 cup (5 oz)	300	8	48	47	0

MAIN MENU SELECTIONS

FOOD	PORTION	CAL	FAT	CARB	SUGAR	FIBER
BBQ Black Beans	1 serv (6 oz)	200	3	38	16	4
Bowl The Original Pollo	1 serv	540	4	85	1	11
Burrito BRC	1 (7.5 oz)	390	10	61	0	6
Burrito Classic Chicken	1 (10.3 oz)	500	14	63	0	6
Burrito Twice Grilled	1 (15 oz)	830	37	58	2	5
Burrito Ultimate Grilled	1 (13.6 oz)	650	20	80	1	8
Chicken Breast	1 (4.3 oz)	220	9	0	0	0
Chicken Breast Skinless	1 (4 oz)	180	4	0	0	0
Chicken Leg	1 (1.8 oz)	90	4	0	0	0
Chicken Thigh	1 (3.1 oz)	220	15	0	0	0
Chicken Wing	1 (1.3 oz)	90	5	0	0	0
Cole Slaw	1 serv (6 oz)	120	9	8	6	2
Corn Cobbette	1 (5 oz)	90	1	19	3	2
French Fries	1 serv (5.5 oz)	440	21	57	0	6

FOOD	PORTION	CAL	FAT	CARB	SUGAR	FIBER
Fresh Vegetables w/ Margarine	1 serv (4.1 oz)	60	3	8	3	3
Fresh Vegetables w/o Margarine	1 serv (4 oz)	35	0	8	3	3
Gravy	1 serv (1 oz)	10	0	2	0	0
Loco Nachos	1 serv	170	14	7	2	1
Macaroni & Cheese	1 serv (5.5 oz)	280	17	28	3	6
Mashed Potatoes	1 serv (5 oz)	100	1	20	tr	2
Pinto Beans	1 serv (6 oz)	140	0	25	0	7
Quesadilla Cheese	1 (4.5 oz)	420	23	35	0	2
Refried Beans w/ Cheese	1 serv (6.3 oz)	270	7	36	2	10
Skinless Breast Meal	1 serv	310	12	17	6	5
Soup Chicken Tortilla w/o Tortilla Strips	1 serv (10 oz)	140	6	8	2	2
Spanish Rice	1 serv (4.5 oz)	160	1	34	0	1
Taco Al Carbon	1 (3.1 oz)	150	5	17	tr	1
Taco Soft Chicken	1 (4.5 oz)	270	13	19	0	2
Taquito Chicken	1	190	9	18	0	1
Tortilla Chips	1 serv (1.5 oz)	210	10	28	tr	3
Tortilla Corn 6 Inches	2	120	2	24	0	2
Tortilla Flour 6.5 Inches	2	210	7	30	2	2
SALAD DRESSINGS AND TOPPINGS						
Creamy Cilantro	1 serv (1.5 oz)	220	23	1	1	0
Creamy Cilantro Light	1 pkg	70	5	6	3	0
Guacamole	1 serv (1 oz)	45	4	4	tr	tr
Hot Sauce Jalapeno	1 pkg	5	0	1	0	0
Jack & Poblano Queso	1 serv (1.8 oz)	100	8	4	1	0
Ketchup	1 pkg	10	0	2	2	0
Light Italian	1 pkg	20	1	2	2	0
Pico De Gallo Medium	1 serv (1 oz)	10	1	1	tr	0
Ranch	1 pkg	230	24	2	2	0
Salsa Avocado Hot	1 serv (1 oz)	30	3	1	0	tr
Salsa Chipotle Hot	1 serv (1 oz)	5	0	1	tr	0

FOOD	PORTION	CAL	FAT	CARB	SUGAR	FIBER
Salsa House Mild	1 serv (1 oz)	5	0	1	tr	0
Sour Cream	1 serv (1 oz)	60	5	1	0	0
Thousand Island	1 pkg	220	21	6	6	0
SALADS						
Caesar Pollo	1 (11.4 oz)	520	38	17	6	4
Ceasar Pollo w/o Dressing	1 (9.4 oz)	220	7	15	4	4
Garden	1 (4.8 oz)	120	4	9	3	2
Tostada Chicken	1 (17.3 oz)	840	40	76	4	7
Tostada Chicken w/o Shell	1 (14.7 oz)	410	11	42	3	5

EMERALD CITY SMOOTHIE

FOOD	PORTION	CAL	FAT	CARB	SUGAR	FIBER
Apple Andie	1 (11 oz)	230	1	46	37	2
Berry Berry	1 (13 oz)	350	0	77	47	9
Blueberry Blast	1 (13 oz)	380	0	78	51	9
Coconut Passion	1 (11 oz)	600	23	80	58	11
Cranberry Delight	1 (10 oz)	550	1	127	114	2
Energizer	1 (10 oz)	350	1	62	36	7
Fruity Supreme	1 (9 oz)	280	1	59	34	6
Grape Escape	1 (10 oz)	480	1	109	102	2
Guava Sunrise	1 (13 oz)	366	1	80	67	6
Kiwi Kic	1 (11 oz)	400	1	88	81	2
Lean Body	1 (11 oz)	330	8	24	6	8
Lean Out	1 (11 oz)	600	26	35	21	5
Low Carb	1 (10 oz)	350	2	27	17	2
Mango Mania	1 (8 oz)	370	0	82	78	2
Marionberry Fuel	1 (13 oz)	380	0	81	50	10
Mega Mass	1 (14 oz)	610	10	103	55	7
Mini Mass	1 (13 oz)	520	11	79	53	6
Mocha Bliss	1 (10 oz)	550	8	63	58	1
Nutty Banana	1 (11 oz)	720	25	97	72	9
Orange Twister	1 (10 oz)	140	0	31	24	2
Pacific Splash	1 (12 oz)	240	0	58	34	6

FOOD	PORTION	CAL	FAT	CARB	SUGAR	FIBER
PB&J	1 (14 oz)	630	25	77	43	12
Peach Pleasure	1 (12 oz)	270	0	54	41	5
Peanut Passion	1 (11 oz)	580	25	61	31	10
Pineapple Bliss	1 (12 oz)	210	1	45	35	4
Power Fuel	1 (11 oz)	450	3	66	29	6
Quick Start	1 (10 oz)	280	0	46	27	4
Raspberry Dream	1 (13 oz)	410	1	80	48	10
Rejuvenator	1 (10 oz)	340	1	62	35	7
Sambazon	1 (15 oz)	410	6	92	69	8
Slim N Fit	1 (10 oz)	350	1	60	35	6
The Builder	1 (18 oz)	1270	46	144	73	10
Zesty Lemon	1 (14 oz)	430	9	67	46	5
Zip Zip	1 (10 oz)	240	3	35	24	3
Zone Zinger	1 (14 oz)	430	3	76	53	4

EVOS

BEVERAGES

FOOD	PORTION	CAL	FAT	CARB	SUGAR	FIBER
Shake Mango Guava	1 reg (16 oz)	180	0	48	44	2
Shake Multi-Berry	1 reg (20 oz)	200	1	52	35	1
Shake Strawberry Banana	1 reg (16 oz)	190	1	47	38	1
Shake Organic Cappuccino	1 reg (16 oz)	230	3	47	44	0
Shake Organic Vanilla	1 reg (16 oz)	180	3	30	30	0

CHILDREN'S MENU SELECTIONS

FOOD	PORTION	CAL	FAT	CARB	SUGAR	FIBER
Kids Champion Burger	1	400	12	48	3	7
Kids Chicken Strips	1 serv	130	3	13	0	0
Kids Freerange Steakburger	1	390	15	39	2	2
Kids Good Corn Dog	1	150	4	27	4	3

MAIN MENU SELECTIONS

FOOD	PORTION	CAL	FAT	CARB	SUGAR	FIBER
Airbaked Chicken Strips	1 serv	260	6	26	0	0
Airfries	1 reg	230	8	35	1	3
American Champion	1	420	12	53	7	6

FOOD	PORTION	CAL	FAT	CARB	SUGAR	FIBER
American DeLite	1	330	6	53	6	7
Burger Bun	1	190	2	39	2	2
Cheddar Cheese Slice	1	80	7	0	0	0
Crispy Mesquite Chicken	1 serv	330	5	53	3	2
Freerange Steakburger	1	400	15	42	4	3
Fresh Fruit Bowl	1 serv	200	1	52	47	4
Good Corn Dog	1	150	4	22	4	3
Herb Crusted Trout	1 serv	440	25	62	7	3
Honey Mesquite Chicken	1 serv	290	3	41	3	2
Spicy Chipotle Turkey	1 serv	370	9	42	3	3
Veggie Chili	1 reg	110	2	20	3	5
Veggie Garden Grill Italian	1	350	5	54	4	8
Wraps Avocado Turkey	1	480	15	51	5	4
Wraps Crispy Buffalo Chicken	1	440	11	64	5	5
Wraps Crispy Thai Trout	1	660	20	96	6	5
Wraps Freerange Beef Taco	1	600	28	53	6	5
Wraps Honey Wheat	1	300	8	49	4	4
Wraps Southwest Soy Taco	1	500	25	58	6	10
Wraps Spicy Thai Chicken	1	510	10	76	3	4
Wraps Spinach Herb	1	310	8	52	3	3
Wraps Tomato Basil Chicken	1	520	11	82	3	4
SALAD DRESSINGS AND TOPPINGS						
Balsamic Vinegar	1 serv (0.5 oz)	5	0	2	2	0
Crispy Noodles	1 serv (7 g)	35	1	5	0	0
Croutons Multi-Grain	1 serv (7 g)	30	2	4	0	0
Dressing Avocado	1 serv (3 oz)	190	21	5	1	2
Dressing Caesar	1 serv (1.7 oz)	300	32	2	0	0

FOOD	PORTION	CAL	FAT	CARB	SUGAR	FIBER
Dressing Fat Free Vinaigrette	1 serv (1 oz)	5	0	2	1	0
Dressing Raspberry	1 serv (2 oz)	50	0	14	12	0
Dressing Spicy Thai	1 serv (1.4 oz)	150	9	15	12	0
Extra Virgin Olive Oil	1 serv (1 oz)	250	28	0	0	0
Herb Spread	1 serv (0.7 oz)	30	3	2	0	0
Ketchup Cayenne Firewalker	1 serv (1.2 oz)	35	0	9	8	0
Ketchup Garlic Gravity	1 serv (1.2 oz)	35	0	9	8	0
Ketchup Mesquite Magic	1 serv (1.2 oz)	35	0	9	8	0
Mustand Mesquite Honey	1 serv (0.7 oz)	80	8	3	2	0
Mustard	1 serv (0.5 oz)	10	0	1	0	0
Southwest Sour Cream	1 serv (1.4 oz)	60	35	4	2	0
Spicy Chipotle Mayo	1 serv (0.7 oz)	30	2	2	0	0
Tomato Basil Sauce	1 serv (1.4 oz)	150	15	5	2	0
SALADS						
Bordeaux Bistro w/o Dressing	1	260	22	7	2	3
For Salads Chicken Strips	1 serv (3 oz)	130	3	13	0	0
For Salads Grilled Chicken	1 serv (3 oz)	90	1	1	0	0
Mediterranean Summer w/o Dressing	1	200	8	22	11	6
Santa Ana Caesar w/o Dressing	1	20	0	4	1	2
Side Salad w/o Dressing	1	35	0	8	3	2
Spicy Thai w/o Dressing	1	35	0	7	4	2
SUPPLEMENTS						
Fat Burner	1 serv (5 g)	16	0	4	0	0
Go Energy	1 serv (5 g)	15	0	4	0	0
Mega Protein	1 serv (0.5 oz)	45	0	0	0	0
Multi-Vitamin	1 serv (5 g)	10	0	3	0	0

FOOD	PORTION	CAL	FAT	CARB	SUGAR	FIBER

FAZOLI'S
BEVERAGES

FOOD	PORTION	CAL	FAT	CARB	SUGAR	FIBER
Lemon Ice All Flavors	1	360	0	90	90	0
Lemon Ice Original	1 reg	180	0	45	45	0
Lemon Ice Strawberry	1	320	0	81	81	0

CHILDREN'S MENU SELECTIONS

Fettuccine Alfredo	1 serv	290	5	50	4	2
Meat Lasagna	1 serv	260	13	21	4	2
Ravioli w/ Marinara	1 serv	290	7	43	5	3
Spaghetti w/ Meatballs	1 serv	350	7	55	5	4
Ziti w/ Meat Sauce	1 serv	190	6	25	4	3

DESSERTS

Cheesecake Original	1 slice	290	22	17	17	0
Cheesecake Turtle	1 slice	450	28	43	31	2
Cookie Chocolate Chunk	1	510	26	68	39	3

MAIN MENU SELECTIONS

Breadstick	1	100	2	20	1	0
Breadstick Garlic	1	150	7	20	1	1
Fettuccine Alfredo	1 sm	520	12	83	8	4
Fettuccine w/ Marinara	1 serv	450	3	88	10	7
Fettuccine w/ Meat Sauce	1 serv	500	7	87	9	7
Oven Baked Chicken Parmesan	1 serv	960	33	117	12	9
Oven Baked Meat Lasagna	1 serv	510	25	43	7	5
Oven Baked Rigatoni Romano	1 serv	1090	54	101	13	11
Oven Baked Spaghetti	1 serv	680	22	90	10	7
Oven Baked Spaghetti w/ Meatballs	1 serv	940	40	100	12	9
Panini Four Cheese & Tomato	1	510	22	53	4	3
Panini Grilled Chicken	1	540	18	56	4	3

FOOD	PORTION	CAL	FAT	CARB	SUGAR	FIBER
Panini Smoked Turkey	1	620	29	54	5	3
Penne w/ Alfredo	1 serv	520	12	83	8	4
Penne w/ Marinara	1 serv	450	3	88	10	7
Penne w/ Meat Sauce	1 serv	500	7	87	9	7
Pizza Slice Cheese	1	270	11	31	2	2
Pizza Slice Pepperoni	1	310	14	31	2	2
Platter Classic Sampler	1	810	25	110	13	8
Platter Ultimate Sampler	1	980	29	134	17	11
Ravioli w/ Marinara	1 serv	500	15	71	10	7
Ravioli w/ Meat Sauce	1 serv	550	20	71	10	7
Spaghetti w/ Alfredo	1 serv	520	12	83	8	4
Spaghetti w/ Marinara	1 sm	450	3	88	10	7
Spaghetti w/ Meat Sauce	1 sm	500	7	87	9	7
Submarinos Club	half	973	34	65	6	3
Submarinos Ham n'Swiss	1	680	30	65	6	3
Submarinos Italian Beef	half	660	24	68	7	3
Submarinos Original	half	940	58	68	6	4
Topping Broccoli	1 serv	25	0	5	1	3
Topping Broccoli & Tomatoes	1 serv	30	0	6	2	3
Topping Garlic Shrimp	1 serv	160	12	3	0	1
Topping Italian Sausage	1 serv	240	21	3	0	1
Topping Meatballs	1 serv	160	18	6	1	1
Topping Peppery Chicken	1 serv	70	1	1	0	0
Ziti w/ Meat Sauce	1 serv	480	15	65	9	6
SALAD DRESSINGS						
Caesar	1 serv	220	25	1	0	0
Fat Free Honey Mustard	1 serv	60	0	15	14	1
Fat Free Italian	1 serv	25	0	6	3	0
Honey French	1 serv	220	18	14	13	0
Italian	1 serv	160	14	7	7	0
Ranch	1 serv	220	24	2	2	0
Ranch Lite	1 serv	120	12	2	1	0

FOOD	PORTION	CAL	FAT	CARB	SUGAR	FIBER
SALADS						
Chicken & Fruit	1	220	2	28	20	4
Chicken & Pasta Caesar	1	440	15	41	8	4
Chicken BLT Ranch	1	270	10	13	5	4
Parmesan Chicken	1	360	15	31	5	4
Side Caesar	1	40	2	4	1	2
Side Garden	1	25	0	4	2	3
Side Pasta	1	320	12	41	7	1
FIVE GUYS BURGERS AND FRIES						
MAIN MENU SELECTIONS						
Bacon Burger	1 (9.8 oz)	780	50	39	8	2
Bacon Cheese Dog	1 (7 oz)	695	48	41	9	2
Bacon Dog	1 (6.4 oz)	625	42	40	8	2
Cheese Dog	1 (6.5 oz)	615	41	41	9	2
Cheeseburger	1 (10.6 oz)	840	55	40	9	2
Cheeseburger Bacon	1 (11 oz)	920	62	40	9	2
Fries	1 reg (8.6 oz)	620	30	78	2	6
Fries	1 lg (16 oz)	1464	71	184	5	14
Grilled Cheese	1 (4 oz)	430	26	41	10	3
Hamburger	1 (9.3 oz)	700	43	39	8	2
Hot Dog	1 (5.9 oz)	545	35	40	8	2
Little Burgers Bacon Burger	1 (6.5 oz)	560	33	39	8	2
Little Burgers Cheeseburger	1 (6.7 oz)	550	32	40	9	2
Little Burgers Cheeseburger Bacon	1 (7.2 oz)	630	39	40	9	2
Little Burgers Hamburger	1 (6 oz)	480	26	39	8	2
Veggie Sandwich	1 (7.3 oz)	440	15	60	14	2
TOPPINGS						
A1 Steak Sauce	1 tbsp (0.6 oz)	15	0	3	2	0

FOOD	PORTION	CAL	FAT	CARB	SUGAR	FIBER
Bacon	2 slices (0.5 oz)	80	7	0	0	0
BBQ Sauce	1 tbsp (0.6 oz)	60	8	16	10	0
Cheese	1 slice (0.7 oz)	70	6	tr	tr	0
Green Peppers	1 serv (0.8 oz)	5	0	2	tr	tr
Hot Sauce	1 tsp (5 g)	0	0	0	0	0
Jalapenos	1 serv (0.4 oz)	3	0	tr	0	0
Ketchup	1 tbsp (0.6 oz)	15	0	4	4	0
Lettuce	1 serv (1 oz)	4	0	1	tr	tr
Mayonnaise	1 serv (0.5 oz)	100	11	0	0	0
Mushrooms	1 serv (0.9 oz)	10	0	1	0	tr
Mustard	1 tbsp (0.6 oz)	0	0	0	0	0
Onions	1 serv (0.9 oz)	10	0	3	1	tr
Pickle Chips	6 (1 oz)	5	0	1	0	0
Relish	1 serv (0.5 oz)	15	0	4	3	0
Tomatoes	1 serv (1.8 oz)	9	0	2	2	tr

GREAT STEAK & POTATO
BEVERAGES

FOOD	PORTION	CAL	FAT	CARB	SUGAR	FIBER
Great Steak Lemonade	1 sm (12 oz)	180	0	48	45	0
Orange Juice	1 (12 oz)	118	0	30	30	0

BREAKFAST SELECTIONS

FOOD	PORTION	CAL	FAT	CARB	SUGAR	FIBER
Potatoes Deluxe Home	1 serv (12 oz)	390	23	44	3	7
Potatoes Fresh Cut Home	1 serv (10.6 oz)	380	23	42	2	6
Sandwich Bacon Egg Cheese	1 (7.6 oz)	600	36	39	2	2
Sandwich Egg Cheese	1 (7 oz)	500	29	39	2	2
Sandwich Ham Cheese	1 (5.5 oz)	430	22	41	4	2
Sandwich Ham Egg Cheese	1 (9 oz)	570	32	42	4	2
Sandwich Sausage Egg Cheese	1 (9 oz)	700	47	39	2	2

FOOD	PORTION	CAL	FAT	CARB	SUGAR	FIBER
Sandwich Steak Egg Cheese	1 (10 oz)	600	34	40	3	2

CHILDREN'S MENU SELECTIONS

FOOD	PORTION	CAL	FAT	CARB	SUGAR	FIBER
Grilled Cheese w/ Fry	1 serv (8.8 oz)	530	28	57	2	6
Kid's Great Fry	1 (6.1 oz)	270	13	36	0	4
Kids Nuggets	1 serv (2.7 oz)	165	9	10	–	1
Slider Chicken w/ Fry	1 serv (11.5 oz)	570	25	60	5	6
Slider Steak w/ Fry	1 serv (11.8 oz)	580	28	60	5	6

MAIN MENU SELECTIONS

FOOD	PORTION	CAL	FAT	CARB	SUGAR	FIBER
Baked Potato Broccoli & Cheese	1 (8.9 oz)	400	24	35	5	4
Baked Potato Cheese & Bacon	1 (7.8 oz)	530	35	29	2	3
Baked Potato Plain	1 (6 oz)	160	0	36	2	4
Baked Potato Sour Cream & Chive	1 (7.3 oz)	350	23	32	2	3
Baked Potato The King	1 (8.8 oz)	590	41	31	2	3
Cheeseburger	1 (10.2 oz)	640	35	41	3	3
Chicagoland Cheesesteak 7 Inch	1 (13.3 oz)	680	29	63	9	5
Coney Island Fry	1 reg (12.7 oz)	570	30	61	5	12
Great Fry	1 reg (10.2 oz)	440	20	60	0	7
Great Steak Cheesesteak 7 Inch	1 (13.6 oz)	740	37	62	8	5
Great Steak Cheesesteak Wrap	1 (13.7 oz)	820	43	67	6	5
Gyro	1 (12 oz)	580	30	52	8	5
Ham Delight 7 Inch	1 (13.1 oz)	710	33	71	16	5
Ham Explosion 7 Inch	1 (14 oz)	710	34	70	13	6

FOOD	PORTION	CAL	FAT	CARB	SUGAR	FIBER
Hamburger	1 (9.7 oz)	590	30	40	3	3
Kansas City BBQ Cheesesteak 7 Inch	1 (12 oz)	680	26	71	14	5
King Fry	1 reg (11.4 oz)	630	39	52	3	5
Nacho Fry	1 reg (11.8 oz)	510	27	53	3	5
Pastrami 7 Inch	1 (13.3 oz)	790	41	65	9	5
Philly Buffalo Chicken 7 Inch	1 (13.8 oz)	660	24	65	9	5
Philly Burger	1 (14.2 oz)	820	50	47	6	4
Philly Chicken Slider	1 (5.4 oz)	300	13	24	5	2
Philly Original Cheesesteak 7 Inch	1 (11.8 oz)	650	26	62	10	5
Philly Original Chicken 7 Inch	1 (11 oz)	620	22	62	10	5
Philly Original Chicken Wrap	1 (11.3 oz)	700	28	67	7	4
Philly Steak Slider	1 (5.6 oz)	310	15	24	5	2
Philly Teriyaki Chicken	1 (14 oz)	290	32	65	11	5
Philly Turkey 7 Inch	1 (13 oz)	670	30	64	8	5
Philly Ultimate Chicken	1 (14.6 oz)	730	33	64	9	6
Philly Ultimate Chicken Wrap	1 (14.7 oz)	810	39	69	6	5
Potato Skins	1 serv (6.4 oz)	390	26	24	4	2
Reuben 7 Inch	1 (12 oz)	690	33	61	7	5
Super Steak Wrap Cheesesteak	1 (15.7 oz)	930	54	69	6	5
The Great Potato Chicken	1 (13 oz)	600	33	37	7	4
The Great Potato Ham	1 (12.8 oz)	520	28	43	11	4
The Great Potato Steak	1 (13.5 oz)	620	38	37	7	4
The Great Potato Turkey	1 (12.8 oz)	490	25	39	7	4
Veggi Delight 7 Inch	1 (12.2 oz)	610	31	66	10	6

FOOD	PORTION	CAL	FAT	CARB	SUGAR	FIBER
Wacker Fry	1 reg (9.8 oz)	490	27	51	3	5
Wisonsin Inside-Out 7 Inch	1 (6.2 oz)	560	27	57	5	4
SALAD DRESSINGS AND SAUCES						
Dressing Ranch	1 oz	170	18	1	1	0
Dressing Thousand Island	1 oz	130	12	4	3	0
Mayonnaise	1 oz	200	22	0	0	0
Mayonnaise Dijon	1 oz	110	11	3	0	0
Oil	1 serv (0.3 oz)	60	7	0	0	0
Sauce Buffalo	1 oz	10	0	2	0	0
Sauce Marinara Dipping	2 oz	15	0	3	1	0
Sauce Teriyaki	1 oz	25	0	3	3	0
Sauce Tzatziki	1 oz	50	4	2	1	0
SALADS						
Chef w/o Dressing	1 (16.1 oz)	260	11	15	8	4
Garden w/o Dressing	1 (12 oz)	60	1	13	7	5
Great Salad Grilled Chicken	1 (18.8 oz)	380	18	18	9	5
Great Salad Grilled Ham	1 (18.8 oz)	360	20	28	13	5
Great Salad Grilled Steak	1 (19.3 oz)	400	23	18	9	5
Great Salad Grilled Turkey	1 (18.8 oz)	330	17	20	9	5
Side w/o Dressing	1 (6 oz)	30	0	6	4	2
Wedge Grilled Chicken	1 (14.8 oz)	270	12	11	6	3
Wedge Grilled Steak	1 (15.3 oz)	290	16	11	6	3

HUNGRY HOWIE'S PIZZA
OTHER MENU SELECTIONS

FOOD	PORTION	CAL	FAT	CARB	SUGAR	FIBER
Cajun Bread	¼ bread	300	9	46	–	1
Chicken Tenders	2	140	5	11	–	0
Cinnamon Bread	¼ bread	313	9	59	–	1
Howie Bread	¼ bread	300	9	46	–	1
Howie Wings	5	180	13	0	0	0

FOOD	PORTION	CAL	FAT	CARB	SUGAR	FIBER
Sub Deluxe Italian	½ sub	506	18	61	–	2
Sub Ham & Cheese	½ sub	475	15	61	–	2
Sub Pizza	½ sub	689	34	67	–	3
Sub Pizza Special	½ sub	606	24	68	–	3
Sub Steak & Cheese	½ sub	491	15	64	–	2
Sub Turkey	½ sub	466	13	63	–	2
Sub Turkey Club	½ sub	556	15	63	–	2
Sub Vegetarian	½ sub	530	21	64	–	3
Three Cheeser Bread	¼ bread	370	14	47	–	1
PIZZA						
Cheese Slice	1 sm	161	4	20	–	1
Cheese Slice	1 extra lg	395	9	42	–	2
Cheese Slice	1 med	191	6	23	–	1
Cheese Slice	1 lg	208	5	25	–	1
Cheese Slice Thin	1 lg	124	6	11	–	1
Cheese Slice Thin	1 med	111	5	10	–	tr
Medium Topping Anchovies	1 serv	44	3	0	0	0
Medium Topping Bacon	1 serv	32	1	tr	–	0
Medium Topping Banana Peppers	1 serv	6	0	1	–	0
Medium Topping Beef	1 serv	30	2	tr	–	tr
Medium Topping Black Olives	1 serv	7	tr	tr	–	tr
Medium Topping Ham	1 serv	7	tr	0	–	0
Medium Topping Mushrooms	1 serv	2	0	tr	–	tr
Medium Topping Pepperoni	1 serv	22	2	0	–	0
Medium Topping Pineapple	1 serv	5	0	2	–	1
Medium Topping Sausage	1 serv	27	2	tr	–	tr

FOOD	PORTION	CAL	FAT	CARB	SUGAR	FIBER
SALAD DRESSINGS AND SAUCES						
Dressing Blue Cheese	1 serv (1 oz)	150	16	1	–	0
Dressing Creamy Italian	1 serv (1 oz)	120	12	2	–	0
Dressing Fat Free Italian	1 serv (1.5 oz)	25	0	5	–	0
Dressing Fat Free Ranch	1 serv (1.5 oz)	45	0	10	–	1
Dressing French Style	1 serv (1 oz)	30	0	7	–	0
Dressing Greek	1 serv (1 oz)	110	11	2	–	0
Dressing Italian	1 serv (1 oz)	80	8	2	–	0
Dressing Ranch	1 serv (1 oz)	180	19	1	–	0
Dressing Thousand Island	1 serv (1 oz)	140	14	4	–	0
Sauce Dipping	1 serv (3 oz)	45	1	9	–	1
SALADS						
Antipasto	1 sm	115	7	3	–	2
Chef	1 sm	114	7	4	–	2
Garden	1 sm	20	tr	3	–	2
Greek	1 sm	126	7	8	–	2
IVAR'S SEAFOOD BARS						
Chicken	3 pieces (4.5 oz)	250	11	14	–	–
Chowder Salmon	1 cup	220	13	22	–	2
Chowder White	1 cup	330	19	24	–	4
Clams	1 serv (5 oz)	400	21	33	–	1
Cocktail Sauce	¼ cup	50	0	12	–	1
Fish	3 pieces	220	9	12	–	1
French Fries	1 serv (3.5 oz)	300	16	34	–	2
Oysters	5	290	14	22	–	1
Prawns	1 serv (5 oz)	290	15	18	–	tr
Salmon Fried	3 pieces (4.5 oz)	210	9	9	–	1
Scallops	1 serv (5 oz)	240	9	14	–	tr
Tartar Sauce	2 tbsp	140	15	1	–	0

FOOD	PORTION	CAL	FAT	CARB	SUGAR	FIBER
JACK IN THE BOX						
BEVERAGES						
Barq's Root Beer	1 (20 oz)	180	0	50	50	0
Chocolate Milk Low Fat Chug	1 (3.5 oz)	200	3	34	33	1
Coca Cola Classic	1 (20 oz)	170	0	46	46	0
Coffee Regular & Decaf	1 (11 oz)	5	0	1	0	0
Diet Coke	1 (20 oz)	0	0	0	0	0
Dr Pepper	1 (20 oz)	150	0	42	42	0
Fanta Orange	1 (20 oz)	150	0	41	41	0
Fanta Strawberry	1 (20 oz)	150	0	41	41	0
Iced Tea	1 (20 oz)	5	0	2	0	0
Lemonade	1 (20 oz)	160	0	42	42	0
Orange Juice	1 (10 oz)	140	0	32	27	2
Reduced Fat Milk Chug	1 (3.5 oz)	130	5	13	13	0
Shake Chocolate	1 (16 oz)	880	45	107	94	1
Shake Oreo	1 (16 oz)	910	49	102	80	1
Shake Strawberry	1 (16 oz)	880	44	105	88	0
Shake Vanilla	1 (16 oz)	790	44	83	70	0
Sprite	1 (20 oz)	160	0	42	42	0
BREAKFAST SELECTIONS						
Biscuit Bacon Egg Cheese	1	430	25	34	3	1
Biscuit Chicken	1	450	24	42	2	2
Biscuit Sausage	1	440	29	32	3	2
Biscuit Sausage Egg Cheese	1	740	55	35	3	2
Biscuit Spicy Chicken	1	460	22	44	2	2
Breakfast Jack	1	290	12	39	4	1
Breakfast Jack Bacon	1	300	14	29	4	1
Breakfast Jack Sausage	1	450	28	29	4	1
Breakfast Sandwich Ciabatta	1	710	30	63	4	3

FOOD	PORTION	CAL	FAT	CARB	SUGAR	FIBER
Breakfast Sandwich Ultimate	1	570	27	49	8	2
Burrito Hearty Breakfast	1	480	29	29	1	2
Burrito Sirloin Steak & Egg w/o Salsa	1	790	48	52	2	6
Croissant Sausage	1	580	39	37	5	2
Croissant Supreme	1	450	25	36	5	1
French Toast Sticks	4 (4.2 oz)	470	23	58	14	4
French Toast Sticks Blueberry	4	450	20	59	15	3
Hash Browns	1 serv	150	10	13	0	2
Sandwich Extreme Sausage	1	670	48	31	5	2
DESSERTS						
Cake Chocolate Overload	1 serv (3.2 oz)	300	7	57	34	2
Cheesecake	1 serv (3.6 oz)	310	16	34	23	0
MAIN MENU SELECTIONS						
Bacon Cheddar Potato Wedges	1 serv (9 oz)	720	48	52	2	4
Cheeseburger Bacon Ultimate	1	1090	77	53	12	2
Cheeseburger Junior Bacon	1	430	25	30	6	1
Cheeseburger Sourdough Ultimate	1	950	73	36	7	2
Cheeseburger Ultimate	1	1010	71	53	12	2
Chicken Fajita Pita	1	280	9	30	3	2
Chicken Sandwich	1	400	21	38	4	2
Chicken Strips Crispy	4	500	25	36	1	3
Chicken Strips Grilled	4 (5 oz)	180	2	3	2	0
Ciabatta Chipotle w/ Grilled Chicken	1	690	28	65	6	4

FOOD	PORTION	CAL	FAT	CARB	SUGAR	FIBER
Ciabatta Chipotle w/ Spicy Crispy Chicken	1	750	34	75	5	5
Ciabatta Sirloin Steak 'N' Cheddar	1	770	38	65	5	4
Ciabatta Burger Bacon 'N Cheese	1	1120	76	66	9	4
Ciabatta Burger Single Bacon 'N' Cheese	1	870	54	66	8	4
Club Sourdough Grilled Chicken	1	530	28	34	5	3
Curly Fries Seasoned	1 sm (3 oz)	270	15	30	1	3
Egg Rolls	1	130	6	15	1	2
Fish & Chips	1 serv (7.6 oz)	570	30	58	1	4
Fries Natural Cut	1 sm	340	17	41	1	5
Fruit Cup	1 serv	90	0	22	18	2
Hamburger	1	310	14	30	6	1
Hamburger Deluxe	1	370	21	31	6	2
Hamburger Deluxe w/ Cheese	1	460	28	33	7	2
Hamburger w/ Cheese	1	350	17	31	7	1
Jack's Spicy Chicken	1 serv	620	31	61	8	4
Jack's Spicy Chicken w/ Cheese	1	700	37	62	8	4
Jumbo Jack	1	600	35	51	11	3
Jumbo Jack w/ Cheese	1	690	42	54	12	3
Mozzarella Cheese Sticks	3	240	12	21	1	1
Onion Rings	8 (4.2 oz)	500	30	51	3	3
Sampler Trio	1 serv	750	39	65	4	5
Sandwich Bacon Chicken	1	440	24	39	4	2

FOOD	PORTION	CAL	FAT	CARB	SUGAR	FIBER
Sirloin Burger w/ American Cheese & Red Onion	1	1120	73	63	11	4
Sirloin Burger w/ Swiss & Grilled Onions	1	1070	71	61	10	4
Sirloin Steak Melt	1	640	40	34	4	2
Sourdough Jack	1	710	51	36	7	3
Spicy Chicken Bites	1 serv	290	14	21	1	3
Stuffed Jalapeno	3 (2.5 oz)	230	13	22	2	2
Taco Monster Beef	1	240	14	20	4	3
Taco Regular Beef	1	160	8	15	4	2
SALAD DRESSINGS AND TOPPINGS						
Asian Sesame	1 serv (2.5 oz)	230	17	20	13	0
Bacon Ranch	1 serv (2.5 oz)	320	33	4	2	0
Creamy Southwest	1 serv (2.5 oz)	270	27	4	1	0
Dipping Sauce Barbeque	1 serv (1 oz)	45	0	11	4	0
Dipping Sauce Buttermilk House	1 serv (0.9 oz)	130	13	3	0	0
Dipping Sauce Frank's Red Hot Buffalo	1 serv (1 oz)	10	0	2	0	0
Dipping Sauce Sweet & Sour	1 serv (1 oz)	45	0	11	6	0
Dipping Sauce Teriyaki	1 serv (1 oz)	60	0	13	11	0
Dipping Sauce Zesty Marinara	1 serv (0.8 oz)	15	0	4	2	0
Low Fat Balsamic	1 serv (2.5 oz)	40	2	6	3	0
Mayo Onion Sauce	1 serv (0.5 oz)	90	10	4	2	0
Ranch	1 serv (2.5 oz)	390	41	4	2	0
Ranch Lite	1 serv (2.5 oz)	190	18	3	2	0

FOOD	PORTION	CAL	FAT	CARB	SUGAR	FIBER
Soy Sauce	1 serv (0.3 oz)	5	0	1	0	0
Syrup Log Cabin	1 serv (2 oz)	190	0	49	18	0
Taco Sauce	1 serv (0.3 oz)	0	0	0	0	0
Tartar Sauce	1 serv (1.5 oz)	210	22	2	1	0
SALADS						
Asian w/ Crispy Chicken w/o Dressing	1 (13.8 oz)	330	13	34	11	7
Asian w/ Grilled Chicken w/o Dressing	1 (12.8 oz)	160	2	18	11	5
Chicken Club w/ Crispy Chicken w/o Dressing	1 (14 oz)	480	27	26	5	6
Chicken Club w/ Grilled Chicken w/o Dressing	1 (13 oz)	320	16	11	5	4
Side w/o Dressing	1 (4.3 oz)	50	3	5	2	2
Southwest w/ Crispy Chicken w/o Dressing	1 (16 oz)	480	23	44	5	9
Southwest w/ w/ Grilled Chicken w/o Dressing	1 (15 oz)	320	12	27	5	7
JAMBA JUICE						
BEVERAGES						
Acai Super Antioxidant	1 (16 oz)	290	5	59	50	4
Acai Topper	1 (12 oz)	440	9	86	55	9
Aloha Pineapple	1 (16 oz)	300	1	70	65	3
Banana Berry	1 (16 oz)	300	1	72	63	3
Berry Fulfilling	1 (16 oz)	160	1	34	26	4
Berry Topper	1 (12 oz)	420	9	80	51	9
Blackberry Bliss	1 (16 oz)	260	1	61	54	4
Boost 3G Charger Super	1 (3 g)	5	0	2	–	2
Boost Flax & Fiber	1 (0.4 oz)	30	2	7	–	7
Boost Soy Protein	1 (8.9 g)	30	0	0	0	0
Boost Weight Burner Super	1 (3.5 g)	30	3	0	0	0

FOOD	PORTION	CAL	FAT	CARB	SUGAR	FIBER
Boost Whey Protein Super	1 (12 g)	45	0	1	–	–
Caribbean Passion	1 (16 oz)	270	1	63	56	3
Carrot Juice	1 (16 oz)	100	1	22	20	0
Chocolate Moo'd	1 (16 oz)	460	6	93	84	2
Chunky Strawberry Topper	1 (12 oz)	480	15	74	44	8
Coldbuster	1 (16 oz)	270	2	63	54	3
Mango-A-Go-Go	1 (16 oz)	310	1	72	65	2
Mango Mantra	1 (16 oz)	170	1	36	33	3
Mango Metabolizer	1 (16 oz)	290	4	63	54	4
Mango Peach Topper	1 (12 oz)	450	9	86	57	8
Matcha Green Tea Blast	1 (16 oz)	290	0	62	55	1
Mega Mango	1 (16 oz)	250	1	62	57	4
Orange Dream Machine	1 (16 oz)	350	2	75	70	tr
Orange Juice	1 (16 oz)	220	1	52	51	tr
Peach Perfection	1 (16 oz)	230	0	57	46	4
Peach Pleasure	1 (16 oz)	290	1	68	56	3
Peanut Butter Moo'd	1 (16 oz)	490	11	85	75	3
Pomegranate Heart Happy	1 (16 oz)	300	1	72	63	3
Pomegranate Paradise	1 (16 oz)	260	1	64	56	4
Pomegranate Pick-Me-up	1 (16 oz)	280	2	67	57	3
Protein Berry Workout w/ Soy Protein	1 (16 oz)	290	1	55	46	4
Protein Berry Workout w/ Whey	1 (16 oz)	300	0	56	46	4
Razzmatazz	1 (16 oz)	300	1	70	57	3
Shot Matcha Energy Orange Juice	1 (4 oz)	60	0	13	13	tr
Shot Matcha Energy Soymilk	1 (4 oz)	70	0	14	12	0
Shot Wheatgrass Detox	1 oz	5	0	tr	0	0

FOOD	PORTION	CAL	FAT	CARB	SUGAR	FIBER
Strawberries Wild	1 (16 oz)	280	0	66	58	3
Strawberry Energizer	1 (16 oz)	300	1	71	63	3
Strawberry Nirvana	1 (16 oz)	170	0	36	30	3
Strawberry Surf Rider	1 (16 oz)	330	1	80	71	3
Strawberry Whirl	1 (16 oz)	240	1	59	50	5
FOOD						
Cheddar Tomato Twist	1 (3.2 oz)	240	5	41	3	2
Cookie Omega-3 Chocolate Brownie	1 (1.5 oz)	150	4	30	24	2
Cookie Omega-3 Oatmeal	1 (1.5 oz)	150	6	26	15	3
Loaf Reduced Fat Blueberry Lemon	1 (3 oz)	290	8	53	30	2
Loaf Reduced Fat Cranberry Orange	1 (3 oz)	310	9	52	21	4
Loaf Zucchini Walnut	1 (3 oz)	270	9	43	26	4
Oatcake Blueberry	1 (3.25 oz)	280	9	46	17	6
Oatmeal Apple Cinnamon	1 serv (9.1 oz)	290	4	60	25	5
Oatmeal Blueberry & Blackberry	1 serv (8.9 oz)	290	4	59	25	6
Oatmeal Fresh Banana	1 serv (9.6 oz)	280	4	57	23	6
Oatmeal w/ Brown Sugar	1 serv (7.6 oz)	220	4	44	12	5
Pretzel Apple Cinnamon	1 (5.2 oz)	380	4	76	14	4
Pretzel Sourdough Parmesan	1 (5 oz)	410	10	67	4	3

JIMMY JOHN'S
BEVERAGES

FOOD	PORTION	CAL	FAT	CARB	SUGAR	FIBER
Coke	1 sm	248	0	68	–	0
Diet Coke	1 sm	0	0	0	0	0
Iced Tea	1 sm	3	0	1	–	0

FOOD	PORTION	CAL	FAT	CARB	SUGAR	FIBER
Iced Tea Raspberry	1 sm	195	0	53	–	0
Lemonade	1 sm	243	0	65	–	0
Lemonade Light	1 sm	13	0	3	–	0
Sprite	1 sm	243	0	65	–	0
SANDWICHES						
Giant Club Beach	1	798	37	78	–	2
Giant Club Billy	1	867	40	77	–	1
Giant Club Bootlegger	1	720	28	74	–	1
Giant Club Country	1	840	38	75	–	1
Giant Club Gourmet Smoked Ham	1	851	40	76	–	1
Giant Club Gourmet Veggie	1	856	46	77	–	2
Giant Club Hunter's	1	854	38	76	–	1
Giant Club Italian Night	1	975	52	77	–	1
Giant Club Lulu	1	790	34	74	–	1
Giant Club Tuna	1	719	29	77	–	2
Giant Club Ultimate Porker	1	843	41	73	–	6
Slim Double Provolone	1	588	19	71	–	0
Slim Ham & Cheese	1	534	12	72	–	0
Slim Salami Capicola Cheese	1	624	21	72	–	0
Slim Tuna Salad	1	577	19	72	–	1
Slim Turkey Breast	1	407	1	70	–	0
Sub Big John	1	564	27	54	–	1
Sub J.J.B.L.T.	1	662	35	54	–	1
Sub Pepe	1	684	37	55	–	1
Sub Totally Tuna	1	502	20	57	–	2
Sub Turkey Tom	1	555	26	54	–	1
Sub Vegetarian	1	640	36	57	–	2
Sub Vito	1	579	25	56	–	1
The J.J. Gargantuan	1	1008	55	60	–	1
Unwich Hunter's Club	1	520	38	8	–	2

FOOD	PORTION	CAL	FAT	CARB	SUGAR	FIBER
Unwich The J.J. Gargantuan	1	769	55	11	–	2
SIDES						
Cookie Chocolate Chunk	1	421	18	62	–	1
Cookie Raisin Oatmeal	1	421	16	65	–	4
Jimmy Chips	1 pkg	160	8	18	–	0
Jimmy Chips BBQ	1 pkg	160	9	17	–	0
Jimmy Chips Jalapeno	1 pkg	150	7	18	–	0
Jimmy Chips Sea Salt & Vinegar	1 pkg	140	8	16	–	0
Pickle Spear	1	4	0	1	–	tr
Pickle Whole	1	15	0	3	–	1

KENTUCKY FRIED CHICKEN

BEVERAGES

FOOD	PORTION	CAL	FAT	CARB	SUGAR	FIBER
Diet Pepsi	1 med (14 oz)	0	0	0	0	0
Mt. Dew	1 med (14 oz)	190	0	54	54	0
Pepsi	1 med (14 oz)	180	0	47	47	0
DESSERTS						
Cake Double Chocolate Chip	1 slice	330	16	41	26	1
Cookie Sweet Life Chocolate Chip	1 (1.2 oz)	160	7	23	14	1
Cookie Sweet Life Oatmeal Raisin	1 (1.2 oz)	150	5	24	12	1
Cookie Sweet Life Sugar	1 (1.2 oz)	160	6	23	10	0
Lil' Bucket Chocolate Cream	1	280	13	38	21	3
Lil' Bucket Lemon Creme	1 serv	410	15	61	53	2
Lil' Bucket Strawberry Short Cake	1 serv	210	7	33	25	1
Pie Mini's Apple	3 (4 oz)	370	20	44	19	2
Teddy Graham Cinnamon Snacks	1 serv	90	3	15	5	1

FOOD	PORTION	CAL	FAT	CARB	SUGAR	FIBER
MAIN MENU SELECTIONS						
Baked Beans	1 serv	220	1	45	20	7
Biscuit	1 (2 oz)	220	11	24	2	1
Bowl Chicken & Biscuit	1	870	44	88	5	7
Bowl Mashed Potato w/ Gravy	1	740	36	80	6	7
Bowl Rice w/ Gravy	1	620	28	67	7	6
Chicken Pot Pie	1 (15 oz)	770	40	70	2	5
Cole Slaw	1 serv	180	10	22	18	3
Corn On The Cob	1 ear (3 inch)	70	2	13	5	3
Crispy Strips	2 (3.5 oz)	240	13	11	0	0
Extra Crispy Breast	1 (5.7 oz)	440	27	15	0	0
Extra Crispy Drumstick	1 (2 oz)	160	10	6	0	0
Extra Crispy Thigh	1 (4 oz)	370	28	12	0	0
Extra Crispy Whole Wing	1 (1.8 oz)	170	11	6	0	1
Green Beans	1 serv	50	2	7	2	2
KFC Snacker	1	290	13	29	5	2
KFC Snacker Buffalo	1	260	8	31	4	1
KFC Snacker Fish	1	330	15	31	6	1
KFC Snacker Fish w/o Sauce	1	290	12	29	4	1
KFC Snacker Honey BBQ	1	210	3	32	12	2
KFC Snacker Ultimate Cheese	1	280	11	30	5	1
Macaroni & Cheese	1 serv	180	8	18	3	0
Mashed Potatoes w/ Gravy	1 serv	140	5	20	1	1
Mashed Potatoes w/o Gravy	1 serv	110	4	17	0	1
Original Recipe Breast	1 (5.6 oz)	360	21	7	0	0
Original Recipe Breast w/o Skin Or Breading	1 (3.8 oz)	140	2	1	0	0
Original Recipe Drumstick	1 (2 oz)	130	8	2	0	0

FOOD	PORTION	CAL	FAT	CARB	SUGAR	FIBER
Original Recipe Thigh	1 (4.4 oz)	330	24	8	0	0
Original Recipe Whole Wing	1 (1.6 oz)	130	8	4	0	0
Popcorn Chicken	1 reg (4 oz)	400	26	22	0	3
Potato Salad	1 serv	180	9	22	6	2
Potato Wedges	1 serv	260	13	33	0	3
Sandwich Crispy Twister	1	550	28	49	5	3
Sandwich Double Crunch	1	470	23	38	4	2
Sandwich Honey BBQ	1	280	4	40	16	3
Sandwich Tender Roast	1	380	13	29	4	2
Sandwich Tender Roast w/o Sauce	1	300	5	28	3	2
Seasoned Rice	1 serv	180	1	32	1	2
Twister Oven Roasted	1	420	17	40	6	3
Twister Oven Roasted w/o Sauce	1	330	7	39	5	3
Wings Boneless Fiery Buffalo	5	420	20	33	1	3
Wings Boneless Honey BBQ	5	450	20	41	11	4
Wings Boneless Sweet & Spicy	5	440	19	38	11	3
Wings Boneless Teriyaki	5	500	21	50	24	3
Wings Fiery Buffalo	5	380	24	19	1	2
Wings Honey BBQ	5	390	24	23	9	3
Wings Hot	5	350	24	14	0	2
Wings Hot & Spicy	5	400	24	24	13	2
Wings Teriyaki	5	480	25	40	30	2
SALAD DRESSINGS						
Creamy Parmesan Caesar	1 serv (2 oz)	260	26	4	2	0
Golden Italian Light	1 serv (1.5 oz)	45	3	6	5	0
Ranch	1 serv (2 oz)	200	20	3	1	0
Ranch Fat Free	1 serv (1.5 oz)	35	0	8	2	0

FOOD	PORTION	CAL	FAT	CARB	SUGAR	FIBER
SALADS						
Crispy BLT w/o Dressing	1 (12 oz)	330	17	18	5	4
Crispy Caesar w/o Dressing & Croutons	1 (11 oz)	350	19	16	3	3
Croutons Parmesan Garlic	1 pkg	60	3	8	1	0
Roasted BLT w/o Dressing	1 (12 oz)	200	6	8	5	4
Roasted Caesar w/o Dressing & Croutons	1 (11 oz)	220	8	6	3	3
Side Caesar w/o Dressing & Croutons	1 (3 oz)	50	3	2	1	1
Side House w/o Dressing	1 (3 oz)	15	0	2	2	1
KOO-KOO-ROO						
MAIN MENU SELECTIONS						
Baked Yam	1 serv (6 oz)	197	tr	47	–	7
Black Beans	1 serv (6 oz)	125	3	23	–	6
Buffalo Wings	6	606	28	42	–	2
Burrito California Chicken	1	810	41	60	–	4
Burrito Fajita Chicken	1	750	33	70	–	4
Burrito Original Chicken	1	709	28	71	–	5
Butternut Squash	1 serv (6 oz)	66	tr	17	–	3
Chicken Bowl Chargrilled w/o Sauce	1	569	19	57	–	4
Chicken Bowl Spicy Garlic Ginger w/o Sauce	1	485	6	63	–	2
Creamed Spinach	1 serv (8 oz)	100	6	10	–	3

FOOD	PORTION	CAL	FAT	CARB	SUGAR	FIBER
Italian Vegetable	1 serv (5.5 oz)	47	2	9	–	2
Kernel Corn	1 serv (4.5 oz)	105	1	26	–	3
Mashed Potatoes	1 serv (6.5 oz)	188	5	32	–	3
Original Breast	1 (4.1 oz)	187	6	tr	–	0
Original Chicken Dark	3 pieces (5 oz)	320	16	5	–	0
Roasted Garlic Potatoes	1 serv (5 oz)	133	5	21	–	2
Rotisserie Chicken Breast & Wing	1 serv (6.5 oz)	355	16	1	–	tr
Rotisserie Chicken Leg & Thigh	1 serv (4.8 oz)	300	18	1	–	tr
Rotisserie Half Chicken	1 serv (11.3 oz)	655	34	2	–	tr
Sandwich BBQ Chicken	1	562	12	71	–	3
Sandwich Chicken Caesar	1	781	36	63	–	2
Sandwich Original Chicken	1	661	29	63	–	3
Sandwich Turkey Hand Carved	1	599	32	31	–	5
Southwestern Bowl w/o Sauce	1	570	19	67	–	8
Tostada Bowl w/o Sauce w/o Shell	1	528	22	45	–	7
Traditional Turkey Dinner	1 serv	692	29	67	–	8
Turkey Breast Sliced	1 serv	182	8	0	0	0
Turkey Pot Pie	1	883	44	83	–	6
Wrap Caesar Chicken	1	757	39	59	–	4
Wrap Chipotle Chicken	1	924	43	89	–	6

FOOD	PORTION	CAL	FAT	CARB	SUGAR	FIBER
SALADS						
BBQ Chicken w/o Dressing	1	365	14	22	–	6
Cantaloupe & Honeydew	1 serv (5 oz)	50	tr	12	–	1
Chicken Caesar w/o Dressing	1	286	11	13	–	4
Chinese Chicken w/o Dressing	1	550	29	39	–	10
Creamy Coleslaw	1 serv (5 oz)	238	20	14	–	2
Cucumber	1 serv (4.5 oz)	41	tr	9	–	2
House	1	113	4	16	–	5
Tangy Tomato	1 serv (4.5 oz)	60	4	6	–	1
Tossed w/ Dressing	1 serv (3 oz)	16	tr	3	–	1
SOUPS						
Chicken Noodle	1 serv (5 oz)	71	3	4	–	tr
Chicken Tortilla	1 serv (5 oz)	112	6	7	–	1
Ten Vegetable	1 serv (5 oz)	94	2	16	–	4
KRISPY KREME						
BEVERAGES						
Chillers Fruity Orange You Glad	1 (12 oz)	180	0	43	43	0
Chillers Fruity Very Berry	1 (12 oz)	170	0	43	43	0
Chillers Kremey Berries & Kreme	1 (12 oz)	620	28	92	71	tr
Chillers Kremey Chocolate Chocolate	1 (12 oz)	970	29	104	62	2
Chillers Kremey Lemon Sherbert	1 (12 oz)	630	28	95	71	tr
Chillers Kremey Lotta Latte	1 (12 oz)	670	28	49	60	tr

FOOD	PORTION	CAL	FAT	CARB	SUGAR	FIBER
Chillers Kremey Mocha Dream	1 (12 oz)	670	28	105	58	1
Chillers Kremey Oranges & Kreme	1 (12 oz)	630	28	92	71	tr
DOUGHNUTS						
Apple Fritter	1	380	20	47	24	2
Caramel Kreme Crunch	1	380	19	40	30	tr
Chocolate Iced Cake	1	280	14	36	20	tr
Chocolate Iced Custard Filled	1	300	17	36	19	tr
Chocolate Iced Glazed	1	250	12	33	21	tr
Chocolate Iced Kreme Filled	1	350	20	39	23	tr
Chocolate Iced w/ Sprinkles	1	270	12	38	24	tr
Cinnamon Apple Filled	1	290	16	32	14	tr
Cinnamon Bun	1	260	16	28	13	tr
Cinnamon Twist	1	240	15	23	7	tr
Dulce De Leche	1	300	18	31	14	tr
Glazed Chocolate Cake	1	300	15	42	27	2
Glazed Cinnamon	1	210	12	24	12	tr
Glazed Creme Filled	1	340	20	39	23	tr
Glazed Cruller	1	240	14	26	14	tr
Glazed Cruller Chocolate	1	290	15	37	25	tr
Glazed Lemon Filled	1	290	16	36	18	tr
Glazed Original	1	200	12	22	10	tr
Glazed Pumpkin Spice	1	300	14	42	27	tr
Glazed Raspberry Filled	1	300	16	36	20	tr
Glazed Sour Cream	1	300	13	43	28	tr
Holes Glazed Blueberry	4	220	12	27	13	tr
Holes Glazed Cake	4	210	10	29	17	tr
Holes Glazed Chocolate Cake	4	210	10	29	17	tr
Holes Glazed Original	4	200	11	25	15	tr

FOOD	PORTION	CAL	FAT	CARB	SUGAR	FIBER
Holes Glazed Pumpkin Spice	4	210	10	29	17	tr
Maple Iced Glazed	1	240	12	32	20	tr
New York Cheesecake	1	340	20	34	17	tr
Powdered Cake	1	290	14	37	19	tr
Powdered Strawberry Filled	1	290	16	33	13	tr
Sugar	1	200	12	21	10	0
Traditional Cake	1	230	13	25	9	tr

KRYSTAL
BEVERAGES

FOOD	PORTION	CAL	FAT	CARB	SUGAR	FIBER
Coca Cola Classic	1 sm (16 oz)	129	0	40	40	0
Coca Cola Classic frzn	1 (16 oz)	130	0	36	36	0
Diet Coke	1 sm (16 oz)	tr	0	tr	0	0
Sprite	1 sm (16 oz)	126	0	39	39	0

BREAKFAST SELECTIONS

FOOD	PORTION	CAL	FAT	CARB	SUGAR	FIBER
4 Carb Scrambler Bacon	1 serv	370	29	4	0	1
4 Carb Scrambler Sausage	1 serv	600	51	3	1	2
Biscuit & Gravy	1	280	14	34	2	0
Biscuit Bacon Egg Cheese	1	390	23	33	2	0
Biscuit Chik	1	360	15	40	2	0
Biscuit Plain	1	270	13	33	2	0
Biscuit Sausage	1	480	33	33	2	0
Country Breakfast	1 serv	660	42	46	3	8
Kryspers	1 serv	190	13	17	0	2
Krystal Sunriser	1	240	14	14	1	2
Scrambler	1 serv	440	26	33	tr	3

DESSERTS

FOOD	PORTION	CAL	FAT	CARB	SUGAR	FIBER
Fried Apple Turnover	1	220	10	31	7	2
Lemon Icebox Pie	1 serv	260	9	41	37	2

FOOD	PORTION	CAL	FAT	CARB	SUGAR	FIBER
MAIN MENU SELECTIONS						
BA Burger	1	470	27	39	6	2
BA Burger Cheese	1	530	32	40	6	2
BA Burger Double Bacon Cheese	1	800	53	41	6	2
Chik'n Bites	1 sm	310	19	16	0	1
Chik'n Bites Salad	1 serv	290	20	12	1	4
Fries	1 reg	470	20	53	0	7
Fries Chili Cheese	1 serv	540	28	59	1	6
Krystal	1	160	7	17	1	1
Krystal Bacon Cheese	1	190	10	16	2	2
Krystal Cheese	1	180	9	17	1	2
Krystal Chik	1	240	11	24	1	2
Krystal Chili	1 serv	200	7	22	2	7
Krystal Double	1	260	13	24	2	2
Krystal Double Cheese	1	310	16	26	2	tr
Pup Chili Cheese	1	210	12	17	2	2
Pup Corn	1	260	19	19	5	1
Pup Plain	1	170	9	15	–	1
MARBLE SLAB CREAMERY						
Cone Honey Wheat	1	130	3	24	12	tr
Cone Sugar	1	130	3	23	12	0
Cone Vanilla Cinnamon	1	130	3	24	12	tr
Frozen Yogurt Nonfat	½ cup	100	tr	22	17	tr
Frozen Yogurt Nonfat No Sugar Added	½ cup	90	tr	17	6	tr
Ice Cream Reduced Fat	1 serv (6.75 oz)	390	20	47	45	0
Ice Cream Superpremium	1 serv (6.75 oz)	450	28	44	43	0
Sorbet	½ cup	90	0	22	19	0

FOOD	PORTION	CAL	FAT	CARB	SUGAR	FIBER

MARCO'S PIZZA
OTHER MENU SELECTIONS

FOOD	PORTION	CAL	FAT	CARB	SUGAR	FIBER
Cheezybread Bran	1 piece	80	2	11	1	0
Chicken Tumblers BBQ	1	67	2	7	3	0
Chicken Tumblers Hot & Spicy	1	57	2	5	0	0
Chicken Tumblers Naked	1	57	2	5	0	0
Chicken Wings BBQ	1	71	4	3	3	0
Chicken Wings Hot & Spicy	1	60	4	0	0	0
Chicken Wings Naked	1	60	4	0	0	0
Cinnasquares	1 piece	60	2	9	5	0
Salad Chicken Ranch	1 serv	240	13	10	2	3
Salad Italian	1 serv	230	17	11	3	3
Sub Chicken Club	½	385	16	34	2	2
Sub Ham & Cheese	½	400	21	33	2	1
Sub Italian	½	430	23	35	3	2
Sub Steak & Cheese	½	380	15	33	2	1
Sub Veggie	½	355	16	39	2	3

PIZZA

FOOD	PORTION	CAL	FAT	CARB	SUGAR	FIBER
Cheese Large	1 slice	280	8	33	3	2
Cheese Medium	1 slice	210	6	24	2	1
Cheese Small	1 slice	200	6	23	2	1
Chicken Fresco Large	1 slice	350	13	35	4	2
Chicken Fresco Medium	1 slice	260	10	26	3	1
Chicken Fresco Small	1 slice	180	7	19	2	1
Deep Pan Cheese	1 slice	290	8	36	3	2
Deep Pan Pepperoni	1 slice	330	12	36	3	2
Deluxe Uno Large	1 slice	380	16	35	3	2
Deluxe Uno Medium	1 slice	280	12	26	2	1
Deluxe Uno Small	1 slice	200	9	18	2	1
Garden Large	1 slice	310	10	36	4	2
Garden Medium	1 slice	230	8	26	3	2
Garden Small	1 slice	160	5	19	2	1

FOOD	PORTION	CAL	FAT	CARB	SUGAR	FIBER
Hawaiian Chicken Large	1 slice	380	15	35	4	2
Hawaiian Chicken Medium	1 slice	260	10	26	3	1
Hawaiian Chicken Small	1 slice	180	6	18	2	1
Meat Supremo Large	1 slice	430	21	34	3	2
Meat Supremo Medium	1 slice	300	15	25	2	1
Meat Supremo Small	1 slice	210	10	18	2	1
Pepperoni Large	1 slice	310	11	33	3	2
Pepperoni Medium	1 slice	230	9	24	2	1
Pepperoni Small	1 slice	210	8	23	2	1
White Cheezy Large	1 slice	340	15	33	2	2
White Cheezy Medium	1 slice	260	11	24	2	1
White Cheezy Small	1 slice	170	7	17	1	1

MAUI WOWI
SMOOTHIES

FOOD	PORTION	CAL	FAT	CARB	SUGAR	FIBER
Fresh Fruit Banana Banana	1 (12 oz)	210	1	50	36	2
Fresh Fruit Black Raspberry	1 (12 oz)	240	0	59	46	0
Fresh Fruit Kiwi Lemon Lime	1 (12 oz)	180	0	42	34	0
Fresh Fruit Lemon Wave	1 (12 oz)	415	tr	108	108	tr
Fresh Fruit Mango Orange Banana	1 (12 oz)	240	1	57	43	tr
Fresh Fruit Passion Papaya	1 (12 oz)	220	1	54	38	tr
Fresh Fruit Pina Colada	1 (12 oz)	240	3	57	46	0

MAX & ERMA'S

FOOD	PORTION	CAL	FAT	CARB	SUGAR	FIBER
Black Bean Roll Up	1 serv	577	10	95	–	10
Caribbean Chicken Lunch Portion	1 serv	536	20	59	–	3
Fruit Smoothie	1	124	tr	29	–	1
Garlic Breadstick	1	156	6	21	–	0

FOOD	PORTION	CAL	FAT	CARB	SUGAR	FIBER
Hula Bowl w/ Fat Free Honey Mustard Dressing w/o Breadsticks	1 serv	823	7	79	–	6
Salad Baby Greens w/o Breadstick	1 serv	119	11	6	–	2
Salad Shrimp Stack	1 serv	322	12	116	–	3
Salad Dressing Bleu Cheese	2 tbsp	201	21	tr	–	0
Salad Dressing French Fat Free	2 tbsp	126	tr	31	–	2
Salad Dressing Honey Mustard Fat Free	2 tbsp	60	0	14	–	0
Salad Dressing Italian	2 tbsp	110	12	1	–	0
Salad Dressing Ranch	2 tbsp	120	13	1	–	0
Salad Dressing Tex Mex Low Fat	2 tbsp	23	tr	2	–	tr

MCALISTER'S DELI
CHILDREN'S MENU SELECTIONS

FOOD	PORTION	CAL	FAT	CARB	SUGAR	FIBER
Kid's Nacho	1 serv	734	43	74	2	3
Mac's Dog	1	307	19	24	2	1
Pita Pizza	1	503	21	54	5	3
Sandwich Ham & Cheese	1	455	22	39	5	4
Sandwich PB&J	1	714	32	86	46	7
Sandwich Toasted Cheese	1	620	38	40	5	4
Sandwich Turkey & Cheese	1	451	21	39	4	4

DESSERTS

FOOD	PORTION	CAL	FAT	CARB	SUGAR	FIBER
Brownie Chocolate	1 (3.5 oz)	424	18	59	48	3
Brownie Delight	1 (11 oz)	917	48	111	81	4

FOOD	PORTION	CAL	FAT	CARB	SUGAR	FIBER
Chocolate Loving Spoon Cake	1 (4 oz)	538	35	54	26	2
Ice Cream Vanilla Bean	1 scoop (5 oz)	160	10	19	16	0
Kentucky Pie	1 slice (12 oz)	807	64	110	32	1
New York Cheesecake	1 slice (5 oz)	505	35	37	34	2
Sundae Topping Caramel	2 tbsp	100	0	20	20	0
Sundae Topping Chocolate	1 tbsp	110	0	21	21	0
MAIN MENU SELECTIONS						
Appetizers Chips & Salsa	1 serv (5 oz)	87	5	9	0	0
Appetizers Dip Cheese & Chili	1 serv (5 oz)	572	35	54	1	3
Appetizers Dip Cheese & Veggie Chili	1 serv (5 oz)	552	31	58	3	5
Appetizers Nacho Basket	1 serv (6 oz)	579	33	61	2	3
Appetizers Nacho Chili	1 serv (6 oz)	564	37	46	2	4
Appetizers Nacho Veggie Chili	1 serv (6 oz)	537	31	52	4	6
Chicken Cordon Bleu	1 serv	810	39	53	11	2
Chili Vegetarian	1 serv (8 oz)	133	1	28	4	15
Cole Slaw	1 serv (4 oz)	190	15	14	10	7
Fruit Cup	1 serv (4 oz)	98	0	12	19	2
Giant Spud Cheese	1 (27 oz)	930	48	139	11	19
Giant Spud Grilled Chicken	1 (27 oz)	839	25	99	14	19
Giant Spud Just A Spud	1 (26 oz)	604	4	123	12	18
Giant Spud Ole	1 (30 oz)	1252	60	110	14	18
Giant Spud Ole w/ Chili	1 (33 oz)	1512	78	134	13	21
Giant Spud Ole w/ Veggie Chili	1 (33 oz)	1457	67	146	18	24
Giant Spud Veggie	1 (28 oz)	668	18	99	11	18
Macaroni & Cheese	1 serv (4 oz)	200	7	17	1	1
Mashed Potatoes	1 serv (4 oz)	136	8	19	1	2

FOOD	PORTION	CAL	FAT	CARB	SUGAR	FIBER
Meatloaf w/ Gravy	1 serv	340	37	21	0	1
Open-Faced Roast Beef	1 serv	751	21	88	6	6
Pot Roast Spud	1 serv	906	30	121	12	17
Potato Salad	1 serv (4 oz)	200	11	22	3	3
Salmon Filet	1 serv	235	4	3	1	1
Steamed Vegetables	1 serv (4 oz)	43	0	7	4	3
SALAD DRESSINGS AND SAUCES						
Au Jus	1 serv (4 oz)	10	0	2	0	0
Comeback Gravy	1 serv (4 oz)	37	2	6	0	0
Dressing Blue Cheese	2 tbsp	140	15	1	1	0
Dressing Greek	2 tbsp	90	9	2	1	0
Dressing Parmesan Peppercorn	2 tbsp	150	16	2	1	0
Dressing Ranch	2 tbsp	100	11	1	1	0
Dressing Tomato Basil	2 tbsp	30	0	6	6	0
Dressing Lite Olive Oil Vinaigrette	2 tbsp	60	6	3	2	0
Dressing Lite Ranch	2 tbsp	100	10	1	1	0
Dressing Low Calorie Italian	2 tbsp	25	2	2	2	0
SALADS						
Caesar w/ Salmon	1 (17 oz)	800	53	42	3	5
Chicken Fiesta	1 (20 oz)	493	22	34	14	8
Chicken Grill	1 (21 oz)	840	15	47	8	4
Garden	1 (15 oz)	264	17	21	8	4
Garden w/ Chicken Salad	1 (18 oz)	537	45	14	16	5
Garden w/ Salmon	1 (17 oz)	315	10	28	4	6
Garden w/ Tuna Salad	1 (18 oz)	373	18	21	8	5
Greek Chicken	1 (19 oz)	584	32	32	8	7
Side Caesar	1 (6 oz)	328	24	19	3	1
Side Garden	1 (8 oz)	138	9	11	4	2
Taco	1 (26 oz)	641	40	33	12	11
Taco w/ Veggie Chili	1 (26 oz)	641	40	33	17	15

FOOD	PORTION	CAL	FAT	CARB	SUGAR	FIBER
SANDWICHES						
BLT	1	654	38	50	11	6
Chicken Salad	1	677	43	58	19	2
Deli Corned Beef On Wheat	1	369	9	39	4	4
Deli Ham On Wheat	1	350	9	43	7	5
Deli Pastrami On Wheat	1	371	10	36	4	4
Deli Roast Beef On Wheat	1	398	12	49	6	5
Deli Salami On Wheat	1	565	32	43	6	5
Deli Turkey On Wheat	1	342	9	43	6	5
French Dip	1	676	34	50	3	2
Grilled Chicken Breast	1	751	36	56	21	2
Grilled Chicken Club	1	1234	64	87	27	7
Ham Melt	1	700	34	52	6	4
McAlisters Club	1	1225	69	86	27	7
Meatloaf Parmesan	1	708	36	49	6	5
Memphian	1	585	26	48	6	4
Muffuletta	¼ (8 oz)	615	35	40	0	2
New Yorker	1	628	25	50	4	4
Orange Cranberry Club	1	954	52	62	18	6
Reuben On Rye	1	492	30	35	8	2
Roast Beef Melt	1	635	32	48	6	4
Salmon	1	608	21	66	10	3
Submarine	1	833	48	53	9	3
Sweetberry Chicken On Wheatberry	1	701	24	67	8	5
Tuna Salad On Wheat	1	452	19	47	7	5
Turkey Melt	1	700	35	52	6	4
Veggie On Pita	1	522	36	33	5	2
Wrap Greek Chicken	1	630	25	57	3	14
Wrap Grilled Chicken Caesar	1	533	25	46	4	13

FOOD	PORTION	CAL	FAT	CARB	SUGAR	FIBER
SOUPS						
Asiago Cheese Bisque	1 (8 oz)	240	17	17	1	0
Broccoli Cheddar	1 (8 oz)	213	15	13	4	0
Cheddar Potato	1 (8 oz)	213	13	19	0	1
Cheesy Chicken Tortilla	1 (8 oz)	150	6	13	4	0
Chicken & Sausage Gumbo	1 (8 oz)	150	5	17	3	2
Clam Chowder	1 (8 oz)	200	11	09	4	0
Country Potato	1 (8 oz)	173	8	23	4	0
Country Vegetable	1 (8 oz)	93	1	17	4	3
French Onion	1 (8 oz)	80	1	11	5	1
Red Beans & Rice	1 (8 oz)	107	3	25	3	11
Southwest Roasted Corn	1 (8 oz)	90	4	20	4	3

MCDONALD'S
BEVERAGES

FOOD	PORTION	CAL	FAT	CARB	SUGAR	FIBER
Apple Juice	1 box (6.8 oz)	90	0	23	21	0
Chocolate Milk 1% Low Fat	8 oz	170	3	26	25	1
Coca Cola Classic	1 sm (16 oz)	150	0	40	40	0
Coffee	1 sm (12 oz)	0	0	0	0	0
Diet Coke	1 sm (16 oz)	0	0	0	0	0
Half & Half Creamer	1 pkg	20	2	0	0	0
Hi-C Orange Lavaburst	1 sm (16 oz)	160	0	44	44	0
Iced Coffee Caramel	1 sm (16 oz)	130	5	21	20	1
Iced Coffee Hazelnut	1 sm (16 oz)	130	5	21	21	0
Iced Coffee Regular	1 sm (16 oz)	140	5	22	22	0
Iced Coffee Vanilla	1 sm (16 oz)	130	5	21	21	0
Iced Tea	1 sm (16 oz)	0	0	0	0	0
Milk Lowfat 1%	1 pkg	100	3	12	12	0
Orange Juice	1 sm (12 oz)	140	0	33	29	0
Powerade Mountain Blast	1 sm (16 oz)	100	0	27	21	0

FOOD	PORTION	CAL	FAT	CARB	SUGAR	FIBER
Shake Triple Thick Chocolate	1 sm (12 oz)	440	10	76	63	1
Shake Triple Thick Strawberry	1 sm (12 oz)	420	10	73	63	0
Shake Triple Thick Vanilla	1 sm (16 oz)	420	10	72	54	0
Sprite	1 sm (16 oz)	150	0	39	39	0
BREAKFAST SELECTIONS						
Big Breakfast Regular Biscuit	1 serv	720	46	49	3	3
Biscuit	1 reg	250	11	32	2	2
Biscuit Regular Bacon Egg Cheese	1	450	25	36	3	2
Biscuit Regular Sausage	1	410	27	33	2	2
Biscuit Regular Sausage w/ Egg	1	500	32	35	2	2
Burrito Sausage	1	300	16	26	2	1
Deluxe Breakfast Regular Biscuit w/o Syrup & Margarine	1 serv	1070	55	109	17	6
English Muffin	1	160	3	27	2	2
Hash Browns	1 serv	140	8	15	0	2
Hotcake Syrup	1 pkg (2 oz)	180	0	45	32	0
Hotcakes & Sausage w/o Syrup & Margarine	1 serv	520	24	61	14	3
Hotcakes w/o Syrup & Margarine	1 serv	350	9	60	14	3
McGriddles Bacon Egg Cheese	1	460	21	48	16	2
McGriddles Sausage	1	420	22	44	15	2
McGriddles Sausage Egg & Cheese	1	560	32	48	15	2
McMuffin Sausage	1	370	22	29	2	2

FOOD	PORTION	CAL	FAT	CARB	SUGAR	FIBER
McMuffin Sausage w/ Egg	1	250	27	30	2	2
McSkillet Burrito w/ Sausage	1	610	36	44	4	3
McSkillet Burrito w/ Steak	1	570	30	44	4	3
Sausage Patty	1	170	15	1	0	0
Scrambled Eggs	2	170	11	1	0	0
DESSERTS						
Apple Dippers	1 pkg	35	0	8	6	0
Apple Pie Baked	1	270	12	36	14	4
Cinnamon Melts	1 serv	460	19	66	32	3
Cookie Chocolate Chip	1	180	7	22	15	1
Cookie Oatmeal	1 (1.1 oz)	150	6	22	13	1
Cookie Sugar	1 (1.1 oz)	150	6	21	11	0
Cookies McDonaldland	1 pkg (2 oz)	250	8	42	14	1
Cookies McDonaldland Chocolate Chip	1 pkg	270	11	39	19	1
Fruit 'n Yogurt Parfait	1 serv	160	2	31	21	1
Ice Cream Cone Reduced Fat Vanilla	1	150	4	24	18	0
Kiddie Cone	1	45	1	8	6	0
McFlurry Oreo	1 (12 oz)	560	16	88	71	0
McFlurry w/ M&M's	1 (12 oz)	620	20	96	85	1
Peanuts For Sundae	1 serv	45	4	2	0	1
Sundae Hot Caramel	1	340	7	60	44	1
Sundae Hot Fudge	1	330	10	54	48	2
Sundae Strawberry	1	280	6	49	45	1
MAIN MENU SELECTIONS						
Apple Sauce Strawberry	1 serv	90	0	23	21	tr
Big Mac	1	540	29	45	9	3
Big N' Tasty	1	460	24	37	8	3
Big N' Tasty w/ Cheese	1	510	28	38	8	3
Cheeseburger	1	300	12	33	6	2

FOOD	PORTION	CAL	FAT	CARB	SUGAR	FIBER
Cheeseburger Double	1	440	23	34	7	2
Cheesy Tots	6 pieces	210	12	20	1	2
Chicken McNuggets	4 pieces	170	10	10	0	0
Chicken Selects	3 pieces	380	20	28	0	0
Filet-O-Fish	1	380	18	38	5	2
French Fries	1 lg	570	30	70	0	7
French Fries	1 sm	250	13	30	0	3
Hamburger	1	250	9	31	6	2
McChicken	1	360	16	40	5	1
McRib	1	500	26	44	11	3
Onion Rings	1 sm	140	7	18	2	2
Quarter Pounder	1	410	19	37	8	3
Quarter Pounder Double w/ Cheese	1	740	42	40	9	3
Quarter Pounder w/ Cheese	1	510	26	40	9	3
Sandwich Chicken Classic Crispy	1	500	17	61	10	3
Sandwich Chicken Classic Grilled	1	420	10	51	11	3
Sandwich Club Chicken Crispy	1	660	28	63	11	4
Sandwich Club Chicken Grilled	1	570	21	52	12	4
Sandwich Ranch BLT Chicken Crispy	1	600	23	64	12	3
Sandwich Ranch BLT Chicken Grilled	1	520	16	53	13	3
Snack Wrap Grilled w/ Chipotle BBQ	1	260	8	28	5	1
Snack Wrap Grilled w/ Honey Mustard	1	260	9	27	4	1
Snack Wrap Grilled w/ Ranch	1	270	10	26	2	1

FOOD	PORTION	CAL	FAT	CARB	SUGAR	FIBER
Snack Wrap w/ Chipotle BBQ	1	320	14	35	4	2
Snack Wrap w/ Honey Mustard	1	320	15	34	4	1
Snack Wrap w/ Ranch	1	140	16	32	2	2
SALAD DRESSINGS AND SAUCES						
Caramel Dip Low Fat	1 pkg	70	1	15	9	0
Dipping Sauce Buffalo	1 serv (1 oz)	80	8	2	1	0
Dipping Sauce Zesty Onion Ring	1 serv (1 oz)	150	15	3	2	tr
Dressing Ken's Light Italian	1 pkg (2 oz)	120	11	5	4	0
Dressing Newman's Own Creamy Caesar	1 pkg (2 oz)	170	18	4	2	0
Dressing Newman's Own Creamy Southwest	1 pkg (1.5 oz)	100	6	11	3	0
Dressing Newman's Own Low Fat Balsamic Vinaigrette	1 pkg (1.5 oz)	40	3	4	3	0
Dressing Newman's Own Low Fat Family Recipe Italian	1 pkg (1.5 oz)	60	3	8	1	0
Dressing Newman's Own Low Fat Sesame Ginger	1 pkg (1.5 oz)	90	3	15	1	0
Dressing Newman's Own Ranch	1 pkg (2 oz)	170	15	9	4	0
Honey	1 pkg (0.5 oz)	50	0	12	11	0
Ketchup	1 pkg	15	0	3	2	0
Sauce Barbecue	1 pkg (1 oz)	50	0	12	10	0
Sauce Creamy Ranch	1 pkg (1.5 oz)	200	22	2	1	0
Sauce Hot Mustard	1 pkg (1 oz)	60	3	9	6	2
Sauce Southwestern Chipotle Barbeque	1 pkg (1.5 oz)	70	0	18	13	1

FOOD	PORTION	CAL	FAT	CARB	SUGAR	FIBER
Sauce Spicy Buffalo	1 pkg (1.5 oz)	60	7	1	0	2
Sauce Sweet'N Sour	1 pkg (1 oz)	50	0	12	10	0
Sauce Tangy Honey Mustard	1 pkg (1.5 oz)	70	3	13	0	0
SALADS						
Asian w/ Crispy Chicken w/o Dressing	1 serv	380	17	33	12	5
Asian w/ Grilled Chicken w/o Dressing	1 serv	300	10	23	12	5
Asian w/o Chicken & Dressing	1 serv	150	7	15	9	5
Bacon Ranch w/ Crispy Chicken	1 serv	350	16	23	4	3
Bacon Ranch w/ Grilled Chicken w/o Dressing	1 serv	260	9	12	5	3
Bacon Ranch w/o Chicken	1 serv	140	7	10	4	3
Caesar w/ Crispy Chicken	1 serv	300	13	22	4	3
Caesar w/ Grilled Chicken	1 serv	220	6	12	5	3
Caesar w/o Chicken	1 serv	90	4	9	4	3
Croutons Butter Garlic	1 pkg	60	2	10	0	1
Fruit & Walnut Snack Size	1 serv	210	8	31	25	2
Side Salad	1 serv	20	0	4	2	1
Southwest w/ Crispy Chicken w/o Dressing	1 serv	400	16	41	10	7
Southwest w/ Grilled Chicken	1 serv	320	9	30	11	7
Southwest w/o Chicken & Dressing	1 serv	140	5	20	5	6

FOOD	PORTION	CAL	FAT	CARB	SUGAR	FIBER

MIMI'S CAFE
BEVERAGES

FOOD	PORTION	CAL	FAT	CARB	SUGAR	FIBER
Cappuccino	1 serv	86	5	7	–	0
Cappuccino Iced	1 serv	86	5	7	–	0
Espresso	1 serv	8	0	1	–	0
Hot Chocolate w/ Whipped Cream	1 serv	986	17	193	–	8
Mocha Iced	1 serv	376	11	70	–	2
Mocha Latte	1 serv	376	11	70	–	2

CHILDREN'S MENU SELECTIONS

FOOD	PORTION	CAL	FAT	CARB	SUGAR	FIBER
Chicken Fingers	1 serv	408	21	21	2	1
Grilled Cheese	1 serv	273	19	14	1	0
Macaroni & Cheese	1 serv	353	13	48	10	2
Mini Burger	1 serv	554	28	48	5	3
Mini Corn Dogs	1 serv	460	32	35	8	0
Pancakes Chocolate Chip	1 serv	563	29	71	33	3
Pancakes Mimi Mouse	1 serv	477	18	69	23	1
PB&J Soldiers	1 serv	730	40	78	29	4
Pepperoni Pizzadillas	1 serv	617	38	39	7	3
Scrambled Eggs & Bacon	1 serv	216	16	1	1	0
Spaghetti	1 serv	343	5	62	17	5
Turkey Dinner	1 serv	337	16	25	1	3

DESSERTS

FOOD	PORTION	CAL	FAT	CARB	SUGAR	FIBER
Apple Crisp Cinnamon	1 serv	898	37	141	–	4
Bread Pudding	1 serv	819	55	69	–	1
Brownie Triple Chocolate	1 serv	1950	87	280	–	6
Cheesecake New York Style	1 serv	1075	42	85	–	4
Pie Banana Foster Mud	1 serv	1245	73	138	–	4
Pie Pecan Chocolate Chip	1 serv	1879	111	220	–	12

FOOD	PORTION	CAL	FAT	CARB	SUGAR	FIBER
MAIN MENU SELECTIONS						
Appetizer Dip Spinach & Artichoke	1 serv	2459	138	191	9	11
Appetizer Fried Chicken Tenders	1 serv	800	33	60	19	3
Appetizer Fried Dill Pickles	1 serv	972	42	132	–	12
Appetizer Jazz Fest	1 serv	1252	72	108	9	8
Appetizer Zucchini Parmesan	1 serv	626	28	73	12	7
Blackened Soul w/ Shrimp Creole	1 serv	852	34	59	–	9
Broiled Flat Iron Steak	1 serv	1026	58	58	–	9
Burger Half Pound	1	684	34	48	–	3
Cafe Fish & Chips	1 serv	1290	57	119	–	10
Cajun Blackened Salmon	1 serv	919	55	55	–	9
Cheeseburger BBQ Ranch	1	999	57	62	–	3
Cheeseburger Half Pound	1	855	48	49	–	3
Chicken Cordon Bleu	1 serv	1360	81	51	–	5
Chicken Feta Penne	1 serv	1879	99	158	–	12
Ciabatta Chicken	1	1251	72	81	–	4
Ciabatta Meatloaf	1	1036	61	83	–	3
Ciabatta Turkey Pesto	1	1248	73	83	–	6
Club Cafe	1	1132	63	73	–	4
Country Fried Steak	1 serv	1061	56	107	–	9
Crab Cake Dinner	1 serv	1662	100	129	–	9
Diablo Center Cut Pork Chops	1 serv	1094	73	55	–	8
Dip Classic Beef	1	521	15	43	–	5
Fillet Of Soul	1 serv	636	26	56	–	7
French Quarter	1	1480	105	68	–	7

FOOD	PORTION	CAL	FAT	CARB	SUGAR	FIBER
Garlic Shrimp Spaghettini	1 serv	860	20	109	–	7
Grilled Beef Liver	1 serv	1003	45	75	–	10
Grilled Chicken Tuscan Style	1 serv	880	36	80	–	12
Hibachi Salmon	1 serv	846	40	75	–	8
Mimi's Meatloaf	1 serv	910	53	68	–	8
Mimi's Pot Roast	1 serv	1291	78	57	–	8
Original Patty Melt	1	976	56	62	–	6
Parmesan Crusted Chicken Breast	1 serv	1820	54	211	–	15
Pasta Jambalaya	1 serv	1223	44	113	–	8
Pot Pie Chicken	1 serv	1403	87	86	–	11
Reuben West Coast	1	2015	138	120	–	11
Sandwich 5 Way Grilled Cheese	1	703	39	49	–	2
Sandwich Albacore & Avocado	1	993	71	58	–	9
Sandwich Bacon Lettuce & Tomato	1	586	34	48	–	7
Sandwich Fresh Roasted Turkey Breast	1	532	27	28	–	1
Sandwich Turkey Walnut Salad On Raisin Bread	1	549	42	36	–	3
Sandwich Veggie Stack	1	836	43	93	–	6
Slow Roasted Turkey Breast	1 serv	851	41	72	–	11
Small Bites Black & Blue Quesadilla	1 serv	1241	80	60	13	7
Small Bites Chicken & Fruit	1 serv	460	9	21	17	3
Small Bites Citrus Salmon	1 serv	699	43	37	21	10
Small Bites Crab Cakes	1 serv	412	25	27	6	2

FOOD	PORTION	CAL	FAT	CARB	SUGAR	FIBER
Small Bites Smokey Chicken Enchiladas	1 serv	1154	72	68	16	8
Small Bites Sweet & Sour Coconut Shrimp	1 serv	608	50	79	38	4
Small Bites Thai Chicken Wrap	1 serv	1004	41	106	16	7
Top Sirloin 12 oz	1 serv	947	48	49	–	7
SALAD DRESSINGS						
Balsamic Vinaigrette	1 serv	316	32	8	–	0
Blue Cheese	1 serv	298	31	1	–	0
Caesar	1 serv	273	29	2	–	0
Chinese Sesame	1 serv	263	25	11	–	0
Dijon Vinaigrette	1 serv	296	32	3	–	0
Honey Mustard	1 serv	243	22	11	–	0
Non Fat French	1 serv	65	0	16	–	1
Ranch	1 serv	194	20	2	–	0
Thousand Island	1 serv	232	23	6	–	0
SALADS						
Asian Chopped	1 serv	751	22	55	–	14
Blue Cheese & Walnut	1 serv	728	53	45	–	10
Caesar Blackened Chicken	1 serv	570	17	41	–	6
Chopped Cobb	1 serv	524	32	18	–	4
Fried Chicken	1 serv	764	67	16	–	3
Zesty Chicken Tostada	1 serv	1046	57	89	–	15
SOUPS						
Broccoli Cheddar	1 serv	270	10	18	4	2
Chicken Gumbo	1 serv	235	12	25	4	2
Clam Chowder	1 serv	240	14	21	2	2
Corn Chowder	1 serv	196	9	28	6	3
Cream Of Chicken	1 serv	337	29	19	3	1
French Market Onion	1 serv	207	12	16	4	2
Red Bean & Andouille Sausage	1 serv	256	10	30	4	5

FOOD	PORTION	CAL	FAT	CARB	SUGAR	FIBER
Split Pea	1 serv	194	3	29	5	11
Vegetarian Vegetable	1 serv	60	0	12	5	2

MR. HERO
DESSERTS

FOOD	PORTION	CAL	FAT	CARB	SUGAR	FIBER
Eli's Cheesecake Oreo Cookie	1 slice (2.5 oz)	260	17	24	–	1
Eli's Cheesecake Original Plain	1 slice (2.6 oz)	280	19	22	–	0
Eli's Cheesecake Snickers	1 slice (2.3 oz)	270	18	23	–	1
Eli's Cheesecake Strawberry Swirl	1 slice (2.6 oz)	280	19	22	–	0

SALADS

FOOD	PORTION	CAL	FAT	CARB	SUGAR	FIBER
Garden Side	1 serv (7.3 oz)	32	0	7	–	2
Grilled Chicken	1 serv (13.4 oz)	166	3	13	–	3
Tuna Delight	1 serv (14.4 oz)	403	48	10	–	3

SANDWICHES

FOOD	PORTION	CAL	FAT	CARB	SUGAR	FIBER
Cheeseburger	1 (10.4 oz)	776	55	47	–	3
Cheesesteak Hot Buttered	1 (9.4 oz)	669	42	45	–	3
Chicken Grilled Philly	1 (9.1 oz)	421	10	48	–	4
Deli Subs Original Italian	1 (9.5 oz)	641	39	47	–	3
Deli Subs Tuna 'N Cheese	1 (9.7 oz)	724	54	44	–	3
Deli Subs Turkey	1 (9.8 oz)	468	20	46	–	3
Deli Subs Ultimate Italian	1 (10.3 oz)	675	40	46	–	3
Romanburger	1 (11.3 oz)	861	62	48	–	3
Steak Tuscan	1 (10.6 oz)	625	31	42	–	2
Steak Zesty Bacon & Swiss	1 (9.8 oz)	616	32	42	–	3

FOOD	PORTION	CAL	FAT	CARB	SUGAR	FIBER
Subs Meatball	1 (9.3 oz)	724	47	47	–	4
Taste Buddies Cheeseburger Bacon	1 (5.9 oz)	264	30	33	–	2
Taste Buddies Grilled Italiano	1 (5.3 oz)	440	32	32	–	2
Taste Buddies Italian Sausage	1 (5.4 oz)	368	22	34	–	1
Taste Buddies Tuna 'N Cheese	1 (6 oz)	483	38	31	–	2
SIDES						
Breadsticks	2 (6 oz)	446	17	64	–	3
Jalapeno Poppers	1 serv (4.5 oz)	432	28	37	–	3
Mozzarella Sticks	1 serv (8.7 oz)	565	43	12	–	1
Onion Petals	1 serv (5.7 oz)	597	37	56	–	2
Potato Babycakes	1 serv (5.9 oz)	477	37	34	–	4
Potato Waffer Fries w/ Cheese Sauce	1 serv (7.2 oz)	482	34	42	–	3

NOAH'S BAGELS
BAGELS AND BREADS

FOOD	PORTION	CAL	FAT	CARB	SUGAR	FIBER
Bagel Asiago Cheese Topped	1 (4.2 oz)	330	6	57	5	2
Bagel Blueberry	1 (3.7 oz)	270	1	59	11	3
Bagel Candy Cane	1 (3.7 oz)	270	3	54	5	2
Bagel Cheddar Stick	1 (4.2 oz)	330	6	57	5	2
Bagel Chocolate Chip	1 (3.7 oz)	290	4	60	12	3
Bagel Chopped Garlic	1 (3.9 oz)	290	3	58	5	2
Bagel Cinnamon Raisin	1 (3.7 oz)	270	1	58	11	3
Bagel Cinnamon Sugar	1 (4.1 oz)	310	3	64	11	2
Bagel Cracked Pepper	1 (3.7 oz)	280	4	55	6	2

FOOD	PORTION	CAL	FAT	CARB	SUGAR	FIBER
Bagel Cranberry Orange	1 (3.5 oz)	250	1	54	6	3
Bagel Dutch Apple	1 (5 oz)	340	3	72	14	3
Bagel Egg	1 (3.7 oz)	290	3	57	5	2
Bagel Everything	1 (3.9 oz)	280	2	57	5	2
Bagel Good Grains	1 (3.9 oz)	280	2	58	6	4
Bagel Jalapeno Cheddar	1 (4.9 oz)	350	7	58	5	2
Bagel Onion	1 (3.7 oz)	270	2	57	5	3
Bagel Plain	1 (3.7 oz)	270	1	57	5	2
Bagel Poppyseed	1 (3.9 oz)	290	3	57	5	2
Bagel Power	1 (4 oz)	310	5	61	16	4
Bagel Pumpernickel	1 (3.7 oz)	260	2	57	4	3
Bagel Sesame Seed	1 (3.9 oz)	290	3	57	5	2
Bagel Six Cheese	1 (4.5 oz)	340	6	57	5	2
Bagel Spinach Florentine	1 (4.9 oz)	350	8	58	6	2
Bagel Sun Dried Tomato	1 (3.7 oz)	270	2	57	6	3
Bagel Whole Wheat	1 (3.7 oz)	260	1	57	6	4
Bagel Whole Wheat Sesame & Sunflower Seeds	1 (4.4 oz)	370	11	61	6	6
Bialy	1 (5.3 oz)	380	4	77	5	4
Bread Ciabatta	1 serv (4.25 oz)	290	3	60	1	2
Bread Corn Meal Rye	1 slice (2 oz)	150	2	31	1	2
Bread Harvest Grain	1 slice (2.3 oz)	180	2	36	7	4
Bread Marble Rye	1 slice (1.7 oz)	160	1	30	1	1
Bread Potato	1 slice (1.7 oz)	140	2	28	3	1
Challah Braided	1 serv (2 oz)	160	3	29	4	1
Challah Roll	1 (3 oz)	230	4	44	6	2
Pizza Bagel Artichoke Tomato & Red Onion	1 (11.1 oz)	550	20	67	8	5

FOOD	PORTION	CAL	FAT	CARB	SUGAR	FIBER
Pizza Bagel Artichoke & Spinach	1 (12 oz)	670	32	70	7	5
Pizza Bagel Cheese	1 (6.2 oz)	420	11	60	6	3
Pizza Bagel Cheesy Garlic & Herb	1 (6.2 oz)	500	19	62	6	2
Pizza Bagel Pepperoni	1 (6.8 oz)	500	19	60	6	3
Pizza Bagel Spinach & Mushroom	1 (9.5 oz)	580	25	68	8	4
Pizza Bagel Tomato & Rosemary	1 (8.7 oz)	540	20	63	7	4
BEVERAGES AND EXTRAS						
Cafe Latte Low Fat	1 reg (12 oz)	160	7	17	17	0
Cafe Latte Nonfat	1 reg (12 oz)	110	0	17	17	0
Cafe Latte Whole	1 reg (12 oz)	200	10	16	16	0
Cappuccino Low Fat	1 reg (12 oz)	120	5	13	13	0
Cappuccino Nonfat	1 reg (12 oz)	90	0	13	13	0
Cappuccino Whole	1 reg (12 oz)	150	8	13	13	0
Chai Tea Low Fat Milk	1 reg (12 oz)	220	2	47	45	0
Chai Tea Non Fat Milk	1 reg (12 oz)	210	0	47	45	0
Chai Tea Whole Milk	1 reg (12 oz)	230	3	47	45	0
Coca Cola	8 oz	99	0	27	27	0
Coca Cola Cherry	8 oz	104	0	28	28	0
Coffee Iced Americano	8 oz	0	0	0	0	0
Coffee Regular & Decaf	1 (12 oz)	0	0	0	0	0
Diet Coke	8 oz	1	0	0	0	0
Espresso	1 reg (2 oz)	0	0	0	0	0
Fanta Orange	8 oz	106	0	29	29	0
Frozen Drinks Cafe Caramel	1 (18 oz)	620	9	100	66	0
Frozen Drinks Cafe Mocha	1 (18 oz)	510	8	102	64	0
Frozen Drinks Strawberry Cream	1 (18 oz)	450	19	75	64	3

FOOD	PORTION	CAL	FAT	CARB	SUGAR	FIBER
Frozen Drinks Wild Berry Fat Free	1 (18 oz)	270	0	62	48	5
Half & Half Creamer	1 oz	40	3	1	1	0
Hi-C Fruit Punch	8 oz	104	0	28	28	0
Hot Chocolate Nonfat	1 reg (12 oz)	220	2	37	36	1
Hot Chocolate Whole	1 reg (12 oz)	290	11	35	34	1
Iced Cappuccino Nonfat	1 reg (12 oz)	90	0	13	13	0
Iced Mocha Low Fat	1 reg (12 oz)	230	5	39	34	0
Iced Tea Raspberry	8 oz	78	0	21	21	0
Iced Tea Unsweetened	8 oz	1	0	0	0	0
Lemonade	1 (16 oz)	200	0	24	24	0
Lemonade Blackberry	1 (16 oz)	310	0	74	74	0
Macchiato Nonfat	1 reg (12 oz)	230	0	49	44	0
Macchiato Whole	1 reg (12 oz)	290	8	47	42	0
Milk Low Fat	8 oz	120	5	12	11	0
Milk Skim	8 oz	80	0	15	13	0
Milk Whole	8 oz	150	8	11	11	0
Mocha Low Fat	1 reg (12 oz)	230	5	39	34	0
Mocha Nonfat	1 reg (12 oz)	190	0	39	34	0
Mocha Whole	1 reg (12 oz)	270	9	38	33	0
Mr. Pibb	8 oz	97	0	26	26	0
On Top Reduced Fat Topping	2 tbsp (0.3 oz)	20	2	2	2	0
Orange Juice	1 (10 oz)	143	0	34	31	2
Sprite	8 oz	97	0	26	26	0
Syrup Blackberry	2 tbsp (1 oz)	100	0	25	25	0
Syrup Caramel	2 tbsp (1 oz)	70	0	18	17	0
Syrup Hazelnut	2 tbsp (1 oz)	100	0	25	25	0
Syrup Vanilla	2 tbsp (1 oz)	100	0	25	25	0
Syrup Vanilla Sugar Free	2 tbsp (1 oz)	116	0	0	0	0
Tea Hamey & Sons All Topping	8 oz	0	0	0	0	0
Whipped Cream Light	2 tbsp (1 oz)	36	3	2	2	0

FOOD	PORTION	CAL	FAT	CARB	SUGAR	FIBER
CREAM CHEESE AND SPREADS						
Butter	1 tbsp (0.5 oz)	110	11	0	0	0
Cream Cheese Whipped Onion & Chive	2 tbsp (0.7 oz)	70	6	3	1	0
Cream Cheese Whipped Plain	2 tbsp (0.7 oz)	70	7	1	1	0
Cream Cheese Whipped Reduced Fat Blueberry	2 tbsp (0.7 oz)	70	5	6	5	0
Cream Cheese Whipped Reduced Fat Garden Vegetable	2 tbsp (0.7 oz)	60	5	3	1	0
Cream Cheese Whipped Reduced Fat Garlic Herb	2 tbsp (0.7 oz)	60	5	3	1	0
Cream Cheese Whipped Reduced Fat Honey Almond	2 tbsp (0.7 oz)	70	5	6	4	0
Cream Cheese Whipped Reduced Fat Jalapeno Salsa	2 tbsp (0.7 oz)	60	5	3	1	0
Cream Cheese Whipped Reduced Fat Plain	2 tbsp (0.7 oz)	60	5	2	1	0
Cream Cheese Whipped Reduced Fat Strawberry	2 tbsp (0.7 oz)	60	5	2	1	0
Cream Cheese Whipped Reduced Fat Sun Dried Tomato & Basil	2 tbsp (0.7 oz)	60	5	2	1	0
Cream Cheese Whipped Smoked Salmon	2 tbsp (0.7 oz)	60	6	2	1	0
Deli Mustard	1 tsp (5 g)	0	0	0	0	0
Garlic Mayo	1 serv (1.5 oz)	270	27	8	1	0
Grape Jam	1 serv (1 oz)	110	0	28	26	0
Honey	1 serv (1 oz)	90	0	23	22	0

FOOD	PORTION	CAL	FAT	CARB	SUGAR	FIBER
Hummus	1 serv (2 oz)	90	4	11	1	2
Mayo	1 tbsp (0.5 oz)	110	12	0	0	0
DESSERTS						
Cinnamon Twists	1 serv (3.8 oz)	370	21	41	18	2
Coffee Cake Apple Cinnamon	1 serv (6.6 oz)	700	28	108	57	1
Coffee Cake Chocolate Chip	1 serv (6.1 oz)	760	34	110	58	2
Coffee Cake Mixed Berry	1 serv (6.9 oz)	710	29	110	59	2
Cookie Chocolate Mudslide	1 (2.75 oz)	320	17	46	38	1
Cookie Chocolate Chip	1 (2.8 oz)	360	18	48	29	2
Cookie Iced Sugar	1 (3.7 oz)	480	15	76	46	1
Cookie Oatmeal Raisin	1 (2.8 oz)	320	11	54	31	2
Cookie Snickerdoodle	1 (2.8 oz)	400	18	56	32	1
Cookie Mini Chocolate Mudslide	1 (1.38 oz)	160	8	23	19	1
Cookie Mini Chocolate Chip	1 (1.38 oz)	180	9	24	14	1
Cookie Mini Iced Sugar	1 (1.87 oz)	230	7	39	24	1
Cookie Mini Oatmeal Raisin	1 (1.38 oz)	160	5	27	16	1
Marshmallow Crispy Treat	1 (3.9 oz)	410	7	86	37	0
Muffin Blueberry	1 (5 oz)	480	22	65	36	2
Muffin Cranberry Orange	1 (4.6 oz)	460	22	63	39	2
Muffin Strawberry White Chocolate	1 (5.5 oz)	550	25	78	49	1
Strudel Cinnamon Walnut	1 serv (5.4 oz)	630	42	56	20	4

FOOD	PORTION	CAL	FAT	CARB	SUGAR	FIBER
SALAD DRESSINGS						
Caesar	2 tbsp (1 oz)	150	16	1	1	0
Harvest Chicken Salad	2 tbsp (1 oz)	90	8	3	2	0
Raspberry Vinaigrette	2 tbsp	160	14	8	8	0
SALADS						
Caesar	1 (10.5 oz)	600	53	23	4	6
Caesar Side	1 (4.5 oz)	280	27	7	2	2
Ceasar Chicken	1 (14 oz)	720	54	23	6	4
City	1 (11.5 oz)	830	68	39	29	7
City w/ Chicken	1 (15 oz)	950	71	40	30	8
Southwestern Chicken	1 (15.2 oz)	710	41	54	14	10
SANDWICHES						
Bagel & Lox	1 (11.2 oz)	520	21	65	11	4
Bagel Dog Asiago	1 (7.1 oz)	510	21	59	6	2
Bagel Dog Everything	1 (7.1 oz)	510	20	59	6	2
Bagel Dog Original	1 (6.9 oz)	490	20	59	6	2
Bagel Plain w/ Peanut Butter & Jelly	1 (6.2 oz)	550	15	90	31	4
Breakfast Wrap Santa Fe	1 (14.5 oz)	750	34	77	8	9
Breakfast Wrap Veggie	1 (15.6 oz)	810	41	77	7	10
California Chicken	1 (9.9 oz)	360	7	49	8	3
Club Blackened Chicken	1 (10.4 oz)	630	33	53	8	2
Club Deli Pesto Turkey	1 (10.9 oz)	670	39	47	9	2
Deli Chicken Salad	1 (11 oz)	1150	95	61	5	5
Deli Cornbeef	1 (14 oz)	740	34	61	5	4
Deli Egg Salad Kosher	1 (11.5 oz)	650	6	68	6	5
Deli Pastrami	1 (14 oz)	750	34	62	6	5
Deli Roast Beef	1 (14 oz)	730	34	60	5	4
Deli Tuna Salad	1 (13 oz)	740	45	53	9	5
Deli Turkey	1 (14.5 oz)	720	29	67	6	5
Deli Whitefish	1 (12.2 oz)	850	55	68	9	6
Deli Melts Hummus	1 (10.2 oz)	570	19	76	7	6
Deli Melts Pastrami	1 (9.6 oz)	530	17	61	7	3
Deli Melts Roast Beef	1 (9.6 oz)	530	17	60	6	3

FOOD	PORTION	CAL	FAT	CARB	SUGAR	FIBER
Deli Melts Tuna	1 (11.6 oz)	700	33	82	7	3
Deli Melts Turkey	1 (9.6 oz)	500	14	60	7	3
Deli Melts Veggie	1 (12.3 oz)	590	25	70	10	5
Egg Mit Artichoke & Tomato	1 (12 oz)	620	28	67	10	4
Egg Mit Bacon & Cheddar	1 (9.2 oz)	620	28	61	8	2
Egg Mit Cheese & Tomato	1 (10 oz)	530	21	61	8	3
Egg Mit Lox & Chives	1 (8.8 oz)	490	17	59	8	2
Egg Mit Plain	1 (7.9 oz)	450	14	59	7	2
Egg Mit Spinach Mushroom & Swiss	1 (9.8 oz)	530	20	61	8	3
Egg Mit Turkey Sausage	1 (9.9 oz)	590	24	61	8	2
Egg Mit w/ Cheese	1 (8.5 oz)	520	20	60	7	2
Kosher Vegetarian On Plain Bagel	1 (13.9 oz)	860	41	79	9	4
Panini Albacore Tuna	1 (13.6 oz)	750	38	62	2	6
Panini Egg Spinach Bacon	1 (11.8 oz)	790	43	65	4	5
Panini Egg Vegetarian Omelet	1 (13.8 oz)	670	31	66	5	6
Panini Italian Chicken	1 (12.5 oz)	810	40	67	3	5
Panini Mediterranean	1 (10.6 oz)	550	18	77	3	9
Panini Tomato Mozzarella	1 (7.9 oz)	440	16	59	1	6
Panini Turkey Club	1 (12.3 oz)	610	21	64	4	6
Sandwich Rachel	1 (13.9 oz)	1030	68	53	14	2
Sandwich Reuben	1 (13.9 oz)	770	41	47	8	3
Sandwich Veg Out	1 (10.1 oz)	490	14	75	9	4
Wrap Albacore Tuna	1 (12.3 oz)	600	28	57	5	8
Wrap Chicken Caesar	1 (12.6 oz)	790	46	62	7	7
Wrap Southwestern Turkey	1 (13.5 oz)	750	37	74	12	9
Wrap Veggie	1 (9.8 oz)	460	17	64	6	9

FOOD	PORTION	CAL	FAT	CARB	SUGAR	FIBER
SIDES						
Cole Slaw	1 serv (3 oz)	120	6	15	2	2
Egg Salad	1 serv (5 oz)	330	29	3	2	0
Fresh Fruit Cup	1 (11 oz)	140	0	36	31	3
Fruit & Yogurt Parfait	1 (12 oz)	220	1	43	25	3
Kosher Pickle	1	5	0	1	1	0
Macaroni & Cheese	1 serv (6 oz)	340	17	32	–	1
Redskin Potato Salad	1 serv (3 oz)	160	12	13	1	1
Tuna Salad	1 serv (5 oz)	280	20	3	1	1
SOUPS						
Broccoli Cheese	1 cup (8.7 oz)	290	20	16	6	2
Chicken Noodle	1 cup (8.7 oz)	110	4	13	1	1
Italian Wedding	1 cup (8.7 oz)	160	6	15	2	2
Tortilla	1 cup (8.7 oz)	300	19	19	6	3
Turkey Chili	1 cup (8.7 oz)	220	7	24	5	5

NOODLES & COMPANY
MAIN MENU SELECTIONS

FOOD	PORTION	CAL	FAT	CARB	SUGAR	FIBER
Bangkok Curry	1 reg	490	13	85	–	7
Bangkok Curry	1 sm	250	6	42	–	3
Beef Braised	1 serv	190	10	0	0	0
Beef Sauteed	1 serv	210	12	0	0	0
Buttered Noodles	1 sm	310	8	42	–	4
Buttered Noodles	1 reg	620	16	84	–	7
Chicken Breast Seasoned	1 serv	130	3	0	0	0
Chicken Parmesan Crusted	1 serv	190	8	17	–	0
Ciabatta Roll	1	160	2	31	–	2
Flatbread	1 serv	210	4	37	–	2
House Marinara	1 sm	330	6	53	–	3
House Marinara	1 reg	650	12	107	–	7
Mushroom Stroganoff	1 reg	780	31	100	–	10
Mushroom Stroganoff	1 sm	390	15	50	–	5

FOOD	PORTION	CAL	FAT	CARB	SUGAR	FIBER
Organic Tofu	1 serv	180	11	4	–	0
Pad Thai	1 reg	700	20	117	–	5
Pad Thai	1 sm	350	10	59	–	3
Pasta Fresca	1 reg	780	22	111	–	6
Pasta Fresca	1 sm	420	12	56	–	3
Penne Rosa	1 sm	420	13	60	–	8
Penne Rosa	1 reg	810	26	119	–	15
Pesto Cavatappi	1 sm	510	21	62	–	4
Pesto Cavatappi	1 reg	910	30	124	–	8
Potstickers	3	200	5	31	–	2
Shrimp Sauteed	1 serv	35	0	0	0	0
Whole Grain Tuscan Linguine	1 reg	770	26	108	–	20
Whole Grain Tuscan Linguine	1 sm	450	20	54	–	10
Wisconsin Mac & Cheese	1 reg	900	31	119	–	13
Wisconsin Mac & Cheese	1 sm	450	16	60	–	7
SALADS						
Caesar	1 sm	160	14	5	–	1
Caesar	1 reg	320	28	11	–	2
Chinese Chopped	1 sm	150	7	11	–	3
Chinese Chopped	1 reg	310	15	23	–	6
Cucumber Tomato Side Salad	1	80	0	18	–	2
The Med	1 sm	150	6	19	–	2
The Med	1 reg	310	13	39	–	4
Tossed Green	1	60	6	3	–	1
SOUPS						
Chicken Noodle	1 reg	300	4	44	–	10
Chicken Noodle	1 sm	150	2	22	–	5
Thai Curry	1 reg	480	19	70	–	3
Thai Curry	1 sm	240	10	35	–	2
Tomato Basil	1 reg	420	23	45	–	13
Tomato Basil	1 sm	210	12	23	–	7

FOOD	PORTION	CAL	FAT	CARB	SUGAR	FIBER
PACIUGO GELATO						
Milk Base Amarena Black Cherry Swirl	1 scoop (3.5 oz)	160	4	30	30	tr
Milk Base Banana Creme Pie	1 scoop (3.5 oz)	80	2	14	13	tr
Milk Base Cheesecake	1 scoop (3.5 oz)	90	4	12	12	tr
Milk Base Chocolate	1 scoop (3.5 oz)	80	3	14	13	tr
Milk Base Chocolate Cookies'N Milk	1 scoop (3.5 oz)	90	3	16	13	tr
Milk Base Coconut	1 scoop (3.5 oz)	80	3	13	12	tr
Milk Base Coffee	1 scoop (3.5 oz)	75	3	12	11	tr
Milk Base Fiordilatte	1 scoop (3.5 oz)	75	2	13	13	tr
Milk Base French Vanilla Bean	1 scoop (3.5 oz)	80	3	13	13	tr
Milk Base Green Tea	1 scoop (3.5 oz)	70	2	12	12	tr
Milk Base Hazelnut	1 scoop (3.5 oz)	85	4	11	11	tr
Milk Base Lemon Custard	1 scoop (3.5 oz)	75	3	12	12	tr
Milk Base Mascarpone Chocolate Rum	1 scoop (3.5 oz)	95	5	11	10	tr
Milk Base Pannacotta Wedding Cake	1 scoop (3.5 oz)	75	2	13	13	tr
Milk Base Peppermint	1 scoop (3.5 oz)	75	2	14	13	1
Milk Base Rose	1 scoop (3.5 oz)	70	2	12	12	tr

FOOD	PORTION	CAL	FAT	CARB	SUGAR	FIBER
Milk Base Tiramisu	1 scoop (3.5 oz)	80	3	12	12	tr
Milk Base Zabajone	1 scoop (3.5 oz)	80	3	12	12	tr
No Sugar Added Chocolate	1 scoop (3.5 oz)	28	1	9	3	1
No Sugar Added Mint	1 scoop (3.5 oz)	25	1	9	3	1
No Sugar Added Mocha	1 scoop (3.5 oz)	28	1	9	3	1
No Sugar Added Strawberry Milk	1 scoop (3.5 oz)	23	1	8	3	1
Soy Banana	1 scoop (3.5 oz)	40	2	6	6	1
Soy Blueberry	1 scoop (3.5 oz)	40	2	6	6	1
Soy Chocolate	1 scoop (3.5 oz)	38	2	5	5	1
Soy Coffee	1 scoop (3.5 oz)	35	2	5	5	1
Soy Hazelnut	1 scoop (3.5 oz)	35	2	5	5	1
Soy Strawberry	1 scoop (3.5 oz)	38	2	6	6	1
Soy Wild Berries	1 scoop (3.5 oz)	40	2	6	6	1
Water Base Blackberry	1 scoop (3.5 oz)	28	0	7	7	tr
Water Base Ginger Lemon	1 scoop (3.5 oz)	25	0	7	7	tr
Water Base Green Apple	1 scoop (3.5 oz)	28	0	7	7	tr
Water Base Lemon Sage	1 scoop (3.5 oz)	25	0	7	7	tr

FOOD	PORTION	CAL	FAT	CARB	SUGAR	FIBER
Water Base Lychee	1 scoop (3.5 oz)	25	0	6	6	tr
Water Base Orange Vidalia	1 scoop (3.5 oz)	25	0	7	7	0
Water Base Passion Fruit	1 scoop (3.5 oz)	23	0	6	6	0
Water Base Pineapple	1 scoop (3.5 oz)	28	0	7	7	tr
Water Base Strawberry Port	1 scoop (3.5 oz)	25	0	6	6	tr
Water Base Watermelon	1 scoop (3.5 oz)	25	0	7	7	tr

PEI WEI ASIAN DINER
CHILDREN'S MENU SELECTIONS

FOOD	PORTION	CAL	FAT	CARB	SUGAR	FIBER
Kid's Wei Honey Seared Chicken w/o Noodles Or Rice	1 serv	290	17	19	8	0
Kid's Wei Lo Mein Chicken w/o Noodles Or Rice	1 serv	180	7	7	3	0
Kid's Wei Teriyaki Chicken w/o Noodles Or Rice	1 serv	240	5	20	18	0

DESSERTS

FOOD	PORTION	CAL	FAT	CARB	SUGAR	FIBER
Cookie Chocolate Chip	1	342	14	53	37	2
Cookie Fortune	1	30	0	7	3	0

MAIN MENU SELECTIONS

FOOD	PORTION	CAL	FAT	CARB	SUGAR	FIBER
Bowl w/ Brown Rice Japanese Teriyaki Beef	1 serv	580	17	66	21	4
Bowl w/ Brown Rice Japanese Teriyaki Chicken	1 serv	460	7	64	21	4

FOOD	PORTION	CAL	FAT	CARB	SUGAR	FIBER
Bowl w/ Brown Rice Japanese Teriyaki Shrimp	1 serv	410	5	64	21	4
Bowl w/ Brown Rice Japanese Teriyaki Vegetables & Tofu	1 serv	410	6	71	24	7
Bowl w/ White Rice Japanese Teriyaki Beef	1 serv	560	16	62	21	3
Bowl w/ White Rice Japanese Teriyaki Chicken	1 serv	440	6	60	21	3
Bowl w/ White Rice Japanese Teriyaki Shrimp	1 serv	390	5	61	21	3
Bowl w/ White Rice Japanese Teriyaki Vegetables & Tofu	1 serv	390	5	68	24	5
Crispy Potstickers	4	130	7	10	1	0
Edamame	1 serv	156	8	12	4	5
Fried Rice Beef	1 serv	630	21	68	9	3
Fried Rice Chicken	1 serv	525	11	68	9	3
Fried Rice Shrimp	1 serv	475	10	67	9	3
Fried Rice Vegetable & Tofu	1 serv	440	7	73	12	5
Ginger Broccoli Beef	1 serv	450	22	19	11	2
Ginger Broccoli Chicken	1 serv	300	9	19	11	2
Ginger Broccoli Shrimp	1 serv	230	7	18	11	2
Ginger Broccoli Vegetables & Tofu	1 serv	170	4	23	14	4
Honey Seared Chicken	1 serv	420	15	45	17	0
Honey Seared Shrimp	1 serv	370	14	43	17	0
Hot & Sour Soup	1 cup	150	9	11	0	2
Lemon Pepper Beef	1 serv	550	31	32	18	2
Lemon Pepper Chicken	1 serv	440	20	34	18	2

FOOD	PORTION	CAL	FAT	CARB	SUGAR	FIBER
Lemon Pepper Shrimp	1 serv	380	18	34	18	2
Lemon Pepper Vegetables & Tofu	1 serv	230	10	29	19	4
Mandarin Kung Pao Beef	1 serv	610	34	31	10	3
Mandarin Kung Pao Chicken	1 serv	450	21	28	10	3
Mandarin Kung Pao Shrimp	1 serv	400	19	28	10	3
Mandarin Kung Pao Vegetables & Tofu	1 serv	290	15	23	10	4
Minced Chicken w/ Cool Lettuce Wraps w/o Rice Sticks	1 serv	250	4	31	15	3
Mongolian Beef	1 serv	420	22	14	8	1
Mongolian Chicken	1 serv	280	9	14	8	1
Mongolian Shrimp	2 serv	210	6	12	8	1
Mongolian Vegetables & Tofu	2 serv	180	6	19	11	3
Noodles Dan Dan Chicken	1 serv	390	7	54	9	3
Noodles Lo Mein Beef	1 serv	570	21	61	9	5
Noodles Lo Mein Chicken	1 serv	460	11	61	9	5
Noodles Lo Mein Shrimp	1 serv	400	8	60	9	5
Noodles Lo Mein Vegetables & Tofu	1 serv	400	8	66	11	7
Noodles Thai Blazing Beef	1 serv	630	32	55	11	4
Noodles Thai Blazing Chicken	1 serv	520	22	55	11	4
Noodles Thai Blazing Shrimp	1 serv	482	22	55	11	4
Noodles Thai Blazing Vegetables & Tofu	1 serv	430	18	59	14	6

FOOD	PORTION	CAL	FAT	CARB	SUGAR	FIBER
Noodles Egg	1 serv	210	3	39	0	2
Noodles Rice	1 serv	130	0	32	0	0
Orange Peel Beef	1 serv	660	31	52	33	3
Orange Peel Chicken	1 serv	520	18	52	33	3
Orange Peel Shrimp	1 serv	460	16	51	33	3
Orange Peel Vegetables & Tofu	1 serv	330	10	46	33	4
Pad Thai Beef	1 serv	670	30	63	19	2
Pad Thai Chicken	1 serv	560	20	61	19	2
Pad Thai Shrimp	1 serv	490	17	60	19	2
Pei Wei Spicy Beef	1 serv	480	26	25	8	2
Pei Wei Spicy Chicken	1 serv	330	13	25	8	2
Pei Wei Spicy Shrimp	1 serv	300	11	29	8	2
Rice Brown	1 serv	170	2	37	0	3
Rice Fried	1 serv	260	5	44	5	2
Rice Sticks	1 cup	130	0	33	0	0
Rice White	1 serv	200	0	44	0	1
Spicy Korean Beef	1 serv	490	24	26	12	3
Spicy Korean Chicken	1 serv	350	11	26	12	3
Spicy Korean Shrimp	1 serv	280	9	24	12	3
Spicy Korean Vegetables & Tofu	1 serv	240	9	27	14	4
Spring Rolls	2	90	5	11	3	1
Sweet & Sour Chicken	1 serv	440	13	61	30	2
Sweet & Sour Shrimp	1 serv	390	11	59	30	2
Thai Coconut Curry Beef	1 serv	550	37	20	10	2
Thai Coconut Curry Chicken	1 serv	380	19	23	10	2
Thai Coconut Curry Shrimp	1 serv	300	17	18	10	2
Thai Coconut Curry Vegetables & Tofu	1 serv	220	14	19	11	2
Thai Dynamite Chicken	1 serv	390	19	20	7	2
Thai Dynamite Shrimp	1 serv	280	16	20	9	2

FOOD	PORTION	CAL	FAT	CARB	SUGAR	FIBER
Thai Dynamite Vegetables & Tofu	1 serv	220	16	15	9	3
Wontons Crab	4	190	13	9	0	0
SALAD DRESSINGS AND SAUCES						
Dressing Sesame Ginger	1 serv (2 oz)	170	16	5	4	0
Lime Vinaigrette	1 serv (2 oz)	230	20	13	11	0
Sauce Lettuce Wrap	1 serv (2 oz)	70	5	2	1	0
Sauce Sweet Chili	1 serv (2 oz)	140	0	34	28	2
Sauce Thai Peanut	1 serv (2 oz)	168	11	15	11	1
SALADS						
Asian Chopped Chicken w/ Dressing	1 serv	280	15	13	4	2
Asian Chopped Chicken w/o Dressing	1 serv	200	8	10	2	2
Pei Wei Spicy Chicken w/ Dressing	1 serv	350	16	28	8	2
Pei Wei Spicy Chicken w/o Dressing	1 serv	210	3	23	3	2
Vietnamese Chicken Salad Rolls	3	53	3	5	3	1

P.F. CHANG'S CHINA BISTRO
DESSERTS

FOOD	PORTION	CAL	FAT	CARB	SUGAR	FIBER
Banana Spring Rolls	1 serv	814	37	130	–	7
Cake The Great Wall Of Chocolate	1 serv	2237	90	376	–	13
Flourless Chocolate Dome Gluten Free	1 serv	572	26	84	–	8
Ice Cream Pineapple Coconut	1 serv	111	12	25	–	0
Mini Dessert Apple Pie	1	170	4	34	–	1
Mini Dessert Banana Split	1	167	6	28	–	1

FOOD	PORTION	CAL	FAT	CARB	SUGAR	FIBER
Mini Dessert Carrot Cake	1	295	14	42	–	1
Mini Dessert Creamy Strawberry Cheesecake	1	239	20	14	–	1
Mini Dessert Great Wall Of Chocolate	1	336	26	24	–	2
Mini Dessert S'mores	1	323	12	50	–	1
Mini Dessert Tiramisu	1	202	14	15	–	0
Mini Dessert Tres Leche Lemon Dream	1	216	8	32	–	1
MAIN MENU SELECTIONS						
Almond & Cashew Chicken	1 serv	815	30	63	–	5
Asian Marinated New York Strip	1 serv	1432	86	68	–	2
Asian Slaw	1 serv	585	57	19	–	5
Beef A La Sichuan	1 serv	1172	64	56	–	5
Beef w/ Broccoli	1 serv	1118	65	38	–	7
Buddha's Feast Steamed	1 serv	137	1	29	–	10
Buddha's Feast Stir Fried	1 serv	367	5	66	–	10
Calamari Salt & Pepper	1 serv	720	11	118	–	3
Cantonese Scallops	1 serv	408	16	26	–	4
Cantonese Shrimp	1 serv	330	12	21	–	4
Cantonese Chow Fun w/ Beef	1 serv	1212	38	142	–	5
Cantonese Chow Fun w/ Chicken	1 serv	1045	23	146	–	5
Chang's Spicy Chicken	1 serv	923	37	88	–	1
Chengdu Spiced Lamb	1 serv	1056	75	34	–	5
Chicken w/ Black Bean Sauce	1 serv	678	23	33	–	1
Chow Fun Vegetable	1 serv	878	8	181	–	26
Chow Mein Combo	1 serv	912	34	86	–	6
Chow Mein w/ Beef	1 serv	793	26	84	–	7

FOOD	PORTION	CAL	FAT	CARB	SUGAR	FIBER
Chow Mein w/ Chicken	1 serv	689	16	84	–	6
Chow Mein w/ Pork	1 serv	898	34	83	–	6
Chow Mein w/ Shrimp	1 serv	625	13	84	–	6
Citrus Soy Salmon w/ Brown Rice	1 serv	1000	59	42	–	4
Citrus Soy Salmon w/ White Rice	1 serv	1025	58	49	–	2
Coconut Curry Vegetables	1 serv	686	46	48	–	12
Crispy Green Beans	1 serv	507	28	59	–	8
Crispy Honey Chicken	1 serv	867	11	121	–	3
Crispy Honey Shrimp	1 serv	1061	44	118	–	2
Dali Chicken	1 serv	1091	52	53	–	6
Double Pan Fried Noodles Combo	1 serv	1384	69	118	–	7
Double Pan Fried Noodles w/ Beef	1 serv	1186	56	112	–	6
Double Pan Fried Noodles w/ Chicken	1 serv	1072	47	115	–	7
Double Pan Fried Noodles w/ Pork	1 serv	1208	60	114	–	7
Double Pan Fried Noodles w/ Shrimp	1 serv	1031	46	115	–	7
Dumplings Peking Pan Fried	1 serv	367	23	21	–	1
Dumplings Peking Steamed	1 serv	327	18	21	–	1
Dumplings Shrimp Pan Fried	1 serv	305	13	25	–	1
Dumplings Shrimp Steamed	1 serv	265	8	25	–	1
Dumplings Vegetable Pan Fried	1 serv	307	11	43	–	2

FOOD	PORTION	CAL	FAT	CARB	SUGAR	FIBER
Dumplings Vegetable Steamed	1 serv	267	7	43	–	2
Eggplant Stir Fried	1 serv	590	34	64	–	10
Fried Rice Combo	1 serv	1539	69	154	–	5
Fried Rice w/ Beef	1 serv	1228	40	150	–	5
Fried Rice w/ Chicken	1 serv	1208	44	151	–	5
Fried Rice w/ Pork	1 serv	1360	57	150	–	5
Fried Rice w/ Shrimp	1 serv	1154	41	149	–	4
Garlic Noodles	1 serv	612	11	111	–	6
Garlic Snap Peas	1 sm	129	7	13	–	4
Ginger Chicken w/ Broccoli	1 serv	656	26	45	–	7
Ginger Chicken w/ Broccoli Gluten Free	1 serv	677	30	43	–	7
Ground Chicken & Eggplant	1 serv	792	40	73	–	9
Harvest Spring Rolls	1 serv	287	15	30	–	2
Hot Fish	1 serv	1338	71	111	–	8
Kung Pao Chicken	1 serv	1228	79	58	–	8
Kung Pao Scallops	1 serv	1136	57	66	–	9
Kung Pao Shrimp	1 serv	977	58	58	–	9
Lemon Pepper Shrimp	1 serv	701	36	59	–	5
Lemon Scallops	1 serv	952	28	100	–	3
Lemongrass Prawns	1 serv	907	58	65	–	4
Lettuce Wraps Chicken	1 serv	377	12	35	–	5
Lettuce Wraps Gluten Free Chicken	1 serv	477	12	63	–	5
Lettuce Wraps Vegetarian	1 serv	281	4	37	–	7
Lo Mein Combo	1 serv	1409	83	98	–	8
Lo Mein w/ Beef	1 serv	1374	80	94	–	8
Lo Mein w/ Chicken	1 serv	1198	67	97	–	8
Lo Mein w/ Pork	1 serv	1400	54	95	–	8
Lo Mein w/ Shrimp	1 serv	1134	64	97	–	8

FOOD	PORTION	CAL	FAT	CARB	SUGAR	FIBER
Lunch Bowl Almond & Cashew Chicken w/ White Rice	1	955	26	112	–	5
Lunch Bowl Beef w/ Broccoli w/ Brown Rice	1	844	27	87	–	8
Lunch Bowl Beef w/ Broccoli w/ White Rice	1	890	26	99	–	5
Lunch Bowl Buddha's Feast w/ Brown Rice	1	541	8	101	–	11
Lunch Bowl Buddha's Feast w/ White Rice	1	587	6	113	–	7
Lunch Bowl Citrus Soy Salmon w/ Brown Rice	1	1047	63	67	–	6
Lunch Bowl Citrus Soy Salmon w/ White Rice	1	1093	62	79	–	2
Lunch Bowl Crispy Honey Chicken w/ Brown Rice	1	943	13	126	–	6
Lunch Bowl Crispy Honey Chicken w/ White Rice	1	989	12	138	–	2
Lunch Bowl Moo Goo Gai Pan w/ Brown Rice	1	545	8	76	–	7
Lunch Bowl Moo Goo Gai Pan w/ White Rice	1	591	6	88	–	3
Lunch Bowl Pepper Steak w/ Brown Rice	1	820	28	82	–	7
Lunch Bowl Pepper Steak w/ White Rice	1 serv	968	39	94	–	3
Lunch Bowl Shrimp w/ Lobster Sauce w/ Brown Rice	1	686	25	75	–	6

FOOD	PORTION	CAL	FAT	CARB	SUGAR	FIBER
Lunch Bowl Shrimp w/ Lobster Sauce w/ White Rice	1	732	23	87	–	2
Mongolian Beef	1 serv	1178	73	29	–	2
Moo Goo Gai Pan	1 serv	661	34	32	–	4
Mu Shu Chicken	1 serv	715	38	49	–	–
Mu Shu Pork	1 serv	871	50	50	–	25
Noodles Dan Dan	1 serv	1087	30	145	–	7
Noodles Tam's	1 serv	1678	93	144	–	6
Oolong Marinated Sea Bass	1 serv	521	12	40	–	3
Orange Peel Beef	1 serv	1568	85	115	–	14
Orange Peel Chicken	1 serv	1151	46	127	–	14
Orange Peel Shrimp	1 serv	1010	41	118	–	14
Pepper Steak	1 serv	971	48	32	–	4
Philip's Better Lemon Chicken	1 serv	1051	42	113	–	5
Rice Brown	1 cup	254	2	53	–	4
Rice Sticks	1 serv	135	0	33	–	0
Rice White	1 cup	295	1	64	–	1
Salt & Pepper Prawns	1 serv	844	50	55	–	5
Seared Ahi Tuna	1 serv	210	9	9	–	1
Shanghai Cucumbers	1 serv	124	6	8	–	4
Shrimp w/ Candied Walnuts	1 serv	1225	80	74	–	2
Shrimp w/ Lobster Sauce	1 serv	480	22	24	–	1
Sichuan Asparagus	1 sm	97	3	16	–	3
Sichuan Chicken Flatbread	1 serv	1160	80	56	–	4
Sichuan From The Sea Calamari	1 serv	1078	36	118	–	4
Sichuan From The Sea Scallops	1 serv	1030	36	98	–	3

FOOD	PORTION	CAL	FAT	CARB	SUGAR	FIBER
Sichuan From The Sea Shrimp	1 serv	728	37	55	–	3
Singapore Street Noodles	1 serv	572	16	81	–	7
Singapore Street Noodles Gluten Free	1 serv	566	15	81	–	4
Spare Ribs Chang's	1 serv	1356	89	43	–	1
Spare Ribs Northern Style	1 serv	720	54	6	–	0
Spicy Green Beans	1 sm	234	13	23	–	6
Spinach w/ Garlic Stir Fried	1 sm	77	3	9	–	6
Sweet & Sour Chicken	1 serv	764	20	107	–	3
Sweet & Sour Pork	1 serv	1095	46	106	–	3
Vegetarian Ma Po Tofu	1 serv	537	19	51	–	6
Wild Alaskan Sockeye Salmon Steamed w/ Ginger	1 serv	646	36	23	–	5
Wild Aslaskan Sockeye Salmon Steamed w/ Ginger Gluten Free	1 serv	672	36	30	–	6
Wok Charred Beef	1 serv	941	63	33	–	8
Wok Seared Lamb	1 serv	1081	80	29	–	8
Wontons Crab	1 serv	440	25	32	–	2
SALAD DRESSINGS AND SAUCES						
Dressing Creamy Wedge	1 serv	443	43	8	–	1
Dressing Signature Ginger	1 serv	483	48	9	–	0
Sauce Chili Bean	1 serv	81	1	12	–	0
Sauce Crispy Green Bean	1 serv	451	48	5	–	0
Sauce Potsticker	1 serv	36	1	6	–	0
Sauce Shrimp Dumpling	1 serv	24	0	1	–	0
Sauce Special	1 serv	55	1	9	–	0

FOOD	PORTION	CAL	FAT	CARB	SUGAR	FIBER
Sauce Spicy Plum	1 serv	110	0	28	–	0
Sauce Sweet & Sour	1 serv	57	0	15	–	0
Vinaigrette Mustard	1 serv	66	2	7	–	0
Vinaigrette Watermelon Citrus	1 serv	240	23	7	–	0
SALADS						
Bikini Shrimp w/o Dressing	1 serv	192	6	30	–	4
Chang's Wedge w/ Chicken w/o Dressing	1 serve	595	35	12	–	5
Chang's Wedge w/o Dressing	1 serv	244	19	12	–	5
Chopped Chicken w/o Dressing	1 serv	401	14	21	–	5
SOUPS						
Chicken Noodle	1 bowl	512	13	30	–	2
Egg Drop	1 cup	48	2	7	–	0
Hot & Sour	1 cup	85	2	11	–	4
Wonton	1 bowl	354	10	44	–	3
PINKBERRY						
Frozen Yogurt Coffee	½ cup	90	0	24	19	0
Frozen Yogurt Green Tea	½ cup	50	0	10	10	0
Frozen Yogurt Original	½ cup	70	0	14	12	0
PIZZA FUSION						
DESSERTS						
Brownies Gluten Free	½ serv	232	16	27	17	1
Calzone Chocolate	½	209	9	30	9	1
Cookies Chocolate Chip	⅓ serv	250	13	33	13	3
Pastry Strawberry Cheese	1 serv	338	10	54	4	2
PIZZA						
BBQ Chicken	1 slice	181	4	26	7	1

FOOD	PORTION	CAL	FAT	CARB	SUGAR	FIBER
Big Kahuna	1 slice	236	9	26	2	2
Bruschetta	1 slice	159	4	23	2	1
Cheese	1 slice	167	5	23	2	2
Eggplant & Mozzarella	1 slice	181	6	24	2	2
Farmer's Market	1 slice	190	6	25	3	2
Founder's Pie	1 slice	201	7	25	3	2
Four Cheese & Sundried Tomato	1 slice	175	5	26	5	2
Greek	1 slice	204	7	25	2	2
Pepperoni	1 slice	220	9	23	2	2
Personal BBQ Chicken	½ pie	272	6	43	10	2
Personal Big Kahuna	½ pie	365	13	39	2	3
Personal Bruschetta	½ pie	234	5	37	1	2
Personal Cheese	½ pie	233	6	35	2	2
Personal Eggplant & Mozzerella	½ pie	304	11	39	2	4
Personal Farmer's Market	½ pie	279	8	40	4	3
Personal Founder's Pie	½ pie	347	14	41	4	3
Personal Four Cheese & Sundried Tomato	½ pie	262	7	39	6	3
Personal Greek	½ pie	299	11	39	2	3
Personal Pepperoni	½ pie	359	15	37	2	2
Personal Philly Steak	½ pie	358	14	42	2	4
Personal Sausage & Tri-Peppers	½ pie	323	12	39	2	3
Personal Spinach & Artichoke	½ pie	270	7	41	3	4
Personal Very Vegan	½ pie	321	15	41	2	4
Philly Steak	1 slice	220	8	26	2	3
Sausage & Tri-Peppers	1 slice	212	8	25	2	2
Spinach & Artichoke	1 slice	184	5	25	2	2
Very Vegan	1 slice	195	8	27	2	3

FOOD	PORTION	CAL	FAT	CARB	SUGAR	FIBER
SALADS						
Caesar & Roasted Chicken	½ serv	358	21	28	5	2
Chicken Bruschetta	½ serv	331	22	22	4	3
Fusion	½ serv	244	8	20	1	4
Pan Roasted Steak	½ serv	388	26	22	3	4
Pear & Gorganzola	½ serv	380	34	12	3	4
Roasted Beet & Feta	½ serv	320	25	19	3	4
Side Salad Arugula	1 serv	48	4	1	0	0
SANDWICHES						
Philly Phusion	½	473	23	39	1	3
Portabello Grill	½	380	20	38	1	3
Roasted Chicken	½	357	14	41	5	4
Roasted Turkey	½	417	19	35	2	2
STARTERS						
Flatbread	1 (2 serv)	198	2	76	2	4
Stuffed Portobello Mushroom	½ serv	140	11	9	3	2
Trio Of Dips	⅓ serv	191	11	30	1	3

PRETZELMAKER

FOOD	PORTION	CAL	FAT	CARB	SUGAR	FIBER
BEVERAGES						
Breezer Coffee	1 (20 oz)	640	21	107	106	0
Breezer Mocha	1 (20 oz)	620	20	106	104	0
Breezer Peach	1 (20 oz)	650	20	117	115	0
Breezer Raspberry	1 (20 oz)	650	20	117	112	0
Breezer Strawberry Banana	1 (20 oz)	650	20	115	108	0
Diet Coke	1 sm (20 oz)	0	0	0	0	0
Lemonade	1 sm (20 oz)	160	0	92	87	0
PRETZELS						
Bites	1 sm (5.3 oz)	450	11	80	15	3
Bites	1 med (7.4 oz)	640	16	112	21	4

FOOD	PORTION	CAL	FAT	CARB	SUGAR	FIBER
Bites Cinnamon Sugar	1 serv (5.8 oz)	520	12	95	28	3
Caramel Nut	1 (4.5 oz)	390	7	74	17	2
Cinnamon Sugar	1 (4.3 oz)	370	8	68	17	2
Garlic	1 (4.1 oz)	350	7	64	12	2
Original	1 (4 oz)	340	7	61	11	2
Parmesan	1 (4.2 oz)	360	9	61	11	2
Plain	1 (4 oz)	209	2	61	11	2
PT Pretzel Dog	1 (6 oz)	440	27	34	8	1
Ranch	1 (4.1 oz)	240	7	63	11	2
TOPPINGS						
Cream Cheese	1 serv (1.5 oz)	200	20	4	2	0
Icing Cream Cheese	1 serv (1.5 oz)	180	9	22	21	0
Ketchup	2 pkg (0.6 oz)	20	0	4	4	0
Mustard	2 pkg (0.4 oz)	5	0	1	0	0
Sauce Caramel	1 serv (1.5 oz)	140	0	35	27	0
Sauce Cheddar Cheese	1 serv (1.5 oz)	70	5	6	2	0
Sauce Nacho Cheese	1 serv (1.5 oz)	80	5	7	2	0
Sauce Pizza	1 serv (1.5 oz)	30	1	6	3	2

QUIZNO'S
COOKIES

FOOD	PORTION	CAL	FAT	CARB	SUGAR	FIBER
Dark Chocolate Chunk	1	380	15	58	32	1
Double Chocolate Chip	1	370	15	58	34	3
Oatmeal Raisin	1	340	11	59	36	2
Snickerdoodle	1	400	16	59	36	0
SANDWICHES						
Breakfast Bacon Egg Cheddar	1	380	21	36	2	4
Breakfast Black Angus Steak & Cheddar	1 sm	330	13	36	2	3

FOOD	PORTION	CAL	FAT	CARB	SUGAR	FIBER
Breakfast Egg & Cheddar	1	240	11	35	2	3
Breakfast Garden Vegetable Cheddar	1	250	11	38	3	4
Breakfast Ham Egg Cheddar	1	290	12	37	3	4
Deli Honey Ham & Swiss	1	260	4	38	5	4
Deli Oven Roasted Turkey & Cheese	1	250	4	39	4	4
Deli Roast Beef & Cheddar	1	230	4	37	3	4
Deli Tuna Melt	1	500	33	37	3	4
Sammie Alpine Chicken	1	200	6	24	1	1
Sammie Balsamic Chicken	1	170	4	24	1	1
Sammie Bistro Steak Melt	1	180	4	25	1	1
Sammie Black Angus Steak	1	180	4	24	1	1
Sammie Italiano	1	240	11	24	1	1
Sammie Sonoma Turkey	1	160	4	25	1	1
Sub Baja Chicken w/ Bacon	1 sm	320	9	37	2	4
Sub Black Angus Steak On Rosemary Parmesan	1 sm	380	8	46	3	5
Sub Chicken Carbonara w/ Bacon	1 sm	360	10	42	3	3
Sub Classic Club w/ Bacon	1 sm	320	9	39	5	5
Sub Classic Italian	1 sm	360	15	38	4	4
Sub Honey Bacon Club	1 sm	320	9	39	5	5
Sub Honey Bourbon Chicken	1 sm	260	4	38	3	4
Sub Honey Mustard Chicken w/ Bacon	1 sm	330	9	38	4	4

FOOD	PORTION	CAL	FAT	CARB	SUGAR	FIBER
Sub Mesquite Chicken w/ Bacon	1 sm	330	9	38	4	4
Sub Prime Rib Cheesesteak	1 sm	360	11	40	4	4
Sub Prime Rib & Peppercorn	1 sm	380	8	46	3	5
Sub Steakhouse Beef Dip	1 sm	260	6	37	3	4
Sub The Traditional	1 sm	260	5	39	5	5
Sub Turkey Bacon Guacamole	1 sm	360	12	43	6	6
Sub Turkey Ranch & Swiss	1 sm	250	4	39	4	5
Sub Tuscan Turkey On Rosemary Parmesan	1 sm	300	5	47	5	4
Sub Veggie	1 sm	270	8	41	5	6
SOUPS						
Bread Bowl Country French	1 serv	720	22	100	7	5
Bread Bowls Chili	1 serv	730	22	104	7	8
Broccoli Cheese	1 cup	150	10	10	5	2
Chicken Noodle	1 cup	130	3	18	1	0
Chili	1 cup	140	7	12	4	4

RANCH 1
BEVERAGES

FOOD	PORTION	CAL	FAT	CARB	SUGAR	FIBER
Barq's Root Beer	1 sm (16 oz)	167	0	45	45	0
Coca-Cola	1 sm (16 oz)	150	0	40	40	0
Diet Coke	1 sm (16 oz)	2	0	0	0	0
Sprite	1 sm (16 oz)	150	0	40	40	0

CHILDREN'S MENU SELECTIONS

FOOD	PORTION	CAL	FAT	CARB	SUGAR	FIBER
Kids Meal Chicken Tenders	1 (2 oz)	111	4	9	0	0
Kids Meal Fries	1 serv (4 oz)	279	15	31	1	4

FOOD	PORTION	CAL	FAT	CARB	SUGAR	FIBER
Kids Meal Popcorn Chicken	1 (2 oz)	112	4	10	0	0
MAIN MENU SELECTIONS						
Bowl Chicken Teriyaki	1 (19.3 oz)	504	7	78	10	1
Chicken Crispy	1 serv (5 oz)	326	15	22	1	1
Chicken Grilled	1 serv (3.9 oz)	146	6	0	0	0
Chicken On Mixed Greens	1 serv (21 oz)	340	19	17	9	7
Chicken Popcorn	1 serv (5.5 oz)	325	12	30	0	1
Chicken Tenders	1 serv (5.6 oz)	387	14	32	1	1
Fajita Mix Tomatoes Onion & Carrot	1 serv (3.2 oz)	20	0	5	3	1
Fajitas Chicken	1 serv (10 oz)	540	24	53	4	3
Fries	1 med	381	21	43	2	6
Fries Cheese	1 reg	493	27	54	2	6
Green Mix For Sandwiches	1 serv (2.5 oz)	31	2	2	1	1
Peppers & Onions	1 serv (1.6 oz)	27	2	3	2	1
Platter Chicken Rice	1 (10.9 oz)	273	6	28	4	3
Popcorn Chicken	1 sm	325	12	30	0	1
Rice	1 serv (4 oz)	97	0	21	0	0
Sandwich Chicken & Cheese	1 (11.2 oz)	389	12	39	5	2
Sandwich Chicken Philly	1 (9.2 oz)	410	13	40	4	2
Sandwich Crispy Chicken	1 (11.4 oz)	711	39	60	4	3
Sandwich Crispy Spicy Chicken	1 (11.4 oz)	543	17	68	7	3
Sandwich Grilled Spicy Chicken	1 (10.3 oz)	363	7	46	7	2
Sandwich Ranch 1 Classic	1 (9.4 oz)	683	47	37	3	2

FOOD	PORTION	CAL	FAT	CARB	SUGAR	FIBER
Steamed Vegetables	1 serv (3 oz)	27	0	6	2	2
Wrap Grilled Chicken Caesar	1 (13.2 oz)	746	41	55	2	4
SALAD DRESSINGS AND SAUCES						
Dressing Balsamic Vinaigrette	1 oz	71	8	1	0	0
Dressing Classic Caesar	1 oz	103	11	1	0	0
Dressing Salad	1 oz	201	22	0	0	0
Sauce Ancho Chili Pepper	1 oz	134	14	1	1	0
Sauce BBQ	1 oz	84	4	12	8	0
Sauce Honey Mustard	1 oz	110	8	9	6	0
Sauce Pepper & Onion Saute	1 oz	143	16	1	0	0
Sauce Roasted Red Pepper	1 oz	232	26	0	–	–
Sauce Teriyaki	1 oz	24	0	5	5	0
SALADS						
Caesar	1 (7 oz)	34	1	7	2	4
Caesar Grilled Chicken	1 (11.3 oz)	223	8	13	2	5
Crispy Chicken Club	1 (13.6 oz)	495	26	29	4	4
Mandarin Chicken	1 (14.5 oz)	553	31	62	19	14
Mixed Greens w/o Cheese	1 (17 oz)	194	14	17	9	7
Salad Blend	1 serv (10.3 oz)	45	1	9	4	5
Southwest Chicken Chop	1 (17.6 oz)	681	43	44	7	7
SAMURAI SAM'S						
BOWLS						
Low Carb	1 reg	230	4	16	9	5
Spicy Beef 'N Broccoli	1 reg	620	13	97	20	3
Spicy Beef 'N Broccoli Brown Rice	1 reg	580	14	85	19	7

FOOD	PORTION	CAL	FAT	CARB	SUGAR	FIBER
Sumo Brown Rice	1	1022	23	111	28	9
Sumo White Rice	1	1083	21	128	28	3
Sweet & Sour Dark Chicken	1 reg	610	10	96	24	6
Sweet & Sour Dark Chicken Brown Rice	1 reg	570	12	84	24	9
Sweet & Sour White Chicken	1 reg	580	5	96	24	6
Sweet & Sour White Chicken Brown Rice	1 reg	540	6	85	24	9
Teriyaki Dark Chicken	1 reg	540	10	79	13	2
Teriyaki Dark Chicken Brown Rice	1 reg	500	11	68	11	12
Teriyaki Dark Chicken & Shrimp	1 reg	492	6	78	12	2
Teriyaki Dark Chicken & Shrimp Brown Rice	1 reg	451	7	67	12	5
Teriyaki Dark Chicken & Steak	1 reg	540	9	83	13	2
Teriyaki Dark Chicken & Steak Brown Rice	1 reg	490	10	71	13	5
Teriyaki Salmon	1 reg	643	3	121	20	3
Teriyaki Shrimp Brown Rice	1 reg	407	3	65	10	5
Teriyaki Steak	1 reg	530	8	86	13	2
Teriyaki Steak Brown Rice	1 reg	490	9	74	13	5
Teriyaki Steak & Shrimp	1 reg	483	5	77	12	2
Teriyaki Steak & Shrimp Brown Rice	1 reg	442	6	66	12	5
Teriyaki Veggie	1 reg	363	1	81	13	3
Teriyaki Veggie Brown Rice	1 reg	323	2	69	13	7
Teriyaki White Chicken	1 reg	520	4	79	13	2

FOOD	PORTION	CAL	FAT	CARB	SUGAR	FIBER
Teriyaki White Chicken Brown Rice	1 reg	470	5	68	13	5
Teriyaki White Chicken & Shrimp	1 reg	478	2	78	12	2
Teriyaki White Chicken & Shrimp Brown Rice	1 reg	437	4	67	12	5
Teriyaki White Chicken & Steak	1 reg	520	6	83	13	2
Teriyaki White Chicken & Steak Brown Rice	1 reg	480	7	71	13	5
Yakisoba Dark Chicken	1	842	24	114	24	6
Yakisoba Dark Chicken & Steak	1	825	22	113	25	6
Yakisoba Shrimp	1	677	10	110	21	6
Yakisoba Steak	1	809	20	112	26	6
Yakisoba Veggie	1	509	8	110	21	6
Yakisoba White Chicken	1	794	14	114	25	6
Yakisoba White Chicken & Steak	1	801	17	113	25	6
SALADS AND SIDES						
Crab Rangoon	1 serv	210	12	20	12	1
Dressing Chinese	1 serv (3.5 oz)	230	7	44	43	–
Dressing Chinese Ginger	1 serv (1 oz)	85	5	9	9	0
Dressing Oriental	1 serv (1 oz)	70	2	12	12	0
Egg Roll Grilled Chicken	1	150	7	17	7	1
Salad Oriental Chicken	1 serv	220	4	9	5	3
Salad Side	1	10	1	2	1	1
Salad Toss Sesame Chicken	1	490	13	57	33	8
Soup Asian Noodle	1 serv	89	2	14	6	1
Teriyaki Sauce	1 serv (1 oz)	40	0	9	8	0
WRAPS						
Teriyaki Dark Chicken	1	670	16	95	13	8

FOOD	PORTION	CAL	FAT	CARB	SUGAR	FIBER
Teriyaki Dark Chicken Brown Rice	1	650	17	90	13	9
Teriyaki Steak	1	650	14	101	14	8
Teriyaki Steak Brown Rice	1	630	15	95	13	9
Teriyaki Veggie	1	510	8	94	12	8
Teriyaki Veggie Brown Rice	1	490	9	89	12	10
Teriyaki White Chicken	1	640	11	96	13	8
Teriyaki White Chicken Brown Rice	1	620	12	90	13	9
Teriyaki White Chicken & Steak	1	649	13	95	13	8
Teriyaki White Chicken & Steak Brown Rice	1	628	13	89	13	9

SCHLOTZSKY'S DELI
CHILDREN'S MENU SELECTIONS

FOOD	PORTION	CAL	FAT	CARB	SUGAR	FIBER
Pizza Cheese	1 serv	479	13	73	3	3
Pizza Pepperoni	1 serv	523	17	73	3	3
Sandwich Cheese	1	394	15	48	2	2
Sandwich Ham & Cheese	1	424	16	49	3	2
Sandwich Turkey	1	300	5	49	2	2

DESSERTS

FOOD	PORTION	CAL	FAT	CARB	SUGAR	FIBER
Carrot Cake	1 serv	717	42	80	56	3
Cookie Chocolate Chip	1	160	8	22	13	1
Cookie Fudge Chocolate Chip	1	160	8	22	14	1
Cookie Oatmeal Raisin	1	150	6	22	14	1
Cookie Sugar	1	160	7	22	11	0
Cookie White Chocolate Macadamia	1	170	9	21	13	1

MAIN MENU SELECTIONS

FOOD	PORTION	CAL	FAT	CARB	SUGAR	FIBER
Salad Caesar	1 serv	103	5	10	3	3

FOOD	PORTION	CAL	FAT	CARB	SUGAR	FIBER
Salad Garden	1 serv	51	1	12	4	4
Salad Grilled Chicken Caesar	1 serv	221	8	12	3	3
Salad Turkey Chef	1 serv	309	18	14	6	4
Sandwich Angus Roast Beef & Cheese	1 sm	534	22	50	3	2
Sandwich Chicken Breast	1 sm	342	4	52	6	3
Sandwich Fresh Veggie	1 sm	342	10	50	6	4
Sandwich Ham & Cheese	1 sm	508	19	54	5	3
Sandwich Smoked Turkey Breast	1 sm	353	6	52	4	2
Sandwich The Original	1 sm	559	26	52	4	3
Sandwich Turkey	1 sm	602	27	54	5	3
Sandwich Turkey Bacon Club	1 sm	561	25	51	4	3
Wraps Asian Chicken	1	537	12	80	26	5
Wraps Parmesan Chicken Caesar	1	556	21	61	5	5

SONIC DRIVE-IN
ADD-ONS

FOOD	PORTION	CAL	FAT	CARB	SUGAR	FIBER
Bacon	1 serv (0.5 oz)	70	5	0	0	0
Cheese	1 serv (0.7 oz)	60	5	2	1	0
Chili	1 serv (1.2 oz)	50	4	2	1	1
Green Chilies	1 serv (1 oz)	5	0	1	0	0
Grilled Onions	1 serv (1 oz)	25	2	2	1	1
Jalapenos	1 serv (0.7 oz)	5	0	1	0	1
Slaw	1 serv (1 oz)	45	3	4	1	1

BEVERAGES

FOOD	PORTION	CAL	FAT	CARB	SUGAR	FIBER
Barqs Root Beer	1 sm (14 oz)	160	0	43	43	0
Coca Cola	1 sm (14 oz)	140	0	39	39	0
Cream Pie Shake Banana	1 reg (14 oz)	590	19	98	83	1

FOOD	PORTION	CAL	FAT	CARB	SUGAR	FIBER
Cream Pie Shake Chocolate	1 reg (14 oz)	660	19	114	96	0
Cream Pie Shake Coconut Cream	1 reg (14 oz)	580	20	93	82	0
CreamSlush Blue Coconut	1 reg (14 oz)	430	13	76	69	0
CreamSlush Cherry	1 reg (14 oz)	440	13	77	71	0
CreamSlush Grape	1 reg (14 oz)	430	13	76	70	0
CreamSlush Orange	1 reg (14 oz)	430	13	77	70	0
CreamSlush Strawberry	1 reg (14 oz)	450	12	84	72	1
CreamSlush Watermelon	1 reg (14 oz)	440	13	77	70	0
Diet Coke	1 sm (14 oz)	0	0	0	0	0
Dr Pepper	1 sm (14 oz)	130	0	37	37	0
Float Barq's Root Beer	1 reg (14 oz)	300	8	56	52	0
Float Coca Cola	1 reg (14 oz)	290	8	54	50	0
Float Dr Pepper	1 reg (14 oz)	310	8	58	54	0
Limeade	1 sm (14 oz)	140	0	38	37	0
Limeade Cherry	1 sm (14 oz)	170	0	45	44	0
Limeade Strawberry	1 sm (14 oz)	170	0	45	41	0
Malt Banana	1 reg (14 oz)	490	17	78	65	1
Malt Caramel	1 reg (14 oz)	550	18	90	78	0
Malt Chocolate	1 reg (14 oz)	550	17	91	76	0
Malt Hot Fudge	1 reg (14 oz)	580	22	87	73	1
Malt Peanut Butter	1 reg (14 oz)	870	36	78	65	0
Malt Peanut Butter Fudge	1 reg (14 oz)	620	29	83	69	1
Malt Pineapple	1 reg (14 oz)	510	17	82	68	0
Malt Strawberry	1 reg (14 oz)	520	17	85	71	1
Malt Vanilla	1 reg (14 oz)	480	18	72	64	0
Milk 1%	8.5 oz	110	3	13	12	0
Milk Chocolate 1%	8.5 oz	160	3	27	25	0
Shake Banana	1 reg (14 oz)	470	16	76	63	1
Shake Chocolate	1 reg (14 oz)	540	16	89	74	0

FOOD	PORTION	CAL	FAT	CARB	SUGAR	FIBER
Shake Hot Fudge	1 reg (14 oz)	570	21	85	71	1
Shake Peanut Butter	1 reg (14 oz)	640	34	75	63	0
Shake Peanut Butter Fudge	1 reg	610	28	81	68	1
Shake Pineapple	1 reg (14 oz)	500	16	80	66	0
Shake Strawberry	1 reg (14 oz)	510	16	83	69	1
Shake Vanilla	1 reg (14 oz)	470	17	71	62	0
Sonic Blast Butterfinger	1 reg (14 oz)	580	22	88	72	0
Sonic Blast M&M's	1 reg (14 oz)	600	24	88	78	1
Sonic Blast Oreo	1 reg (14 oz)	540	21	80	67	1
Sonic Blast Reese's Peanut Butter Cup	1 reg (14 oz)	560	19	89	74	1
Sprite	1 sm (14 oz)	104	0	37	37	0
Sprite Zero	1 sm (14 oz)	5	0	0	0	0
BREAKFAST SELECTIONS						
Breakfast Burrito Jr.	1 (4.1 oz)	330	21	25	1	2
Breakfast Burrito Sausage Egg Cheese	1 (5.9 oz)	480	31	38	2	1
Breakfast Toaster Bacon Egg Cheese	1 (5.6 oz)	530	32	40	7	2
Breakfast Toaster Ham Egg Cheese	1 (6.5 oz)	490	26	40	6	2
Breakfast Toaster Sausage Egg Cheese	1 (6.8 oz)	620	42	40	6	2
CroisSonic Bacon	1 (5.3 oz)	510	36	29	5	0
CroisSonic Sausage	1 (6.2 oz)	600	46	29	5	0
DESSERTS						
Apple Slice w/ Fat Free Caramel Dipping Sauce	1 serv (3.4 oz)	120	0	27	23	2
Apple Slices	1 serv (2.4 oz)	35	0	9	7	2
Banana Split	1 (10.8 oz)	420	9	80	57	2
Cone Vanilla	1 (4.7 oz)	180	6	30	22	0
Dish Vanilla	1 (6.5 oz)	240	9	36	32	0

FOOD	PORTION	CAL	FAT	CARB	SUGAR	FIBER
Sundae Chocolate	1 (8.9 oz)	410	13	67	55	0
Sundae Hot Fudge	1 (8.9 oz)	440	18	63	52	1
Sundae Pineapple	1 (8.8 oz)	370	13	58	47	0
Sundae Strawberry	1 (8.8 oz)	380	13	61	49	1
MAIN MENU SELECTIONS						
California Cheeseburger	1 (9.3 oz)	690	39	57	13	5
Ched 'R' Bites	12 (3 oz)	280	15	22	0	1
Ched'R'Peppers	4 (4.2 oz)	330	17	36	2	2
Chicken Strip Dinner	1 serv (13.5 oz)	930	43	100	7	7
Chicken Strips	2 (2.5 oz)	200	11	10	0	1
Chili Cheeseburger	1 (7.9 oz)	660	35	56	11	5
Coney Extra Long Chili Cheese	1 (9 oz)	660	39	55	7	4
Coney Regular	1 (5.2 oz)	390	23	32	4	2
Corn Dog	1 (2.6 oz)	210	11	23	4	2
Crispy Chicken Bacon Ranch	1 serv (8.9 oz)	610	34	48	10	4
French Fries	1 sm (2.5 oz)	200	8	30	0	2
French Fries w/ Cheese	1 sm (3 oz)	270	13	32	1	2
French Fries w/ Chili & Cheese	1 sm (4.1 oz)	300	16	33	1	3
Fritos Chili Pie	1 med (4.8 oz)	470	32	36	1	3
Green Chili Cheeseburger	1 (10 oz)	630	31	56	12	5
Grilled Chicken Bacon Ranch	1 serv (8.9 oz)	470	22	35	10	3
Hickory Cheeseburger	1 (8.3 oz)	640	31	61	17	5
Jalapeno Burger	1 (7.6 oz)	550	26	53	10	5
Jalapeno Cheeseburger	1 (8.3 oz)	620	31	54	11	5
Jr. Bacon Cheeseburger	1 (5 oz)	410	23	31	8	3
Jr. Burger	1 (4.1 oz)	310	15	30	7	3
Jr. Burger Deluxe	1 (4.7 oz)	350	20	28	4	3

FOOD	PORTION	CAL	FAT	CARB	SUGAR	FIBER
Jr. Double Cheeseburger	1 (6.7 oz)	570	35	33	9	3
Jumbo Popcorn Chicken	1 sm (4 oz)	380	22	27	1	3
Mozzarella Sticks	1 serv (5 oz)	440	22	40	1	2
Onion Rings Onion Rings	1 med (5.5 oz)	440	21	55	14	3
Pickle-O's	1 serv (4 oz)	310	16	36	2	2
Sandwich Breaded Pork Fritter	1 (8.5 oz)	640	33	66	11	7
Sandwich Crispy Chicken	1 (7.9 oz)	550	32	46	8	4
Sandwich Fish	1 (8.6 oz)	650	31	71	12	7
Sandwich Grilled Cheese	1 (3.9 oz)	380	20	39	6	2
Sandwich Grilled Chicken	1 (7.8 oz)	400	19	32	8	3
Sonic Bacon Cheeseburger w/ Mayonnaise	1 (9.8 oz)	780	48	57	12	5
Sonic Burger w/ Ketchup	1 (8.7 oz)	560	26	57	14	5
Sonic Burger w/ Mayonnaise	1 (8.7 oz)	650	37	55	11	5
Sonic Burger w/ Mustard	1 (8.5 oz)	560	26	54	11	5
Sonic Cheeseburger w/ Ketchup	1 (9.3 oz)	630	31	59	15	5
Sonic Cheeseburger w/ Mayonnaise	1 (9.3 oz)	720	42	56	12	5
Sonic Cheeseburger w/ Mustard	1 (9.1 oz)	620	31	55	12	5
SuperSonic Cheeseburger w/ Ketchup	1 (12 oz)	900	53	60	16	5
SuperSonic Cheeseburger w/ Mayonnaise	1 (12 oz)	980	64	58	13	5

FOOD	PORTION	CAL	FAT	CARB	SUGAR	FIBER
SuperSonic Cheeseburger w/ Mustard	1 (11.8 oz)	890	53	57	13	5
Thousand Island Burger	1 (8.7 oz)	610	32	56	13	5
Toaster Sandwich Bacon Cheeseburger	1 (8.5 oz)	670	39	52	13	3
Toaster Sandwich BLT	1 (5.2 oz)	500	29	45	7	2
Toaster Sandwich Chicken Club	1 (9 oz)	740	46	55	7	4
Toaster Sandwich Country Fried Steak	1 (8.5 oz)	670	37	71	6	4
Tots	1 sm (1.5 oz)	130	8	13	0	1
Tots w/ Cheese	1 sm (2.2 oz)	190	13	14	1	1
Tots w/ Chili & Cheese	1 sm (3.2 oz)	220	16	16	1	2
Wrap Crispy Chicken	1 (8.2 oz)	490	23	49	5	3
Wrap Fritos Chili Cheese	1 (8.5 oz)	670	39	66	3	4
Wrap Grilled Chicken	1 (8.8 oz)	390	14	39	5	2
SALAD DRESSINGS AND SAUCES						
Dressing Honey Mustard	1 serv (1.5 oz)	180	16	10	8	0
Dressing Italian Fat Free	1 serv (1.5 oz)	40	0	10	3	0
Dressing Original Ranch	1 serv (1.5 oz)	190	20	2	1	0
Dressing Original Ranch Light	1 serv (1.5 oz)	110	5	14	3	0
Dressing Thousand Island	1 serv (1.5 oz)	190	19	7	5	0
Sauce BBQ	1 serv (1 oz)	45	0	11	7	0
Sauce Honey Mustard	1 serv (1 oz)	90	7	7	5	0
Sauce Marinara	1 serv (1 oz)	15	0	3	2	1
Sauce Ranch	1 serv (1 oz)	140	16	1	1	0
SALADS						
Crispy Chicken	1 serv (11.4 oz)	340	19	24	6	5
Grilled Chicken	1 serv (12 oz)	250	10	12	6	3

FOOD	PORTION	CAL	FAT	CARB	SUGAR	FIBER
SOUPER SALAD						
BEVERAGES						
Lemonade	1 (24 oz)	190	0	49	46	0
Lemonade Mango	1 (24 oz)	220	0	58	55	0
Lemonade Raspberry	1 (24 oz)	220	0	58	54	0
Lemonade Strawberry	1 (24 oz)	220	0	57	53	0
Smoothie Mango	1 tall	250	0	64	62	0
Smoothie Peach	1 tall	230	0	62	60	0
Smoothie Raspberry	1 tall	230	0	62	58	0
Smoothie Strawberry	1 tall	230	0	60	55	0
DESSERTS						
Blueberry Bread	1 piece	150	3	29	13	1
Brownies	2 pieces	120	5	21	14	0
Cornbread	1 piece	170	5	30	9	1
Cottage Cheese	½ cup	90	2	5	4	0
Gingerbread	1 piece	180	6	30	14	1
Peaches	½ cup	70	0	17	13	0
Pineapple Tidbits	¼ cup	60	0	15	13	1
Pudding Banana	½ cup	160	6	26	19	0
Pudding Chocolate	½ cup	170	5	30	23	0
Soft Serve Cone Chocolate	1	120	2	22	16	0
Soft Serve Cone Vanilla	1	120	3	22	14	0
Sponge Cake	4 pieces	80	2	14	8	0
Strawberry Parfait	½ cup	100	2	19	18	0
Vanilla Wafers	4	70	2	13	6	0
Whipped Topping	½ cup	100	8	8	8	0
PASTA AND PIZZA						
Chicken Alfredo	1 cup	320	9	40	3	1
Macaroni & Cheese	1 cup	380	18	38	2	1
Pizza Slice Cheese	1	70	3	8	1	0
Pizza Slice Garden	1	80	3	9	1	1
Pizza Slice Pepperoni	1	90	4	8	1	0
Pizza Slice Sausage	1	80	4	9	1	1
Spaghetti & Meatballs	1 cup	280	9	38	2	4

FOOD	PORTION	CAL	FAT	CARB	SUGAR	FIBER
SALAD DRESSINGS AND SAUCES						
Balsamic Vinegar	1 oz	60	0	15	15	0
Bleu Cheese	2 oz	220	23	1	1	0
Caesar	2 oz	280	30	4	4	0
Chipotle Ranch	2 oz	280	28	8	4	0
Fat Free French	2 oz	60	0	18	10	1
Fat Free Italian w/ Cheese	2 oz	30	0	6	4	0
Green Goddess	2 oz	260	24	4	4	0
Honey Mustard	2 oz	240	26	2	1	0
Mayonnaise	2 tbsp	200	22	20	0	0
Olive Oil	1 oz	240	28	0	0	0
Peppercorn Ranch	2 oz	220	23	2	2	0
Pesto Basil	1 tbsp	45	5	0	0	0
Ranch	2 oz	220	23	2	2	0
Reduced Calorie Ranch	2 oz	120	11	3	2	0
Sauce Alfredo	1 ½ tbsp	45	4	2	1	0
Sauce Chipotle Pepper	¼ tsp	0	0	0	0	0
Sauce Cholula Hot	¼ tsp	0	0	0	0	0
Sauce Jalapeno Cheese	1 serv (2 oz)	35	2	5	0	1
Sauce Marinara	1 ½ tbsp	10	0	2	1	0
Sauce Meaty Marinara	1 ½ tbsp	40	1	2	1	0
Sauce Sriracha Hot	¼ tsp	0	0	0	0	0
Sour Cream Light	2 tbsp	40	3	3	2	0
Tangy Oriental	2 oz	160	12	10	8	0
Thousand Island	1 oz	300	30	6	4	0
Vinaigrette Cranberry	2 oz	100	0	24	20	0
Vinaigrette House	2 oz	220	22	4	4	0
SALADS						
Apple Walnut	1 cup	130	11	7	5	1
Asian Chicken	1 cup	80	3	10	7	2
Asian Shrimp	1 cup	100	4	13	7	2
Buffalo Chicken	1 cup	70	6	3	2	1
Caesar Chicken	1 cup	90	7	4	1	1

FOOD	PORTION	CAL	FAT	CARB	SUGAR	FIBER
Caesar Chicken Salsa	1 cup	80	5	4	1	1
Caesar Shrimp	1 cup	90	7	3	1	1
California Chicken Salad	1/3 cup	80	6	4	3	0
Capri	1 cup	50	2	8	3	0
Chicago Chopped	1 cup	120	10	3	2	1
Chickpea	1/3 cup	110	6	11	1	4
Cobb	1 cup	100	8	2	2	1
Coleslaw Broccoli	1/3 cup	80	6	6	4	1
Edamame	1/3 cup	70	5	4	2	2
Fisherman's Kettle Shrimp & Crab	1/3 cup	120	8	15	9	1
Gazpacho	1/3 cup	30	3	3	2	1
Green Goddess Crab	1 cup	70	5	4	2	1
Italian Antipasto	1 cup	70	5	3	2	1
Mango Berry	1 cup	110	6	13	11	1
Marinated Mushrooms	1/3 cup	60	7	1	0	0
Marinated Oriental Cucumber	1/3 cup	10	0	2	1	0
Marinated Tomato	1 cup	60	2	11	10	1
Melon Couscous	1/3 cup	50	1	10	4	1
Mustard Potato	1/3 cup	80	5	7	1	1
Paco's Taco	1/3 cup	100	5	12	1	2
Pasta De Garden	1/3 cup	80	5	8	1	0
Pasta Fettuccine	1/3 cup	100	5	11	1	1
Pasta Primavera	1/3 cup	45	3	4	1	0
Pasta Thai Chicken	1/3 cup	100	5	11	2	1
Pasta Tuna Skroodle	1/3 cup	130	9	10	1	1
Red Potato	1/3 cup	50	4	5	1	1
Rice Florentine	1/3 cup	90	5	11	0	0
Roasted Mushrooms & Artichokes w/ Feta Cheese	1/3 cup	40	3	3	1	1
Roasted Vegetables	1/3 cup	20	2	2	1	1
Salad Of The Sea	1/3 cup	50	2	6	1	0

FOOD	PORTION	CAL	FAT	CARB	SUGAR	FIBER
Salmon Medley	1 cup	70	2	10	8	1
Santa Fe Corn	⅓ cup	100	4	13	2	3
Shrimp & Crab Louie	1 cup	130	10	5	2	1
Southwest Chicken Chipotle	1 cup	90	7	4	2	1
Sweet Garden Slaw	⅓ cup	35	2	4	3	1
Tropical Tuxedo	⅓ cup	60	3	7	2	0
Tuna Fish	⅓ cup	70	5	1	1	0
SOUPS						
Adobe Rice & Chicken	1 (5 oz)	100	5	10	2	1
Alaskan Salmon Chowder	1 (5 oz)	70	2	9	1	1
Beef Mushroom Barley	1 (5 oz)	80	2	11	1	2
Beef Noodle	1 (5 oz)	80	3	10	2	1
Beef Shellini	1 (5 oz)	90	3	11	3	1
Beef Stroganoff	1 (5 oz)	120	5	13	2	1
Black Bean	1 (5 oz)	80	2	20	2	11
Broccoli Cheese	1 (5 oz)	70	2	10	2	1
Cajun Gumbo	1 (5 oz)	110	4	13	1	1
Cauliflower Cheese	1 (5 oz)	70	2	11	2	1
Cheddar Chicken Broccoli Stew	1 (5 oz)	140	6	15	3	2
Cherokee Joe Cornbread	1 (5 oz)	70	2	13	5	2
Chicken Creole	1 (5 oz)	100	4	12	3	1
Chicken Enchilada	1 (5 oz)	180	12	13	3	1
Chicken Gumbo	1 (5 oz)	90	4	10	2	1
Chicken Mushroom Barley	1 (5 oz)	80	3	9	2	1
Chicken Noodle	1 (5 oz)	80	3	9	2	1
Chicken Tetrazini	1 (5 oz)	120	5	13	2	1
Chicken Tortilla	1 (5 oz)	60	2	7	2	1
Cream Of Asparagus	1 (5 oz)	140	10	7	3	1
Cream Of Broccoli	1 (5 oz)	60	2	9	2	1
Cream Of Cauliflower	1 (5 oz)	60	2	10	2	1

FOOD	PORTION	CAL	FAT	CARB	SUGAR	FIBER
Cream Of Chicken	1 (5 oz)	100	5	9	2	1
Cream Of Mushroom	1 (5 oz)	80	4	10	1	1
Holiday Harvest	1 (5 oz)	90	6	5	1	0
Vegan Split Pea	1 (5 oz)	90	1	16	2	5
Vegetable Beef	1 (5 oz)	80	3	11	3	2
Vegetable Cheese	1 (5 oz)	80	3	12	2	1
Vegetable Lentil	1 (5 oz)	70	0	16	2	5
Vegetarian Butter Bean	1 (5 oz)	70	0	21	2	10
Vegetarian Vegetable	1 (5 oz)	50	1	11	2	2

STARBUCKS
BAKED SELECTIONS

FOOD	PORTION	CAL	FAT	CARB	SUGAR	FIBER
Apple Fritter	1	480	22	64	27	1
Bagel French Toast	1	280	1	62	10	2
Bagel Multigrain	1	280	3	60	12	4
Bagel Plain	1	280	0	62	8	2
Bar Cranberry Bliss	1	320	16	41	28	1
Bar Toffee Almond	1	400	19	53	34	1
Brownie Espresso	1	340	19	40	27	2
Cinnamon Roll	1	470	26	56	29	1
Cocoa Crispy Square	1	420	17	66	30	1
Cookie Chocolate Chunk	1	420	20	56	28	6
Cookie Coffee Ginger	1	470	18	70	40	3
Cookie Penguin	1	370	18	50	31	tr
Cookie Rainbow	1	420	19	61	33	1
Cookies Mini Black & White	2	240	12	32	22	1
Croissant Butter	1	370	23	35	4	3
Dougnut Glazed	1	490	23	65	39	1
Loaf Banana Nut	1 serv	470	24	56	32	2
Loaf Iced Lemon	1 serv	500	18	78	53	1
Loaf Marble	1 serv	410	22	52	31	tr
Loaf Pumpkin	1 serv	380	14	59	36	2
Mallorca Sweet Bread	1	420	24	43	14	2

FOOD	PORTION	CAL	FAT	CARB	SUGAR	FIBER
Muffin Blueberry	1	310	11	55	31	1
Muffin Pumpkin Cream Cheese	1	490	24	63	42	1
Muffin Reduced Fat Chocolate	1	290	5	53	31	2
Muffin Walnut Bran	1	430	18	62	26	4
Reduced Fat Coffee Cake Banana Chocolate Chip	1	390	8	76	50	3
Reduced Fat Coffee Cake Blueberry	1 serv	320	6	54	33	1
Reduced Fat Coffee Cake Cinnamon Swirl	1 serv	290	4	52	33	1
Reduced Fat Coffee Cake Pumpkin Chocolate Chip	1	300	6	58	36	3
Rustic Apple Tart	1	190	5	37	30	3
Scone Blueberry	1	480	22	64	24	2
Scone Cran Apple Crumb	1	490	20	74	30	4
Scone Raspberry	1	470	21	64	25	2
BEVERAGES						
Apple Juice	1 grande	250	0	64	57	0
Cafe Americano	1 grande	15	0	3	0	0
Cafe Au Lait Nonfat Milk	1 grande	70	0	10	10	0
Caffe Mocha No Whip Nonfat Milk	1 grande	220	3	42	32	2
Caffe Mocha Whip Nonfat Milk	1 grande	290	10	44	34	2
Cappuccino Nonfat Milk	1 grande	80	0	12	10	0
Caramel Apple Cider Whipe	1 grande	380	8	76	68	0
Caramel Apple Spice No Whip	1 grande	310	tr	74	66	0
Caramel Macchiato Nonfat Milk	1 grande	190	1	35	32	0

FOOD	PORTION	CAL	FAT	CARB	SUGAR	FIBER
Chocolate Milk Nonfat	1 grande	280	3	53	45	2
Cinnamon Dolce Creme No Whip Nonfat Milk	1 grande	220	0	41	41	0
Cinnamon Dolce Whip Nonfat Milk	1 grande	290	7	43	43	0
Coffee Of The Week	1 grande	5	tr	0	0	0
Coffee Of The Week Decafe	1 grande	5	0	0	0	0
Frappaccino Light Blended Creme White Chocolate No Whip Nonfat Milk	1 grande	480	7	89	77	0
Frappuccino Blended Coffee Cafe Vanilla Whip Nonfat Milk	1 grande	430	14	70	60	0
Frappuccino Blended Coffee Cafe Vanilla Whip Soy	1 grande	430	14	70	60	0
Frappuccino Blended Coffee Cafe Vanilla No Whip Soy	1 grande	310	3	67	58	0
Frappuccino Blended Coffee Caffe Vanilla No Whip Nonfat Milk	1 grande	310	3	67	58	0
Frappuccino Blended Coffee Caramel No Whip Nonfat Milk	1 grande	270	4	53	45	0
Frappuccino Blended Coffee Caramel No Whip Soy	1 grande	270	4	53	45	0
Frappuccino Blended Coffee Caramel Whip Soy	1 grande	380	15	57	48	0

FOOD	PORTION	CAL	FAT	CARB	SUGAR	FIBER
Frappuccino Blended Coffee Cinnamon Dolce No Whip Nonfat Milk	1 grande	260	3	52	45	0
Frappuccino Blended Coffee Cinnamon Dolce No Whip Soy	1 grande	260	3	52	45	0
Frappuccino Blended Coffee Cinnamon Dolce Whip Soy	1 grande	370	14	55	47	0
Frappuccino Blended Coffee Espresso Nonfat Milk	1 grande	190	3	38	31	0
Frappuccino Blended Coffee Java Chip No Whip Nonfat Milk	1 grande	340	8	64	52	2
Frappuccino Blended Coffee Java Chip No Whip Soy	1 grande	190	3	38	31	0
Frappuccino Blended Coffee Java Chip Whip Nonfat Milk	1 grande	460	19	67	55	2
Frappuccino Blended Coffee Java Chip Whip Soy	1 grande	460	19	67	55	2
Frappuccino Blended Coffee Mocha No Whip Nonfat Milk	1 grande	260	4	54	45	0
Frappuccino Blended Coffee Mocha No Whip Soy	1 grande	260	4	54	45	0

FOOD	PORTION	CAL	FAT	CARB	SUGAR	FIBER
Frappuccino Blended Coffee Mocha Whip Nonfat Milk	1 grande	380	15	57	47	0
Frappuccino Blended Coffee Pumpkin Spice No Whip Nonfat Milk	1 grande	290	4	59	51	0
Frappuccino Blended Coffee Pumpkin Spice No Whip Soy	1 grande	290	4	59	51	0
Frappuccino Blended Coffee Pumpkin Spice Whip Nonfat Milk	1 grande	400	15	62	53	0
Frappuccino Blended Coffee Pumpkin Spice Whip Soy	1 grande	400	15	62	53	0
Frappuccino Blended Coffee Whip Nonfat Milk	1 grande	370	14	55	47	0
Frappuccino Blended Coffee White Chocolate Mocha No Whip Nonfat Milk	1 grande	300	5	59	51	0
Frappuccino Blended Coffee White Chocolate Mocha No Whip Soy	1 grande	300	5	59	51	0
Frappuccino Blended Coffee White Chocolate Mocha Whip Nonfat Milk	1 grande	410	16	62	54	0
Frappuccino Blended Coffee White Chocolate Mocha Whip Soy	1 grande	410	16	62	54	0
Frappuccino Blended Creme Tazo Chai No Whip Nonfat Milk	1 grande	330	2	67	56	0

FOOD	PORTION	CAL	FAT	CARB	SUGAR	FIBER
Frappuccino Blended Creme Tazo Chai Whip Nonfat Milk	1 grande	570	15	95	83	1
Frappuccino Blended Creme Vanilla Bean No Whip Nonfat Milk	1 grande	350	3	72	60	0
Frappuccino Blended Creme Vanilla Bean Whip Nonfat Milk	1 grande	470	14	75	62	0
Frappuccino Light Blended Coffee Cafe Vanilla Nonfat Milk	1 grande	190	1	42	32	3
Frappuccino Light Blended Coffee Caramel	1 grande	160	2	30	21	3
Frappuccino Light Blended Coffee Cinnamon Dolce Nonfat Milk	1 grande	140	1	29	21	3
Frappuccino Light Blended Coffee Java Chip Nonfat Milk	1 grande	200	5	36	24	4
Frappuccino Light Blended Coffee Mocha Nonfat Milk	1 grande	140	1	29	19	3
Frappuccino Light Blended Coffee Nonfat Milk	1 grande	130	1	25	16	3
Frappuccino Light Blended Coffee Pumpkin Spice Nonfat Milk	1 grande	150	1	31	22	3

FOOD	PORTION	CAL	FAT	CARB	SUGAR	FIBER
Frappuccino Light Blended Creme Double Chocolaty Chip Whip Nonfat Milk	1 grande	510	19	78	59	2
Frappuccino Light Blended Creme Pumpkin Spice No Whip Nonfat Milk	1 grande	360	3	71	61	0
Frappuccino Light Blended Creme Pumpkin Spice Whip Nonfat Milk	1 grande	470	13	74	63	0
Frappuccino Light Blended Creme Tazo Green Tea No Whip Nonfat Milk	1 grande	380	3	78	67	1
Frappuccino Light Blended Creme Tazo Green Tea Whip Nonfat Milk	1 grande	440	13	71	59	0
Frappuccino Light Blended Creme Tazo Green Tea Whip Nonfat Milk	1 grande	490	14	82	69	1
Frappuccino Light Blended Creme White Chocolate Whip Nonfat Milk	1 grande	610	19	92	79	0
Frappuccino Light Espresso Nonfat Milk	1 grande	110	1	20	12	2
Hot Chocolate No Whip Nonfat Milk	1 grande	240	3	48	40	2
Hot Chocolate Whip Nonfat Milk	1 grande	320	10	50	41	2

FOOD	PORTION	CAL	FAT	CARB	SUGAR	FIBER
Iced Brewed Coffee	1 grande	90	0	21	20	0
Iced Cafe Mocha Whip Nonfat Milk	1 grande	290	14	39	29	2
Iced Caffe Americano	1 grande	15	0	3	0	0
Iced Caffe Latte Nonfat Milk	1 grande	90	0	13	11	0
Iced Caffe Mocha No Whip Nonfat Milk	1 grande	170	3	36	26	2
Iced Caramel Macchiato Nonfat Milk	1 grande	190	2	34	31	0
Iced Latte Pumpkin Spice No Whip Nonfat Milk	1 grande	220	0	44	42	0
Iced Latte Pumpkin Spice Whip Nonfat Milk	1 grande	330	11	48	44	0
Iced Latte Skinny Cinnamon Dolce No Whip Nonfat Milk	1 grande	80	0	12	10	0
Iced Latte Sugar Free Flavored Syrup Nonfat Milk	1 grande	80	0	12	10	0
Iced Latte Syrup Flavored Nonfat Milk	1 grande	160	0	31	28	0
Iced Latte Vanilla Nonfat Milk	1 grande	160	0	31	28	0
Iced Peppermint White Chocolate Mocha No Whip Nonfat Milk	1 grande	370	6	72	68	0
Iced Peppermint White Chocolate Mocha Whip Nonfat Milk	1 grande	490	17	75	71	0
Iced Tazo Latte Black Tea Nonfat Milk	1 grande	170	0	35	34	0

FOOD	PORTION	CAL	FAT	CARB	SUGAR	FIBER
Iced Tazo Latte Black Tea Soy	1 grande	200	3	38	34	1
Iced Tazo Latte Chai Nonfat Milk	1 grande	200	0	44	42	0
Iced Tazo Latte Green Tea Nonfat Milk	1 grande	220	5	45	43	1
Iced Tazo Latte Green Tea Soy	1 grande	260	4	48	44	2
Iced Tazo Latte Red Tea	1 grande	200	3	38	34	1
Iced Tazo Latte Red Tea Nonfat Milk	1 grande	170	0	35	34	0
Iced White Chocolate Mocha No Whip Nonfat Milk	1 grande	310	6	55	52	0
Iced White Chocolate Mocha Whip Nonfat Milk	1 grande	430	17	59	55	0
Latte Caffe Nonfat Milk	1 grande	130	5	19	18	0
Latte Cinnamon Dolce No Whip Nonfat Milk	1 grande	210	0	41	39	0
Latte Cinnamon Dolce w/ Sugar Free Syrup Nonfat Milk	1 grande	130	0	19	17	0
Latte Cinnamon Dolce Whip Nonfat Milk	1 grande	280	7	43	40	0
Latte Pumpkin Spice No Whip Nonfat Milk	1 grande	260	0	50	48	0
Latte Pumpkin Spice Whip Nonfat Milk	1 grande	330	7	52	50	0
Latte Skinny Caramel No Whip Nonfat Milk	1 grande	130	0	19	17	0
Latte Skinny Cinnamon Dolce No Whip Nonfat Milk	1 grande	130	0	19	17	0

FOOD	PORTION	CAL	FAT	CARB	SUGAR	FIBER
Latte Skinny Hazelnut No Whip Nonfat Milk	1 grande	130	0	19	17	0
Latte Skinny Vanilla No Whip Nonfat Milk	1 grande	130	0	19	17	0
Latte Syrup Flavored Nonfat Milk	1 grande	200	0	37	35	0
Milk Nonfat	1 grande	180	0	26	26	0
Peppermint White Chocolate Mocha No Whip Nonfat Milk	1 grande	420	6	78	75	0
Peppermint White Chocolate Mocha Whip Nonfat Milk	1 grande	490	13	80	76	0
Pumpkin Spice Creme No Whip Nonfat Milk	1 grande	270	0	51	51	0
Pumpkin Spice Creme Whip Nonfat Milk	1 grande	340	7	53	52	0
Shaken Black Iced Tea & Lemonade	1 grande	130	0	33	33	0
Shaken White Iced Tea Blueberry	1 grande	80	0	21	20	0
Steamed Apple Juice	1 grande	230	0	56	50	0
Tazo Black Shaken Iced Tea & Lemonade	1 grande	130	0	33	33	0
Tazo Chai Latte Iced Tea Soy	1 grande	230	3	47	43	1
Tazo Chai Latte Nonfat Milk	1 grande	200	0	44	42	0
Tazo Chai Latte Soy	1 grande	230	3	47	42	1
Tazo Latte Black Tea Nonfat Milk	1 grande	170	0	34	32	0
Tazo Latte Black Tea Soy	1 grande	190	3	36	32	1
Tazo Latte Green Tea Nonfat Milk	1 grande	200	0	42	41	1

FOOD	PORTION	CAL	FAT	CARB	SUGAR	FIBER
Tazo Latte Green Tea Soy	1 grande	220	3	44	40	2
Tazo Latte Red Tea Nonfat Milk	1 grande	170	0	34	32	0
Tazo Latte Red Tea Soy	1 grande	190	3	36	32	1
Tazo Shaken Iced Tea Green	1 grande	80	0	21	20	0
Tazo Shaken Iced Tea Green & Lemonade	1 grande	130	0	33	33	0
Tazo Shaken Iced Tea Orange Passion	1 grande	70	0	19	18	0
Tazo Shaken Iced Tea Passion	1 grande	80	0	21	20	0
Tazo Shaken Iced Tea Passion & Lemonade	1 grande	130	0	33	33	0
Tazo Tea	1 grande	0	0	0	0	0
Vanilla Creme Whip Nonfat Milk	1 grande	270	7	39	38	0
Vanilla Creme No Whip Nonfat Milk	1 grande	200	0	37	37	0
Vivanno Blend Banana Chocolate	1 grande (20 oz)	270	2	44	28	6
Vivanno Blend Orange Mango Banana	1 grande (20 oz)	250	2	47	32	5
White Chocolate Mocha No Whip Nonfat Milk	1 grande	360	6	62	61	0
White Chocolate Mocha Whip Nonfat Milk	1 grande	430	13	64	62	0
SALADS						
Fiesta	1 (9.4 oz)	320	10	44	12	8
Fruit & Cheese Plate	1 (8.6 oz)	400	20	44	26	2
Vegetable Vinaigrette	1 (10.7 oz)	310	15	40	8	10

FOOD	PORTION	CAL	FAT	CARB	SUGAR	FIBER
SANDWICHES						
Club Chicken Cheddar Bacon w/ Mayo	1	480	18	48	8	2
Club Turkey & Avocado	1	390	19	33	5	7
Egg Salad On Multigrain	1	470	21	53	11	2
Turkey & Swiss w/ Mayo	1	310	13	26	3	2
TOPPINGS						
Caramel	1 tbsp	15	1	2	2	0
Chocolate	1 tsp	5	0	1	1	0
Flavored Sugar Free Syrup	1 pump	0	0	0	0	0
Flavored Syrup	1 pump	20	0	5	5	0
Mocha Syrup	1 pump	25	1	5	4	0
Sprinkles	1 serv	0	0	0	0	0
TACO BELL						
Border Bowl Southwest Steak	1 serv	600	24	68	3	9
Border Bowl Zesty Chicken	1 serv	640	35	60	4	10
Border Bowl Zesty Chicken w/o Dressing	1 serv	440	15	57	3	10
Burrito 7 Layer	1	490	18	65	5	9
Burrito Bean	1	350	9	54	4	8
Burrito Grilled Stuft Chicken	1	640	23	73	6	7
Burrito Supreme Beef	1	420	17	51	5	7
Burrito ½ Lb Beef & Potato	1	530	23	68	4	6
Burrito ½ Lb Combo Beef	1	440	18	51	4	8
Burrito Fiesta Chicken	1	360	10	47	4	3
Burrito Fiesta Steak	1	370	13	49	4	4

FOOD	PORTION	CAL	FAT	CARB	SUGAR	FIBER
Burrito Stuft Grilled Stuft Steak	1	630	25	72	5	7
Burrito Supreme Chicken	1	400	13	49	5	6
Burrito Supreme Steak	1	390	14	49	5	6
Chalupa Baja Beef	1	410	27	30	4	4
Chalupa Baja Chicken	1	390	23	29	4	3
Chalupa Baja Steak	1	390	24	28	3	3
Chalupa Nacho Cheese Beef	1	370	22	32	4	3
Chalupa Nacho Cheese Chicken	1	360	18	30	4	2
Chalupa Nacho Cheese Steak	1	340	19	30	4	2
Chalupa Supreme Beef	1	380	20	30	4	3
Chalupa Supreme Chicken	1	360	20	29	4	2
Chalupa Supreme Steak	1	360	21	28	4	2
Cheesy Fiesta Potatoes	1 serv	290	17	29	2	2
Cinnamon Twists	1 serv	170	7	26	12	1
Crunchwrap Supreme	1	560	24	68	7	5
Crunchwrap Supreme Spicy Chicken	1	540	24	67	7	4
Crunchy Taco	1	170	25	13	1	3
Crunchy Taco Supreme	1	210	10	15	2	3
Empanada Caramel Apple	1	290	14	37	13	1
Enchirito Beef	1	360	17	34	3	7
Enchirito Chicken	1	340	13	33	3	6
Fresco Border Bowl Zesty Chicken w/o Dressing	1 serv	350	8	51	4	10
Fresco Burrito Bean	1 (7.5 oz)	340	8	56	4	11

FOOD	PORTION	CAL	FAT	CARB	SUGAR	FIBER
Fresco Burrito Fiesta Chicken	1	330	8	48	4	3
Fresco Burrito Supreme Chicken	1 (8.5 oz)	340	8	50	4	8
Fresco Burrito Supreme Steak	1 (8.5 oz)	330	8	49	4	8
Fresco Crunchy Taco	1 (3.2 oz)	150	7	13	1	3
Fresco Soft Taco Beef	1 (4 oz)	180	7	22	2	3
Fresco Soft Taco Grilled Steak	1 (4.5 oz)	160	4	21	3	2
Fresco Soft Taco Ranchero Chicken	1 (4.7 oz)	170	4	22	3	2
Gordita Baja Beef	1	340	19	29	8	4
Gordita Baja Chicken	1	320	16	28	6	3
Gordita Baja Steak	1	320	17	27	5	3
Gordita Nacho Cheese Beef	1	300	14	31	6	3
Gordita Nacho Cheese Chicken	1	280	11	29	6	2
Gordita Nacho Cheese Steak	1	270	12	29	6	2
Gordita Supreme Beef	1	310	16	29	6	3
Gordita Supreme Chicken	1	290	12	28	6	2
Gordita Supreme Steak	1	290	13	28	6	2
Guacamole Side	1 serv	70	5	5	1	2
Mexican Pizza	1	530	30	46	3	6
Mexican Rice	1 serv	180	7	23	0	1
MexiMelt	1 serv	260	14	22	2	3
Nacho Supreme	1 serv	440	26	41	3	7
Nachos	1 serv	330	21	32	3	2
Nachos Bellgrande	1 serv	770	44	77	5	12
Pintos 'n Cheese	1 serv	160	6	19	1	7
Quesadilla Cheese	1	470	26	39	4	2

FOOD	PORTION	CAL	FAT	CARB	SUGAR	FIBER
Quesadilla Chicken	1	520	28	40	4	3
Quesadilla Steak	1	520	28	39	4	3
Salsa Side	1 serv	15	0	3	2	0
Soft Taco Grande	1	430	20	43	5	5
Soft Taco Grilled Steak	1	270	16	20	3	2
Soft Taco Ranchero Chicken	1	270	14	21	3	2
Soft Taco Supreme Beef	1	250	13	23	3	3
Taco Double Decker	1	320	13	38	2	6
Taco Double Decker Supreme	1	370	17	40	4	7
Taco Spicy Chicken	1	170	8	20	2	2
Taco Salad Express	1	610	32	56	8	14
Taco Salad Fiesta	1	840	45	80	10	15
Taco Salad Fiesta w/o Shell	1	470	24	41	9	13
Taco Salad Fiesta Chicken	1	790	38	77	10	13
Taco Salad Fiesta Chicken w/o Shell	1	430	18	38	9	11
Taquitos Chicken Grilled	1 serv	310	11	37	3	2
Taquitos Steak Grilled	1 serv	310	11	36	3	2
Tostada	1	240	10	27	2	7

TACO BUENO
MAIN MENU SELECTIONS

FOOD	PORTION	CAL	FAT	CARB	SUGAR	FIBER
Bueno Chilada Beef	1 (7.9 oz)	523	32	42	6	2
Bueno Chilada Beef w/o Chili	1 (5.5 oz)	412	26	29	6	1
Bueno Chilada Beef w/o Queso	1 (5.6 oz)	337	18	36	2	2
Bueno Chilada Chicken	1 (7.4 oz)	477	26	43	7	2
Bueno Chilada Chicken w/o Chili	1 (5 oz)	366	20	30	6	1

FOOD	PORTION	CAL	FAT	CARB	SUGAR	FIBER
Bueno Chilada Chicken w/o Queso	1 (5.1 oz)	290	12	30	2	2
Burrito Bean	1 (6.4 oz)	490	29	45	1	5
Burrito Bean w/o Cheddar Cheese	1 (5.9 oz)	412	23	44	1	5
Burrito Bean w/o Chili	1 (5.2 oz)	434	26	39	1	4
Burrito Beef	1 (6.9 oz)	510	29	41	1	3
Burrito Beef Potato	1 (4.8 oz)	350	21	32	3	3
Burrito Beef Potato w/o Queso	1 (4.1 oz)	305	17	30	1	3
Burrito Beef Potato w/o Sour Cream	1 (4.3 oz)	330	18	31	2	3
Burrito Beef w/o Cheddar Cheese	1 (6.4 oz)	432	22	40	1	3
Burrito Beef w/o Chili	1 (5.7 oz)	455	25	36	1	2
Burrito Big Ol' Beef	1 (10.6 oz)	772	46	57	2	3
Burrito Big Ol' Beef w/o Cheddar Cheese	1 (9.6 oz)	615	33	56	2	3
Burrito Big Ol' Beef w/o Chili	1 (9.4 oz)	716	43	51	2	2
Burrito Big Ol' Beef w/o Sour Cream	1 (9.6 oz)	715	40	55	1	3
Burrito Big Ol' Chicken	1 (8.4 oz)	607	30	53	3	5
Burrito Big Ol' Chicken w/o Cheddar Cheese	1 (7.4 oz)	450	17	52	3	2
Burrito Big Ol' Chicken w/o Sour Cream	1 (7.4 oz)	551	24	51	2	2
Burrito Chicken Potato	1 (4.5 oz)	327	18	33	3	3
Burrito Chicken Potato w/o Queso	1 (3.8 oz)	274	14	31	2	3
Burrito Chicken Potato w/o Sour Cream	1 (4 oz)	299	15	32	2	3
Burrito Combination	1 (6.8 oz)	507	29	43	1	4

FOOD	PORTION	CAL	FAT	CARB	SUGAR	FIBER
Burrito Combination w/o Cheddar Cheese	1 (6.3 oz)	429	23	42	1	4
Burrito Combination w/o Chili	1 (5.6 oz)	452	26	37	1	3
Burrito Combination w/o Refried Beans	1 (5.7 oz)	440	23	40	1	3
Burrito Party	1 (4 oz)	298	18	29	1	3
Burrito Party w/o Cheddar Cheese	1 (3.8 oz)	259	14	29	1	3
Chimichanger Cheesecake	1 (2 oz)	210	11	24	4	1
Cinnamon Chips	1 serv (4.5 oz)	676	31	95	54	4
Corn Tortilla Chips	1 serv (1.5 oz)	219	11	27	1	4
Guacamole	1 serv (0.9 oz)	55	5	2	0	1
Jalapenos	1 serv (0.7 oz)	3	0	1	0	1
Mexican Rice	1 serv (4.2 oz)	469	12	83	4	2
Muchaco Beef	1 (5.2 oz)	449	25	40	2	3
Muchaco Beef w/o Cheddar Cheese	1 (4.9 oz)	410	22	40	2	3
Muchaco Beef w/o Refried Beans	1 (4.2 oz)	392	20	38	2	2
Muchaco Chicken	1 (4.6 oz)	387	18	40	2	2
Muchaco Chicken w/o Cheddar Cheese	1 (4.4 oz)	348	14	39	2	2
Nachos Cheese	1 serv (5.5 oz)	572	35	47	8	6
Quesadilla Beef	1 (8.5 oz)	823	51	49	1	2
Quesadilla Cheese	1 (6.5 oz)	709	42	48	1	2
Quesadilla Chicken	1 (7.9 oz)	761	44	50	1	2
Quesadilla Kids Cheese	1 (2.2 oz)	219	11	23	1	1
Quesadilla Mini Cheese	1 (2.7)	274	15	23	1	1

FOOD	PORTION	CAL	FAT	CARB	SUGAR	FIBER
Refried Beans Powdered	1 serv (6.3 oz)	406	34	17	1	5
Refried Beans w/o Cheddar Cheese	1 serv (5.8 oz)	327	28	16	1	5
Refried Beans w/o Chili	1 serv (5.1 oz)	360	31	11	0	4
Salsa Red	1 serv (2 oz)	14	0	3	0	1
Soup Tortilla	1 bowl	237	11	19	3	2
Soup Tortilla w/o Tortilla Strips & Cheese	1 bowl	148	6	11	3	2
Sour Cream	1 serv (1 oz)	57	6	2	1	0
Taco Party	1 (1.9 oz)	143	10	5	0	0
Taco w/o Cheddar Cheese	1 (1.5 oz)	104	7	5	0	0
Taco Crispy Beef	1 (2.6 oz)	200	14	7	0	0
Taco Crispy Chicken	1 (1.9 oz)	140	7	8	1	0
Taco Crispy Chicken w/o Cheddar Cheese	1 (1.7 oz)	100	4	7	1	0
Taco Crispy w/o Cheddar Cheese	1 (2.4 oz)	161	11	6	0	0
Taco Soft Beef	1 (3.5 oz)	245	14	18	0	1
Taco Soft Beef w/o Cheddar Cheese	1 (3.2 oz)	206	11	17	0	1
Taco Soft Chicken	1 (2.9 oz)	184	8	19	1	1
Taco Soft Chicken w/o Cheddar Cheese	1 (2.5 oz)	145	5	18	1	1
Tostada	1 (4.1 oz)	324	24	18	1	3
Tostada w/o Cheddar Cheese	1 (3.3 oz)	207	15	17	1	3
Tostada w/o Chili	1 (2.9 oz)	269	21	12	0	3
Tostada w/o Refried Beans	1 (2.5 oz)	234	16	15	1	2
SALADS						
Nacho Beef	1 (9.3 oz)	759	48	58	6	8

FOOD	PORTION	CAL	FAT	CARB	SUGAR	FIBER
Nacho Beef w/o Cheddar Cheese	1 (8.8 oz)	681	42	57	6	8
Nacho Beef w/o Chili	1 (6.9 oz)	648	41	45	5	6
Nacho Chicken	1 (8.9 oz)	713	43	59	7	8
Nacho Chicken w/o Cheddar Cheese	1 (8.4 oz)	634	37	58	7	8
Nacho Chicken w/o Chili	1 (6.5 oz)	601	36	46	6	6
Taco Beef	1 (12.7 oz)	1043	75	58	2	12
Taco Beef w/o Cheddar Cheese	1 (11.7 oz)	886	62	56	2	12
Taco Beef w/o Chili	1 (11.5 oz)	987	72	51	2	12
Taco Beef w/o Guacamole	1 (11.7 oz)	988	70	56	2	11
Taco Beef w/o Sour Cream	1 (11.7 oz)	986	70	56	2	12
Taco Beef w/o Tortilla Bowl	1 (9.7 oz)	564	45	15	2	2
Taco Chicken	1 (9.6 oz)	838	57	53	3	12
Taco Chicken w/o Cheddar Cheese	1 (8.6 oz)	680	44	52	3	12
Taco Chicken w/o Guacamole	1 (8.6 oz)	783	52	51	3	11
Taco Chicken w/o Sour Cream	1 (8.6 oz)	781	51	51	2	12
Taco Chicken w/o Tortilla Bowl	1 (6.6 oz)	359	26	10	2	1

TACOTIME
DESSERTS

FOOD	PORTION	CAL	FAT	CARB	SUGAR	FIBER
Churro Plain	1 (1.5 oz)	205	15	16	4	0
Churro w/ Cinnamon & Sugar	1 (2 oz)	245	15	26	14	0
Crustos	1 serv	294	6	58	19	3
Empanada Apple	1 (4 oz)	234	7	40	10	2

FOOD	PORTION	CAL	FAT	CARB	SUGAR	FIBER
Empanada Cherry	1 (4 oz)	240	7	41	4	2
Empanada Pumpkin	1 (4 oz)	256	8	42	16	2
MAIN MENU SELECTIONS						
Burrito Big Juan Chicken	1 (13 oz)	594	19	68	5	10
Burrito Big Juan Seasoned Ground Beef	1 (13 oz)	651	28	71	6	12
Burrito Big Juan Shredded Beef	1 (13 oz)	633	25	67	5	10
Burrito Casita Chicken	1 (12 oz)	494	18	43	4	5
Burrito Casita Seasoned Ground Beef	1 (12 oz)	552	25	46	5	6
Burrito Casita Shredded Beef	1 (12 oz)	533	25	42	4	5
Burrito Chicken & Black Bean	1 (10 oz)	478	16	51	3	9
Burrito Chicken BLT	1 (10 oz)	721	41	44	4	8
Burrito Chicken Ranchero	1 (10.8 oz)	654	32	52	3	7
Burrito Crisp Chicken	1 (5.5 oz)	336	10	32	0	2
Burrito Crisp Meat	1 (5.8 oz)	450	22	36	1	4
Burrito Crisp Pinto Bean	1 (6 oz)	394	16	50	1	6
Burrito Soft Meat	1 (6.7 oz)	426	16	43	2	8
Burrito Soft Pinto Bean	1 (6.7 oz)	377	11	54	1	10
Burrito Veggie	1 (11 oz)	534	18	74	4	12
Cheddar Fries	1 sm (6 oz)	374	26	29	1	3
Cheddar Melt	1 (2.8 oz)	250	12	25	0	4
Mexi-Fries	1 sm (5 oz)	290	19	29	1	2
Mexi-Rice	1 serv (4 oz)	87	1	19	1	0
Nachos Grande	1 serv (16.5 oz)	1132	57	114	8	11
Refritos w/ Chips	1 serv (7 oz)	304	11	35	2	6
Refritos w/o Chips	1 serv (6.7 oz)	285	11	32	2	6
Stuffed Fries	1 sm (5 oz)	321	7	29	3	3

FOOD	PORTION	CAL	FAT	CARB	SUGAR	FIBER
Taco Crisp Seasoned Ground Beef	1 (4.3 oz)	225	12	12	1	2
Taco Super Soft Chicken	1 (11 oz)	540	18	56	3	10
Taco Super Soft Seasoned Ground Beef	1 (11 oz)	598	25	59	4	12
Taco Super Soft Shredded Beef	1 (11 oz)	579	25	55	3	10
Taco Value Soft	1 (5.3 oz)	314	13	28	2	6
Taco ½ Lb Shredded Beef	1 (9 oz)	440	18	42	3	7
Taco ½ Lb Soft Chicken	1 (9 oz)	401	11	43	3	7
Taco ½ Lb Soft Seasoned Ground Beef	1 (9 oz)	459	18	46	4	9
Taco Chips	1 serv (2 oz)	150	3	27	0	1
SALAD DRESSINGS AND TOPPINGS						
Cheddar Cheese	1 serv (2 oz)	223	18	1	0	0
Dressing Chipotle Ranch	1 serv (1 oz)	165	18	1	1	0
Dressing Ranch	1 serv (1 oz)	181	20	1	1	–
Dressing Thousand Island	1 serv (1 oz)	132	12	5	3	0
Guacamole	1 serv (1 oz)	50	5	2	1	1
Salsa Nuevo	1 serv (1 oz)	8	0	2	1	0
Salsa Verde	1 serv (1 oz)	6	0	2	0	0
Sour Cream	1 serv (1.5 oz)	85	7	1	1	0
SALADS						
Taco Chicken	1 reg (9.2 oz)	351	15	24	4	2
Taco Seasoned Ground Beef	1 reg (7.8 oz)	396	23	24	3	4
Taco Shredded Beef	1 reg (7.8 oz)	377	22	21	2	2
Tostada Delight Chicken	1 (10.5 oz)	565	29	36	3	4
Tostada Delight Seasoned Ground Beef	1 (10.5 oz)	623	36	39	4	6
Tostada Delight Shredded Beef	1 (10.5 oz)	604	36	35	3	5

FOOD	PORTION	CAL	FAT	CARB	SUGAR	FIBER
TCBY						
FROZEN YOGURT AND SORBET						
Hand Scooped Butter Pecan Perfection	½ cup	110	5	14	11	tr
Hand Scooped Chocolate Chocolate Swirl	½ cup	120	4	19	16	tr
Hand Scooped Chocolate Chunk Cookie Dough	½ cup	160	6	24	18	0
Hand Scooped Cookies & Cream	½ cup	140	4	22	17	0
Hand Scooped Cotton Candy	½ cup	120	4	20	16	0
Hand Scooped Mint Chocolate Chunk	½ cup	140	5	22	18	0
Hand Scooped Mocha Almond	½ cup	150	5	22	18	tr
Hand Scooped No Sugar Added Chocolate Chocolate Swirl	½ cup	90	1	23	5	6
Hand Scooped No Sugar Added Vanilla	½ cup	80	1	19	6	5
Hand Scooped No Sugar Added Vanilla Fudge Brownie	½ cup	100	2	22	5	5
Hand Scooped Pralines & Cream	½ cup	140	5	23	19	0
Hand Scooped Psychedelic Sorbet	½ cup	290	0	75	55	0
Hand Scooped Rainbow Cream	½ cup	120	4	20	16	0
Hand Scooped Rocky Road	½ cup	220	7	36	27	1

FOOD	PORTION	CAL	FAT	CARB	SUGAR	FIBER
Hand Scooped Strawberries & Cream	½ cup	120	3	21	18	0
Hand Scooped Vanilla Chocolate Chunk	½ cup	140	5	22	18	0
Hand Scooped Vanilla Bean	½ cup	120	4	19	16	0
Soft Serve Frozen Yogurt All Flavors 96% Fat Free	½ cup	140	3	23	20	0
Soft Serve Frozen Yogurt All Flavors Low Carb	½ cup	110	7	16	3	7
Soft Serve Frozen Yogurt All Flavors Nonfat	½ cup	110	0	23	20	0
Soft Serve Frozen Yogurt All Flavors Nonfat No Sugar Added	½ cup	90	0	20	7	0
Soft Serve Sorbet All Flavors Nonfat Nondairy	½ cup	100	0	24	19	0
SMOOTHIES						
Berrylicious	1 (16 oz)	290	3	65	54	3
Black 'N Blueberry	1 (16 oz)	280	3	63	54	2
Mango Tango	1 (16 oz)	330	3	76	66	2
Mangolada	1 (16 oz)	340	6	70	60	2
Mondo Mango	1 (16 oz)	310	3	70	63	2
Pina Paradise	1 (16 oz)	350	12	58	48	1
Pink Pineapple	1 (16 oz)	340	9	63	52	2
Straight Up Strawberry	1 (16 oz)	280	4	44	54	1
Strawberry Bonanza	1 (16 oz)	320	4	74	61	2
Strawberry Fling	1 (16 oz)	340	3	78	67	2

TIM HORTONS
BAKED SELECTIONS

FOOD	PORTION	CAL	FAT	CARB	SUGAR	FIBER
Bagel Blueberry	1	270	1	55	7	2
Bagel Cinnamon Raisin	1	270	1	55	12	3
Bagel Everything	1	280	2	53	7	3

FOOD	PORTION	CAL	FAT	CARB	SUGAR	FIBER
Bagel Flax Seed	1	290	5	53	4	4
Bagel Onion	1	260	2	53	8	3
Bagel Plain	1	260	2	52	7	2
Bagel Poppy Seed	1	270	2	53	7	3
Bagel Sesame Seed	1	270	3	53	7	3
Bagel Sun Dried Tomato	1	310	4	59	4	2
Bagel Twelve Grain	1	330	9	52	5	6
Cinnamon Roll Frosted	1	470	25	57	20	2
Cinnamon Roll Glazed	1	420	23	50	15	2
Cookie Caramel Chocolate Pecan	1	230	11	32	17	1
Cookie Chocolate Chip	1	230	9	34	19	1
Cookie Oatmeal Raisin Spice	1	220	8	35	21	1
Cookie Peanut Butter Chocolate Chunk	1	260	15	28	18	2
Cookie Triple Chocolate	1	250	13	31	20	2
Cookie White Chocolate Macadamia Nut	1	240	12	31	17	1
Croissant Butter	1	340	18	38	7	1
Croissant Cheese	1	370	20	37	6	0
Danish Cherry Cheese	1	330	13	46	24	1
Danish Chocolate	1	430	24	51	27	1
Danish Maple Pecan	1	380	20	46	21	1
Donut Apple Fritter	1	300	11	49	16	2
Donut Chocolate Dip	1	210	9	30	8	1
Donut Chocolate Glazed	1	260	10	39	20	2
Donut Honey Dip	1	210	8	33	11	1
Donut Maple Dip	1	210	8	31	9	1
Donut Old Fashion Glazed	1	320	19	35	22	1
Donut Old Fashion Plain	1	260	19	20	7	1
Donut Sour Cream Plain	1	270	17	27	10	1
Donut Walnut Crunch	1	360	23	35	19	1

FOOD	PORTION	CAL	FAT	CARB	SUGAR	FIBER
Donut Filled Angel Cream	1	310	13	46	21	1
Donut Filled Blueberry	1	230	8	36	11	1
Donut Filled Boston Cream	1	250	9	38	12	1
Donut Filled Canadian Maple	1	260	9	41	16	1
Donut Filled Strawberry	1	230	8	36	12	1
Honey Cruller	1	320	19	37	23	0
Muffin Blueberry	1	330	11	54	27	2
Muffin Blueberry Bran	1	300	10	53	25	5
Muffin Carrot Wheat	1	400	19	55	26	4
Muffin Chocolate Chip	1	430	16	69	40	2
Muffin Cranberry Blueberry Bran	1	290	10	51	24	5
Muffin Cranberry Fruit	1	350	12	59	31	2
Muffin Fruit Explosion	1	360	11	61	32	2
Muffin Raisin Bran	1	360	10	65	37	6
Muffin Strawberry Sensation	1	350	11	61	31	1
Muffin Low Fat Blueberry	1	290	3	62	32	2
Muffin Low Fat Cranberry	1	290	3	62	31	2
Tea Biscuit Plain	1	250	9	35	4	1
Tea Biscuit Raisin	1	290	10	45	12	2
Timbits Apple Fritter	1	50	2	9	4	0
Timbits Chocolate Glazed	1	70	3	10	5	0
Timbits Honey Dip	1	60	2	9	4	0
Timbits Old Fashion Plain	1	70	5	5	2	0
Timbits Filled Banana Cream	1	60	2	9	3	0

FOOD	PORTION	CAL	FAT	CARB	SUGAR	FIBER
Timbits Filled Lemon	1	60	2	9	4	0
Timbits Filled Strawberry	1	60	2	10	4	0
BEVERAGES						
Cafe Mocha	1 (10 oz)	160	7	25	21	1
Cappuccino Iced	1 (12 oz)	300	15	41	40	0
Coffee Decaffeinated Sugar & Cream	1 (10 oz)	75	4	9	9	0
Coffee Sugar & Cream	1 (10 oz)	75	4	9	9	0
English Toffee	1 (10 oz)	220	6	40	30	0
Flavor Shot	1 serv	5	0	1	0	0
French Vanilla	1 (10 oz)	240	7	39	31	0
Hot Chocolate	1 (10 oz)	240	6	45	35	2
Hot Smoothie	1 (10 oz)	260	10	39	28	2
Iced Cappuccino w/ Milk	1 (12 oz)	180	2	39	35	0
Tea Sugar & Milk	1 (10 oz)	50	1	10	10	0
CREAM CHEESE						
Garden Vegetable	1.5 oz	120	11	3	2	1
Light Plain	1.5 oz	60	5	3	3	0
Plain	1.5 oz	130	12	2	2	0
Strawberry	1.5 oz	120	10	6	6	0
SANDWICHES						
B.L.T.	1	450	18	53	9	2
Breakfast Bacon Egg Cheese	1	410	25	31	4	1
Breakfast Egg Cheese	1	360	21	30	3	1
Breakfast Sausage Egg Cheese	1	520	37	30	3	1
Chicken Salad Salad	1	380	9	55	6	3
Egg Salad	1	390	13	52	7	2
Ham & Swiss	1	440	12	56	7	3
Toasted Chicken Club	1	460	7	70	14	2
Turkey Breast	1	390	5	59	6	4

FOOD	PORTION	CAL	FAT	CARB	SUGAR	FIBER
SOUPS						
Beef Stew	1 serv (10 oz)	236	8	25	3	3
Chicken Noodle	1 serv (10 oz)	120	2	18	2	1
Chili	1 serv (10 oz)	300	16	18	5	5
Country Field Mushroom	1 serv (10 oz)	150	3	28	3	1
Cream Of Broccoli	1 serv (10 oz)	160	9	16	6	1
Minestrone	1 serv (10 oz)	120	3	24	4	2
Potato Bacon	1 serv (10 oz)	180	6	30	5	2
Split Pea w/ Ham	1 serv (10 oz)	150	3	27	3	5
Turkey Rice	1 serv (10 oz)	120	2	21	2	1
Vegetable Beef Barley	1 serv (10 oz)	110	2	21	2	2
YOGURT						
Low Fat Creamy Vanilla w/ Berries	1 (6 oz)	160	3	32	26	2
Low Fat Strawberry w/ Berries	1 (6 oz)	150	3	28	23	2
TJ CINNAMONS						
Chocolate Twist	1	250	12	34	12	2
Cinnamon Twist	1	280	14	33	11	1
Mocha Chill w/ Whipped Cream	1 (12.5 oz)	306	7	48	48	1
Mocha Chill w/o Whipped Cream	1 (12.5 oz)	264	4	48	44	1
Original Roll w/o Icing	1	507	10	73	31	4
Pecan Sticky Bun	1	688	22	91	45	5
TJ Icing	1 serv (1 oz)	117	5	18	16	0
TOGO'S						
SALAD DRESSINGS						
Asian	1 serv (2.5 oz)	380	33	19	10	0
Blue Cheese	1 serv (2.5 oz)	260	26	3	3	0

FOOD	PORTION	CAL	FAT	CARB	SUGAR	FIBER
Buttermilk Ranch	1 serv (2.5 oz)	250	26	3	3	0
Caesar	1 serv (2.5 oz)	150	12	8	3	0
Fat Free Serano Grape Vinaigrette	1 serv (2.5 oz)	90	0	23	21	0
Low Fat Basalmic Vinaigrette	1 serv (2.5 oz)	90	4	16	6	0
SALADS						
Asian Chicken w/o Dressing	1 full serv	200	9	17	5	3
Chicken Caesar w/o Dressing	1 full serv	210	6	17	3	3
Cobb w/o Dressing	1 full serv	330	20	12	4	6
Santa Fe Chicken w/o Dressing	1 full serv	370	16	33	6	10
Taco w/o Dressing	1 full serv	600	39	36	8	9
SANDWICHES						
Albacore Tuna	1 reg	660	28	73	9	4
Avocado & Cucumber	1 reg	560	25	75	7	9
Black Forest Ham & Cheese	1 reg	670	31	67	7	4
Capicolla Dry Salami & Provolone	1 reg	1080	59	69	12	4
Cheese	1 reg	800	45	68	6	4
Chef's Creations Pacific Cobb	1 reg	710	36	68	8	6
Chef's Creations Pastrami Reuben	1 reg	990	55	67	9	3
Chicken Salad	1 reg	650	29	74	10	5
Egg Salad & Cheese	1 reg	750	39	70	8	4
Hot BBQ Beef	1 reg	670	19	85	29	3
Hot Meatball	1 reg	690	27	78	6	5
Hot Pastrami	1 reg	750	33	69	6	4

FOOD	PORTION	CAL	FAT	CARB	SUGAR	FIBER
Hot Roast Beef	1 reg	730	25	67	6	4
Hummus	1 reg	650	27	90	6	9
Salami & Cheese	1 reg	1100	53	73	15	4
Turkey & Cranberry	1 reg	670	19	95	33	4
Turkey & Avocado	1 reg	640	26	74	7	9
Turkey & Cheese	1 reg	670	28	68	6	4
Turkey Bacon Club	1 reg	680	32	68	6	4
Turkey Ham & Cheese	1 reg	690	29	68	7	4

WHATABURGER
BEVERAGES

FOOD	PORTION	CAL	FAT	CARB	SUGAR	FIBER
Barq's Root Beer	1 sm (16 oz)	220	0	61	61	0
Cherry Coke	1 sm (16 oz)	210	0	56	56	0
Coca Cola	1 sm (16 oz)	207	0	56	56	0
Coffee	1 sm (8 oz)	5	0	1	0	0
Coffee Decafe	1 sm (8 oz)	5	0	1	0	0
Diet Coke	1 sm (16 oz)	0	0	0	0	0
Dr Pepper	1 sm (16 oz)	190	0	51	51	0
Fanta Orange	1 sm (16 oz)	210	0	56	56	0
Fanta Strawberry	1 sm (16 oz)	230	0	61	61	0
Iced Tea Sweetened	1 (34 oz)	430	0	114	114	0
Iced Tea Unsweetened	1 sm (19 oz)	0	0	0	0	0
Lemonade Hi-C Poppin' Pink	1 sm (16 oz)	200	0	51	51	0
Malt Chocolate	1 sm (16 oz)	670	15	123	115	2
Malt Strawberry	1 sm (16 oz)	670	15	123	117	0
Malt Vanilla	1 sm (16 oz)	600	17	98	92	0
Milk Reduced Fat	8 oz	120	5	11	11	0
Orange Juice Tropicana	1 (10 oz)	140	0	33	28	0
Powerade Fruit Punch	1 sm (16 oz)	130	0	33	28	0
Shake Chocolate	1 sm (16 oz)	630	16	111	103	2
Shake Strawberry	1 sm (16 oz)	630	16	111	105	0
Shake Vanilla	1 sm (16 oz)	560	17	87	80	0
Sprite	1 sm (16 oz)	200	0	51	51	0

FOOD	PORTION	CAL	FAT	CARB	SUGAR	FIBER
CHILDREN'S MENU SELECTIONS						
Kid's Meal Chicken Strips	1 serv	770	51	53	0	2
Kid's Meal Justaburger	1 serv	570	29	60	2	3
DESSERTS						
Apple Pie A La Mode	1 serv	520	20	75	43	2
Apple Pie Hot	1	230	11	29	1	2
Cinnamon Roll	1	400	7	80	16	2
Cookie Chocolate Chunk	1 (2 oz)	230	11	33	21	1
Cookie White Chocolate Chunk Macadamia	1 (2 oz)	250	14	30	20	0
Peach Pie A La Mode	1 serv	570	23	82	52	2
MAIN MENU SELECTIONS						
Biscuit	1	300	17	32	2	1
Biscuit Sandwich Bacon Egg & Cheese	1	500	32	33	2	1
Biscuit Sandwich Egg & Cheese	1	450	28	33	2	1
Biscuit Sandwich Honey Butter Chicken	1	610	38	51	9	1
Biscuit Sandwich Sausage Egg & Cheese	1	690	49	33	2	1
Biscuit w/ Bacon	1	355	20	32	2	1
Biscuit w/ Gravy	1	530	36	52	7	1
Biscuit w/ Sausage	1	540	37	32	2	1
Breakfast Platter w/ Bacon	1 serv	730	45	53	3	2
Breakfast Platter w/ Sausage	1 serv	930	62	53	3	2
Breakfast On A Bun w/ Bacon	1	380	22	29	2	1
Breakfast On A Bun w/ Sausage	1	570	39	29	2	1
Chicken Strips	1	200	12	11	0	0
Chicken Strips w/ Gravy	4	840	54	53	2	0

FOOD	PORTION	CAL	FAT	CARB	SUGAR	FIBER
French Fries	1 sm	260	13	31	0	2
Gravy White Peppered	1 serv	60	5	8	2	0
Hashbrown Sticks	4	200	12	20	0	1
Justaburger	1	329	16	30	2	1
Onion Rings	1 med	420	28	36	17	3
Pancakes Plain	1 serv	580	8	112	27	5
Pancakes w/ Bacon	1 serv	630	12	112	27	5
Pancakes w/ Sausage	1 serv	820	20	112	27	5
Sandwich Chicken Strip Honey BBQ	1	1110	59	102	16	3
Sandwich Chicken Strip Junior Honey BBQ	1	720	41	59	9	1
Sandwich Egg	1	330	18	29	2	1
Sandwich Grilled Chicken	1	450	18	45	8	6
Taquito w/ Bacon & Egg	1	370	21	27	2	3
Taquito w/ Bacon Egg & Cheese	1	420	24	27	2	3
Taquito w/ Potato & Egg	1	430	23	37	2	3
Taquito w/ Potato Egg & Cheese	1	470	27	37	2	3
Taquito w/ Sausage & Egg	1	410	24	27	2	3
Taquito w/ Sausage Egg & Cheese	1	450	28	27	2	3
Texas Toast	1 slice	180	8	25	3	1
Whataburger	1	640	32	61	10	3
Whataburger Double Meat	1	890	51	61	10	3
Whataburger Jr.	1	330	16	32	3	1
Whataburger Triple Meat	1	1140	70	61	10	3
Whataburger w/ Bacon & Cheese	1	800	45	62	10	3
Whatacatch	1	480	30	42	3	2

FOOD	PORTION	CAL	FAT	CARB	SUGAR	FIBER
Whatacatch Dinner	1 serv	1095	92	161	88	8
Whatachick'n	1	530	20	61	8	7
SALADS						
Chicken Strips	1 serv	570	38	34	6	4
Garden Salad	1	60	0	12	6	4
Grilled Chicken	1 serv	230	7	19	6	4

WHITE CASTLE
BEVERAGES

FOOD	PORTION	CAL	FAT	CARB	SUGAR	FIBER
Barq's Red Cream Soda	1 sm (21 oz)	260	0	69	69	0
Barq's Root Beer	1 sm (21 oz)	250	0	68	68	0
Coca Cola	1 sm (21 oz)	220	0	61	61	0
Coffee Black	1 sm (12 oz)	<5	0	1	0	0
Crave Cooler Coke	1 sm (21 oz)	150	0	41	41	0
Diet Coke	1 sm (21 oz)	0	0	0	0	0
Fanta Orange	1 sm (21 oz)	240	0	64	64	0
Hi-C Flashing Fruit Punch	1 sm (21 oz)	240	0	63	63	0
Hot Chocolate	1 sm (12 oz)	220	6	40	32	tr
Hot Tea	1 sm (12 oz)	0	0	0	0	0
Iced Tea Sweetened w/ Lemon	1 sm (21 oz)	170	0	46	46	0
Iced Tea Unsweetened	1 sm (21 oz)	0	0	0	0	0
Lemonade Raspberry	1 sm (21 oz)	290	0	78	73	0
Pibb Xtra	1 sm (21 oz)	220	0	59	59	0
Powerade Mountain Blast	1 sm (21 oz)	140	0	38	33	0
Sprite	1 sm (21 oz)	220	0	59	59	0
MAIN MENU SELECTIONS						
Cheeseburger	1	170	9	15	2	tr
Cheeseburger Bacon	1	200	11	15	2	tr
Cheeseburger Bacon Double	1	370	22	23	4	1
Cheeseburger Double	1	300	17	23	4	1

FOOD	PORTION	CAL	FAT	CARB	SUGAR	FIBER
Cheeseburger Jalapeno	1	180	10	15	2	tr
Cheeseburger Jalapeno Double	1	320	19	23	4	1
Chicken Rings	6	210	23	15	0	0
Clam Strips	1 reg	250	22	5	1	0
Fish Nibblers	1 reg	280	16	24	0	5
French Fries	1 reg	310	15	39	1	4
Mozzarella Cheese Sticks	3	250	14	22	2	1
Onion Chips	1 reg	480	23	62	9	2
Sandwich Chicken Breast w/ Cheese	1	200	8	21	2	1
Sandwich Chicken Ring	1	180	8	19	2	tr
Sandwich Chicken Ring w/ Cheese	1	200	10	19	2	tr
Sandwich Fish w/ Cheese	1	180	8	19	2	tr
White Castle	1	140	7	14	2	tr
White Castle Double	1	250	13	22	4	1
SAUCES AND SPREADS						
Dressing Ranch	1 serv (1 oz)	150	17	0	0	0
Ketchup	1 pkg	10	0	3	2	0
Lemon Juice	1 pkg	0	0	0	0	0
Mayonnaise	1 pkg	60	7	0	0	0
Sauce BBQ	1 serv (1 oz)	35	1	8	7	0
Sauce Hot	1 pkg	0	0	0	0	0
Sauce Marinara	1 serv (1 oz)	15	0	4	3	0
Sauce Seafood	1 serv (1 oz)	30	0	7	6	0
Sauce Tartar	1 pkg	30	3	2	1	0
Sauce Zesty Zing	1 serv (1 oz)	110	11	3	3	0
Sauce Fat Free Honey Mustard	1 serv (1 oz)	50	0	12	10	0

FOOD	PORTION	CAL	FAT	CARB	SUGAR	FIBER
WINCHELL'S DONUTS						
Chocolate Bar	1	240	16	29	–	–
Chocolate Round	1	240	16	29	–	–
Chocolate Twist	1	240	16	29	–	–
Croissant	1	260	17	28	–	–
Glazed Round	1	230	15	27	–	–
Glazed Twist	1	230	15	27	–	–
Iced Chocolate	1	230	15	28	–	–
Traditional	1	215	14	26	–	–
YOGEN FRUZ						
Blend It No Sugar Added Vanilla	1 sm	110	0	24	8	0
Blend It Probiotic Low Fat Chocolate	1 sm	121	2	22	21	0
Blend It Probiotic Low Fat Vanilla	1 sm	121	2	22	21	4
Blend It Probiotic Non Fat Vanilla	1 sm	110	0	24	21	0
Smoothie Dairy Blueberry Breeze	1 sm	180	0	45	36	2
Smoothie Dairy Peach Berry Sunset	1 sm	150	0	36	30	2
Smoothie Dairy Strawberry Banana	1 sm	180	0	42	33	3
Smoothie Non Dairy Raspberry Blast	1 sm	208	0	51	45	3
Smoothie Non Dairy Tropical Storm	1 sm	224	0	56	46	2
Smoothie Non Dairy Very Berry	1 sm	192	0	50	40	3
Top It Probiotic Soft Serve	1 sm	132	0	28	25	0

FOOD	PORTION	CAL	FAT	CARB	SUGAR	FIBER
YOGURTLAND						
Arctic Vanilla	½ cup (3 oz)	108	0	24	14	0
Blueberry Tart	½ cup (3 oz)	127	0	16	15	0
Cafe Con Leche	½ cup (3 oz)	108	0	24	14	0
Chocolate Mint	½ cup (3 oz)	100	0	23	15	0
Double Cookies & Cream	½ cup (3 oz)	121	0	27	14	0
Dutch Chocolate	½ cup (3 oz)	118	0	27	14	0
French Vanilla No Sugar Added	½ cup (3 oz)	89	0	19	9	0
Fresh Strawberry	½ cup (3 oz)	108	0	24	14	0
Green Tea	½ cup (3 oz)	107	tr	24	15	0
Heath Bar	½ cup (3 oz)	132	3	25	14	0
Mango	½ cup (3 oz)	96	0	22	16	0
Mango Tart	½ cup (3 oz)	127	0	16	15	0
NY Cheesecake	½ cup (3 oz)	100	0	23	16	0
Peach	½ cup (3 oz)	100	0	23	15	0
Peach Tart	½ cup (3 oz)	127	0	16	15	0
Peanut Butter	½ cup (3 oz)	119	3	24	14	0
Pineapple Tart	½ cup (3 oz)	127	0	16	15	0
Pistachio	½ cup (3 oz)	100	0	22	16	0
Plain Tart	½ cup (3 oz)	108	0	19	19	0
Strawberry Tart	½ cup (3 oz)	127	0	16	15	0
Taro	½ cup (3 oz)	102	0	23	14	0
ZOUP!						
DESSERTS						
Cookie Chocolate Chunk	1	410	19	57	–	1
Cookie Peanut Butter	1	420	21	43	–	1
SANDWICHES						
Grilled Turkey Club	½	470	28	22	–	1
Panini Italian Chicken	½	370	21	22	–	1
Pesto Three Cheese	1	720	42	42	–	2
Tuna Melt	1	600	23	42	–	2
Wrap American Farm	½	435	29	30	–	5

FOOD	PORTION	CAL	FAT	CARB	SUGAR	FIBER
Wrap Asian	½	615	33	54	–	7
Wrap Chicken Caesar w/o Dressing	½	505	19	43	–	5
Wrap Greek w/o Dressing	½	485	33	33	–	6
Wrap Sonoma	½	595	37	38	–	8
Wrap Tuna	½	365	13	35	–	4
Zesty Southwest Turkey	½	310	16	22	–	1
SOUPS						
Chicken & Dumplings	1 (8 oz)	130	3	22	–	1
Chicken Potpie	1 (8 oz)	200	8	21	–	3
Italian Wedding w/ Turkey Meatballs	1 (8 oz)	120	4	13	–	1
Jamaican Bay Gumbo	1 (8 oz)	140	3	20	–	2
Lobster Bisque	1 (8 oz)	260	18	14	–	0
Pepper Steak	1 (8 oz)	160	6	19	–	1
Potato Cheddar	1 (8 oz)	210	13	16	–	1
Sesame Noodle Bowl	1 (8 oz)	80	3	7	–	1
Shrimp & Crawfish Etouffee	1 (8 oz)	130	4	17	–	1
Sicilian Pizza	1 (8 oz)	150	7	18	–	2
Spicy Crab & Rice	1 (8 oz)	110	2	21	–	1
Turkey Chili	1 (8 oz)	120	2	19	–	3
Wild Mushroom Barley	1 (8 oz)	108	3	18	–	2

INDEX

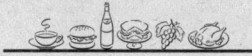